# SOCIAL IDENTITY PROCESSES
# IN ORGANIZATIONAL CONTEXTS

Sue Kinsey

# SOCIAL IDENTITY PROCESSES IN ORGANIZATIONAL CONTEXTS

*Edited by*

## Michael A. Hogg and
## Deborah J. Terry
*University of Queensland*

| **USA** | Publishing Office: | PSYCHOLOGY PRESS |
| | | A member of the Taylor & Francis Group |
| | | 325 Chestnut Street |
| | | Philadelphia, PA 19106 |
| | | Tel: (215) 625-8900 |
| | | Fax: (215) 625-2940 |
| | Distribution Center: | PSYCHOLOGY PRESS |
| | | A member of the Taylor & Francis Group |
| | | 7625 Empire Drive |
| | | Florence, KY 41042 |
| | | Tel: 1 (800) 634-7064 |
| | | Fax: 1 (800) 248-4724 |
| **UK** | | PSYCHOLOGY PRESS |
| | | A member of the Taylor & Francis Group |
| | | 27 Church Road |
| | | Hove |
| | | E. Sussex, BN3 2FA |
| | | Tel.: +44 (0) 1273 207411 |
| | | Fax: +44 (0) 1273 205612 |

**SOCIAL IDENTITY PROCESSES IN ORGANIZATIONAL CONTEXTS**

1  2  3  4  5  6  7  8  9  0

Printed by Sheridan Books, Ann Arbor, MI, 2001.
Cover design by Carolyn O'Brien.

A CIP catalog record for this book is available from the British Library.
∞ The paper in this publication meets the requirements of the ANSI Standard Z39.48-1984 (Permanence of Paper)

**Library of Congress Cataloging-in-Publication Data**

Social identity processes in organizational contexts / edited by Michael A. Hogg and Deborah J. Terry.
    p. cm.
    Includes bibliographical references and index.
    ISBN 1-84169-007-4 (case : alk. paper)—ISBN 1-84169-057-0 (paper : alk. paper)
    1. Group identity. 2. Organizational behavior. I. Hogg, Michael A., 1954–
II. Terry, Deborah J.

    HM753 .S62 2000
    302.3'5—dc21

                                                          2001019213

ISBN: 1-84169-007-4 (case)
ISBN: 1-84169-057-0 (paper)

# Contents

# About the Editors

**Michael A. Hogg** is professor of social psychology and director of the Centre for Research on Group Processes at the University of Queensland. He is also director of research for the Faculty of Social and Behavioural Sciences and is a fellow of the Academy of the Social Sciences in Australia. His research interests are in group processes, intergroup relations, collective self-conception, and social identity and self-categorization processes. He has published 15 books and over 140 research articles, chapters, and other scholarly works. He is the founding editor, with Dominic Abrams, of the journal *Group Processes and Intergroup Relations* and serves on the editorial board of a number of journals including *Journal of Personality and Social Psychology*, *Personality and Social Psychology Bulletin*, and *European Review of Social Psychology*. His most recent books include, with Abrams, *Social Identity and Social Cognition* (1999) and *Intergroup Relations: Essential Readings* (2001); with Foddy, Smithson, and Schneider, *Resolving Social Dilemmas* (1999); and, with Tindale, *Blackwell Handbook of Social Psychology: Group Processes* (2001).

**Deborah J. Terry** is professor of social psychology and head of the School of Psychology at the University of Queensland. Her main research interests are attitudes, social influence, persuasion, group processes, and intergroup relations. She also has applied research interests in organizational and health psychology. She has published more than 90 journal articles and book chapters in these areas, and is editor, with Gallois and McCamish, of *The Theory of Reasoned Action: Its Application to AIDS-Preventive Behaviour* (1993) and, with Hogg, of *Attitudes, Behavior, and Social Context: The Role of Group Norms and Group Membership* (1999). She is on the editorial board of the journals *Group Dynamics: Theory, Research, Practice*, and *Group Processes and Intergroup Relations*.

# Contributors

**Dominic Abrams,** University of Kent, UK
**Blake E. Ashforth,** Arizona State University, USA
**Betty A. Bachman,** Siena College, USA
**Brenda S. Banker,** University of Delaware, USA
**Caroline Bartel,** New York University, USA
**Marilynn Brewer,** Ohio State University, USA
**Shelley Brickson,** Harvard University, USA
**Richard J. Crisp,** University of Birmingham, UK
**Jack Dovidio,** Colgate University, USA
**Jane Dutton,** University of Michigan, USA
**Naomi Ellemers,** Leiden University, The Netherlands
**Kimberly D. Elsbach,** University of California, Davis, USA
**Samuel L. Gaertner,** University of Delaware, USA
**Claudia Hammer-Hewstone,** Fischer-Gaertner Gruppe Management
    Consultants, UK
**S. Alexander Haslam,** University of Exeter, UK
**Miles Hewstone,** University of Wales, Cardiff, UK
**Michael A. Hogg,** University of Queensland, Australia
**Scott A. Johnson,** Arizona State University, USA
**John T. Jost,** Stanford University, USA
**Roderick M. Kramer,** Stanford University, USA
**John M. Levine,** University of Pittsburgh, USA
**Robin Martin,** University of Queensland, Australia
**Jamie G. McMinn,** University of Pittsburgh, USA
**Richard L. Moreland,** University of Pittsburgh, USA
**Michael J. Platow,** LaTrobe University, Australia
**Michael G. Pratt,** University of Illinois, Urbana-Champaign, USA
**Georgina Randsley de Moura,** University of Kent, UK
**Deborah J. Terry,** University of Queensland, Australia
**Tom Tyler,** New York University, USA
**Daan van Knippenberg,** University of Amsterdam, The Netherlands
**Esther van Leeuwen,** Leiden University, The Netherlands
**Alberto Voci,** Università degli Studi di Padova, Italy

# Preface and Acknowledgments

This book is an exciting landmark for a process that has been gathering momentum for a number of years. Since about 1970, social identity theory has developed, within social psychology, as an increasingly influential perspective on group processes, intergroup relations, and the collective self. Social identity researchers have largely focused on intergroup relations, prejudice, discrimination, stereotyping, collective action, and other such behaviors. In 1989 Ashforth and Mael published an influential article, in *Academy of Management Review*, entitled Social Identity Theory and the Organization that introduced social identity theory to organizational psychologists. Organizational psychologists have not turned back; rather, they have found social identity ideas very useful in a growing focus on organizational commitment, organizational identification, and so forth. Social identity theorists started paying systematic attention to organizational contexts a few years ago—a trend which has gathered momentum. And yet, there has been only very limited interaction between organizational and social psychologists who employ and develop social identity theory to understand organizational behavior. The two groups seem to have rarely met. This book is an attempt to remedy this situation and to provide an integrative platform on which new developments can be founded.

From a social psychological perspective the background to our venture lies in 10 years of collaborative research between Deborah Terry and Michael Hogg. In developing the Center for Research on Group Processes at the University of Queensland, we adopted an explicitly eclectic and inclusive approach to research that was conceptually framed by social identity theory. We felt that theory development was best achieved by diversity. We and our colleagues, visitors, and students explored the limits of social identity in a wide range of arenas, including attitudes, roles, dissonance, deviance, health behaviors, self-presentation, leadership, mass communication, language, ethnicity, and so forth. Among these, organizational contexts has been a major focus.

During the mid-1990s we started to convene symposia on social identity and organizations at various conferences, for example, the 1997 and 1999 international organizational psychology conferences in Melbourne and Brisbane. In 1999 there was a similar symposium organized by Daan van Knippenberg at the meeting of the European Association of Experimental Social Psychology in Oxford. In 1997 Daan van Knippenberg, then at Leiden University, and Michael Hogg ran a Kurt Lewin Institute workshop in Leiden on social identity processes in organizational contexts. We ran the workshop again in 2000 in Amsterdam, but this time it was followed by a European Association of Experimental Social Psychology Small Group Meeting on the same topic, which brought together many of the authors of chapters of this book and also spawned a special issue of the journal *Group Processes and Intergroup Relations*.

The plan for this book was hatched in 1997 and finalized in early 1998 while Michael Hogg was spending a year as visiting professor of social psychology at Princeton University. We were wonderfully gratified by the enthusiasm we received from those we invited to take part, and from our publishers, Psychology Press. In particular we would like to thank Alison Mudditt at Psychology Press for her wonderful support and breathtaking efficiency—and also her willingness to scoot up from Philadelphia to Princeton to humor Michael Hogg by sitting in bars to discuss the project. A special thanks also goes to Kelly Fielding who organized the references and tidied up all the final loose ends, and to Alicia Svensson who helped with the indexes.

Michael A. Hogg and Deborah J. Terry
Brisbane, January 2001

*1*

# Social Identity Theory and Organizational Processes

MICHAEL A. HOGG
DEBORAH J. TERRY
*University of Queensland*

*T*his book is about the role of social identity processes in organizational contexts. It is about how collective self-conception influences and is influenced by organizational processes. More specifically, it brings together two literatures that have much to learn from one another, but which, until recently, have not often appeared together on the same stage: social psychology research on social identity theory, and organizational psychology research on identity processes in organizations and work groups. Since about 1989, organizational psychologists have increasingly incorporated social identity concepts in their thinking but have tended to focus more on early emphases of the theory. Social identity theorists finally started paying systematic attention to organizational contexts only a few years ago—a trend which has gathered momentum. In this brief introductory chapter we provide some background to these developments, give a basic description of key features of the social identity approach, and then overview the ensuing chapters in order to identify controversies, integrative themes, and future directions for research.

## SOME BACKGROUND

Organizational contexts provide a near-perfect arena for the operation of social identity processes. Organizations are internally structured groups, which are located in complex networks of intergroup relations that are characterized by power, status, and prestige differentials. To varying degrees people derive part of their identity and sense of self from the organizations or work groups to which they belong. Indeed, for many people their professional and/or organizational identity may be more pervasive and important than ascribed identities based on gender, age, ethnicity, race, or nationality.

The relevance of organizational contexts for social identity processes was not lost on early social identity researchers (e.g., R. J. Brown, 1978; Skevington, 1981), however, it was only a few years ago that social identity theorists began to pay systematic attention to organizational contexts (e.g., Haslam, 2001; Hogg & Terry, 2000). Social identity researchers have tended to be more focused on social-cognitive processes and on intergroup behavior between social categories and, for example, on the study of stereotyping (e.g., Oakes, Haslam, & Turner, 1994), categorization processes (e.g., Hogg, 2001), motivational processes (e.g., Hogg, 2000d), social influence and norms (e.g., J. C. Turner, 1991), solidarity and cohesion (e.g., Hogg, 1992), attitudes, behavior, and norms (e.g., Terry & Hogg, 1999), collective behavior (e.g., Reicher, 2001), and intergroup relations (e.g., Ellemers, 1993; Hornsey & Hogg, 2000a). (For general developments, see books by Abrams & Hogg, 1990b, 1999; Ellemers, Spears, & Doosje, 1999; Hogg & Abrams, 1988; Oakes et al., 1994; Robinson, 1996; Spears, Oakes, Ellemers, & Haslam, 1997; Terry & Hogg, 1999; J. C. Turner, Hogg, Oakes, Reicher, & Wetherell, 1987; Worchel, Morales, Páez, & Deschamps, 1998.)

Organizational psychologists were quicker and more determinedly off the mark regarding the relevance of social identity concepts to organizational life. Ashforth and Mael (1989) first systematically introduced the theory to organizational psychology (also see Ashforth & Humphrey, 1993; Nkomo & Cox, 1996) and subsequently published some related empirical work (e.g., Mael & Ashforth, 1992, 1995). Others have also applied it to organizational settings (e.g., Dutton, Dukerich, & Harquail, 1994; Pratt, 1998; Riordan & Shore, 1997; Tsui, Egan, & O'Reilly, 1992). This literature has, however, often only touched the surface of social identity theory. It has focused on some aspects, but has not systematically incorporated significant theoretical developments made since 1987 that focus on self-categorization, group prototypicality, contextual salience, and depersonalization processes (see Hogg & Terry, 2000; Pratt, 1998).

## THE SOCIAL IDENTITY APPROACH

The social identity approach is an integrated theoretical perspective on the relationship between self-concept and group behavior, which contains a number of distinct but compatible and dynamically interrelated conceptual components (subtheories or hypotheses; Abrams & Hogg, 2001; Hogg, 2001; Hogg & Abrams, 1988, 1999; J. C. Turner, 1999). Two of the main components are the original social identity theory and the more recent self-categorization theory.

Tajfel (1972) first introduced the concept of social identity, "the individual's knowledge that he belongs to certain social groups together with some emotional and value significance to him of this group membership" (p. 292), to extend his earlier consideration of social, largely intergroup, perception (i.e., stereotyping and prejudice) to consideration of how self is conceptualized in intergroup contexts; how a system of social categorizations "creates and defines an individual's *own* place in society" (Tajfel, 1972, p. 293). Social identity rests on intergroup social comparisons which seek to confirm or establish ingroup-favoring evaluative distinctiveness between ingroup and outgroup, motivated by an underlying need for self-esteem (J. C. Turner, 1975; also see Hogg, 2000c). Tajfel (1974a, 1974b) quickly developed the theory to specify how beliefs about the nature of relations between groups (status, stability, permeability, legitimacy) influence the way that individuals or groups pursue positive social identity. This emphasis is retained in Tajfel and Turner's (1979) classic statement of social identity theory. The emphasis on social identity as part of the self-concept was explored more fully by J. C. Turner (1982). Intergroup, self-conceptual, and motivational emphases were integrated and grounded in a comprehensive coverage of relevant research by Hogg and Abrams (1988). At about the same time, Turner and his colleagues (J. C. Turner, 1985; J. C. Turner et al., 1987) extended social identity theory through the development of self-categorization theory. Self-categorization theory specified in detail how social categorization produces prototype-based depersonalization of self and others and thus generates social identity phenomena.

The social identity approach, or aspects of it, have been described by social identity theorists in detail elsewhere (e.g., Hogg, 2001; Hogg & Abrams, 1988; Hogg, Terry, & White, 1995; Tajfel & Turner, 1986; J. C. Turner, 1999; J. C. Turner et al., 1987), but will be summarized here.

## Social Identity Theory

The basic idea of social identity theory is that a social category (e.g., nationality, political affiliation, organization, work group) within which one falls, and to which one feels one belongs, provides a definition of who one is in terms of the defining characteristics of the category—a self-definition that is a part of the self-concept. People have a repertoire of such discrete category memberships that vary in relative overall importance in the self-concept. Each category membership is represented in the individual member's mind as a social identity that both describes and prescribes one's attributes as a member of that group, i.e. what one should think and feel and how one should behave. Thus, when a specific social identity becomes the salient basis for self-regulation in a particular context, self perception and conduct become ingroup stereotypical and normative, perceptions of relevant outgroup members become outgroup stereotypical, and intergroup behavior acquires, to varying degrees depending on the nature of relations between the groups, competitive and discriminatory properties. Social identities are not only descriptive and prescriptive, they are also evaluative. They furnish an evaluation (generally widely shared or consensual) of a social category and thus of its members, relative to other relevant social categories. Because social identities have these important self-evaluative consequences, groups and their members are motivated to adopt behavioral strategies for achieving or maintaining ingroup-outgroup comparisons that favor the ingroup, and thus of course the self.

To account for social identity phenomena, social identity theory invokes the operation of two underlying sociocognitive processes: (a) *Categorization*, which sharpens intergroup boundaries by producing group-distinctive stereotypical and normative perceptions and actions and assigns people, including self, to the contextually relevant category. Categorization is a basic cognitive process which operates on social and nonsocial stimuli alike, to highlight and bring into focus those aspects of experience that are subjectively meaningful in a particular context (see Hogg, 2001). Social categorization of self and others reduces people's uncertainty about themselves and others and about how they and others may or ought to behave in specific social contexts (Hogg, 2000d; Hogg & Mullin, 1999). (b) *Self-enhancement*, which guides the social categorization process such that ingroup norms and stereotypes are largely ingroup-favoring. It is assumed that people have a very basic need to see themselves in a positive light in relation to relevant others (i.e., to have an evaluatively positive self-concept), and that in group contexts, self-enhancement can be achieved by making comparisons between ingroup and relevant outgroups in ways that favor the ingroup (but see Hogg & Abrams, 1993; Hogg & Mullin, 1999; Long & Spears, 1997). For example, comparisons can be made on stereotypical dimensions that favor the ingroup rather than on those that are less flattering to the ingroup.

An important feature of social identity theory is that in order to explain the behavior of group members, it formally articulates these basic sociocognitive processes of categorization and self-enhancement with *subjective belief structures* (see Ellemers, 1993; D. M. Taylor & McKirnan, 1984; A. van Knippenberg & Ellemers, 1993). The latter refer to people's beliefs about the nature of relations between their own group and relevant outgroups. These beliefs (which are not necessarily accurate reflections of reality because they can be, and often are, ideological constructs) concern the stability and legitimacy of intergroup status relations and the possibility of social mobility (psychologically passing from one group to another) or social change (psychologically changing the self-evaluative consequences of existing ingroup membership). Subjective belief structures influence the specific behaviors that group members adopt in the pursuit of self-enhancement through evaluatively positive social identity. For example, a lower status group that believes its position is relatively legitimate and stable but also believes that it is quite possible to pass psychologically into the dominant group (i.e., acquire a social identity as a member of the higher status group) will be unlikely to show much solidarity or engage in much direct intergroup competition. Instead, members will attempt, as individuals, to disidentify and gain psychological entry to the dominant group. In contrast, a lower status group that believes its position is illegitimate and unstable, that passing is not viable, and that a different social order is achievable, will show marked solidarity and engage in direct intergroup competition.

## Self-Categorization Theory

Self-categorization theory evolves directly from Tajfel and Turner's earlier ideas on social identity. It specifies in detail the operation of the social categorization process as the cognitive basis of group behavior. Social categorization of self and others into ingroup and outgroup accentuates the perceived similarity of the target to the relevant ingroup or outgroup prototype (cognitive representation of features that describe and prescribe attributes of the group). Targets are no longer represented as unique individuals, but rather as embodiments of the relevant prototype: a process of *depersonalization*. Social categorization of self, self-categorization, cognitively assimilates self to the ingroup prototype and thus depersonalizes self-conception. This transformation of self is the process underlying group phenomena, because it brings self-perception and behavior in line with the contextually relevant ingroup prototype. It produces, for instance, normative behavior, stereotyping, ethnocentrism, positive ingroup attitudes and cohesion, cooperation and altruism, emotional contagion and empathy, collective behavior, shared norms, and mutual influence. Depersonalization refers simply to a change in self-conceptualization and the basis of perception of others; it does not have the negative connotations of terms such as "deindividuation" or "dehumanization."

**Representation of groups as prototypes.** The notion of prototypes, which is not part of the earlier intergroup focus of social identity theory, is central to self-categorization theory. People cognitively represent the defining and stereotypical attributes of groups in the form of prototypes. Prototypes are typically not checklists of attributes, but are fuzzy-sets that capture the context-dependent features of group membership often in the form of representations of exemplary members (actual group members who best embody the group) or ideal types (an abstraction of group features). Prototypes embody all attributes that characterize groups and distinguish them from other groups, including beliefs, attitudes, feelings, and behaviors. A critical feature of prototypes is that they maximize similarities within and differences between groups and thus define groups as distinct entities. Prototypes form according to the principle of *metacontrast*: maximization of the ratio of intergroup differences to intragroup differences. Because members of the same group are exposed to similar social information, their prototypes will usually be similar, and thus shared.

Prototypes are stored in memory but are constructed, maintained, and modified by features of the immediate or more enduring social interactive context. They are context dependent and are particularly influenced by which outgroup is contextually salient. Enduring changes in prototypes and thus changes in self-conception can therefore arise if the relevant comparison outgroup changes over time; for instance, if a car manufacturer compares itself to a computer software manufacturer rather than another car manufacturer. Such changes are also transitory in that they are tied to whatever outgroup is salient in the immediate social context. For instance, a psychology department may experience a contextual change in self-definition if it compares itself with a management school rather than a history department. Thus social identity is dynamic. It is responsive, in type and content, to intergroup dimensions of immediate comparative contexts.

Self-categorization theory's focus on prototypes allows some important conceptual developments in social identity theory, which have direct implications for organizational contexts. When group membership is salient, cognition is attuned to and guided by prototypicality. Thus, within groups people are able to distinguish among themselves and others in terms of how well they match the prototype. An intragroup prototypicality gradient exists; some people are or are perceived to be more prototypical than others (Hogg, 1996b, in press). This idea allows social identity theory now to explicate intragroup processes that are social identity based, such as cohesion and social attraction, deviance and overachievement, and leadership and intragroup structural differentiation.

**Self-enhancement and uncertainty reduction motivations.** According to social identity theory, social identity and intergroup behavior is guided by the pursuit of evaluatively positive social identity through positive intergroup distinctiveness, which in turn is motived by the need for positive self-esteem. This is referred to as *the self-esteem hypothesis* (e.g., Abrams & Hogg, 1988). Self-categorization theory's focus on the categorization process hints at an additional (perhaps more fundamental), epistemic motivation for social identity, which has only recently been described and is termed *the uncertainty reduction hypothesis* (e.g., Hogg, 2000b, 2000d; Hogg & Mullin, 1999). In addition to being motivated by self-enhancement, social identity processes are also motivated by a need to reduce subjective uncertainty about one's perceptions, attitudes, feelings, and behaviors, and ultimately one's self-concept and place within the social world. Uncertainty reduction, particularly about subjectively important matters that are generally self-conceptually relevant, is a core human motivation. Certainty renders existence meaningful and confers confidence in how to behave and what to expect from the physical and social environment within which one finds oneself. Self-categorization reduces uncertainty by transforming self-conception and assimilating self to a prototype that describes and prescribes perceptions, attitudes, feelings, and behaviors. Because prototypes are relatively consensual, they also furnish moral support and consensual validation for one's self-concept and attendant cognitions and behaviors. It is the prototype that actually reduces uncertainty. Hence, uncertainty is better reduced by prototypes that are simple, clear, highly focused, and consensual, and that thus describe groups that have pronounced entitativity (Campbell, 1958; also see Brewer & Harasty, 1996; Hamilton & Sherman, 1996), are very cohesive (e.g., Hogg, 1992), and provide a powerful social identity. Such groups and prototypes will be attractive to individuals who are contextually or more enduringly highly uncertain or during times of, or in situations characterized by, great uncertainty.

Uncertainty reduction and self-enhancement are probably independent motivations for social identity processes, and in some circumstances it may be more urgent to reduce uncertainty than to pursue self-enhancement (e.g., when group entitativity is threatened), whereas in others it may be the opposite (e.g., when group prestige is threatened). However, uncertainty reduction may be more fundamentally adaptive because it constructs a self-concept that defines who we are and prescribes what we should perceive, think, feel, and do.

**Salience of social identity.** The responsiveness of social identity to immediate social contexts is an important feature of social identity theory, and of self-categorization theory within it. The cognitive system, governed by uncertainty reduction and self-enhancement motives, matches social categories to properties of the social context and brings into active use (i.e., makes salient) that category which renders the social context and one's place within it subjectively most meaningful. Specifically, there is an interaction between category accessibility and category fit, such that people draw on accessible categories and investigate how well they fit the social field. The category that best fits the field becomes salient in that context (e.g., Oakes & Turner, 1990; Oakes et al. 1994). Categories can be accessible because they are valued, important, and frequently employed aspects of the self-concept (i.e., chronic accessibility) and/or because they are perceptually salient (i.e., situational accessibility). Categories fit the social field because they account for situationally relevant similarities and differences among people (i.e., structural fit) and/or because category specifications account for context-specific behaviors (i.e., normative fit). Once fully activated (as opposed to merely "tried on") on the basis of optimal fit, category specifications organize themselves as contextually relevant prototypes and are used as a basis for the perceptual accentuation of intragroup similarities and intergroup differences, thereby maximizing separateness and clarity. Self-categorization in terms of the activated ingroup category then depersonalizes behavior in terms of the ingroup prototype.

Salience is not, however, a mechanical product of accessibility and fit (see Hogg, 1996a; Hogg & Mullin, 1999). Social interaction involves the motivated manipulation of symbols (e.g., through speech, appearance, behavior) by people who are strategically competing with one another to influence the frame of reference within which accessibility and fit interact. People are not content to have their identity determined by the social-cognitive context. On the contrary, they say and do things to try to change the parameters so that a subjectively more meaningful and self-favoring identity becomes salient.

This dynamic perspective on identity and self-conceptual salience has clear implications for organizational contexts. Manipulation of the intergroup social comparative context can be a powerful way to change organizational identity (self-conception as a member of a particular organization) and thus attitudes, motives, goals, and practices. Organizations or divisions within organizations that have poor work practices or organizational attitudes can be helped to reconstruct themselves through surreptitious or overt changes in the salience of relevant intergroup comparative contexts (different levels of categorization or different outgroups at the same level of categorization). Such changes affect contextual self-categorization and thus people's internalized attitudes and behaviors (e.g., Terry & Hogg, 1996b). One way in which organizations may deliberately manipulate the intergroup social comparative context is by "benchmarking." An organization selects specific other organizations as a legitimate comparison set, which threatens the group's prestige. This motivates upward redefinition of organizational identity and work practices to make the group evaluatively more competitive.

## THE CHAPTERS

The social identity approach has quite obvious relevance for organizational contexts. The chapters in this book represent a rare and diverse mix of scholars who address the social identity–organizational behavior nexus from different angles. Some chapters adhere closely to the relatively formal outline of the approach given above, whereas others adopt a more broad-based social identity or identity perspective.

Chapters 2, 3, 4, and 5 all share a focus on organizational diversity. In Chapter 2, Michael Pratt overviews social identity theory from the perspective of organizational psychology and organizational behavior, with an emphasis on the explanation of the management of conflict and diversity in organizations. Pratt makes the point that organizations contain multiple social identities with which people can identify, and that one task for successful organizations is to ensure that members identify with the "right" organizational identity. He asks why people identify with low status and undesirable organizations, which he believes is quite a common practice, and discusses the growing prevalence of virtual or distributed groups in organizations.

In Chapter 3, Blake Ashforth and Scott Johnson remind us that organizational members have many different hats or identities and asks what makes different identities within the organization salient at different times. Organizations have a hierarchy of identities that stretches from inclusive, abstract, and distal to exclusive and more concrete and proximal—the latter identities tend to represent organizational members' primary groups (higher order identities tend to provide the general comparative frame for making salient these lower order identities). How, therefore, do you encourage organizational identification when the natural level of identification is at the subgroup or work group level? Ashforth and Johnson suggest that modern job insecurity encourages people to construct a portable personal identity that works even more strongly against organizational identification.

The multiple identity theme is continued in Chapter 4 by Shelley Brickson and Marilynn Brewer, who focus on multiple identities and roles in organizations and the impact of demographic categories such as gender, race, and ethnicity. Brickson and Brewer adopt their new identity orientation framework that distinguishes between personal, relational, and collective identification, and then relate this theory to other theories to prescribe interventions to improve intergroup relations within organizations. They champion the view that an interpersonal relational identity orientation is the key to harmonious intergroup relations within an organization.

The final chapter with a focus on diversity is Chapter 5, by Miles Hewstone, Robin Martin, Claudia Hammer-Hewstone, Richard Crisp, and Alberto Voci. Hewstone and his associates take a slightly different perspective. They focus on numerical proportions within groups and the effects that minority/majority status has on organizational creativity and productivity. The vehicle for their intergroup analysis is primarily gender relations and gender proportions within organizations.

Chapters 6, 7, 8, and 9 share a general focus on people's commitment and identification with an organization and how this may relate to the effort they exert on behalf of the group or the extent to which they may feel like leaving the organization. In Chapter 6, Richard Moreland, John Levine, and Jamie McMinn argue that the reality of modern organizational life is such that people are generally more committed to their work groups within the organization than to the organization as a whole, a point that Ashforth and Johnson also emphasize in Chapter 3. Thus, the critical issue of how one raises organizational commitment hinges on work group socialization and the relationship between the work group and the superordinate organization. Moreland and his colleagues suggest that this places an understanding of small group socialization processes center stage in the analysis of organizational socialization and commitment. They describe their group socialization model and relate it closely to self-categorization processes, noting a number of possible limitations of self-categorization theory in the context of small, ongoing, interactive groups. In particular, they suggest a more textured analysis of group prototypes and strategic self-categorization processes.

In Chapter 7 Naomi Ellemers uses social identity theory to try to understand how to connect people's self-interest to the interest of the organization under modern circumstances of low job security, changed work content, and new life expectations. How do you get people to exert effort on behalf of the organization? She also focuses on identification as a multidimensional construct with cognitive, evaluative, and affective dimensions—different dimensions may be important in different contexts. Ellemers reports research on how effort exertion on behalf of the group (mediated by commitment) is affected by the type and legitimacy of power exerted by organizational supervisors.

Chapter 8, by Caroline Bartel and Jane Dutton, focuses on the problem of having unclear, vague, or unstable membership status in an organization—not knowing if one is in or out and/or to what extent one is in or out. They suggest that this may be a particularly acute problem for modern organizations in which people work from home and there are virtual or computer mediated communication (CMC) groups. Bartel and Dutton describe the relatively deliberate actions organizational members can take to clarify their membership status; these are actions that operate at a discursive level in which people claim and grant membership mainly through talk.

In Chapter 9, Dominic Abrams and Georgina Randsley de Moura focus directly on the role played by organizational identification in the relationship between attitudes and behavior regarding employee turnover. The argue that in order to understand employee turnover, we need to know not only about employee attitudes, but also about the extent to which employees identify with the organization. Abrams and Randsley de Moura describe a program of correlational research and present a model of organizational context and participative intentions and behavior.

Chapters 10, 11, and 12 focus on how people relate to one another within an organization based upon perceptions of trust, respect, and people's pride in the organization. Tom Tyler, in Chapter 10, discusses how people in organizations engage in cooperative group-serving behaviors and limit behaviors that are self-serving but detrimental to the organization. Whereas organizationally desirable behavior can be shaped by rules and regulations, Tyler argues that it is more effective to create conditions under which people identify strongly enough with the organization that they voluntarily and perhaps automatically engage in such behaviors. Tyler discusses in detail the role that pride in the organization and respect received from the organization play in organizational identification and pro-organizational behaviors. He describes how pride-based and respect-based organizations may differ.

In Chapter 11, Roderick Kramer discusses trust. He argues that the development and maintenance of trust within organizations is more problematic than in small groups or dyads, partly because organizations are too big and can be too political. Kramer argues that organizational identification is the basis for trust within an organization: if members all identify with the organization, then they are likely to trust one another even if there is no opportunity to test for evidence of others' trustworthiness. Being a deviant or token member of an organization can make one feel uncertain and in the limelight, which can cause one to have a fragile sense of trust for others, to actively distrust them, or even to feel paranoid. Kramer's chapter is about the negative personal and organizational consequences of being a deviant or marginal member, as mediated by feelings of distrust and even paranoia.

John Jost and Kimberly Elsbach focus more on status-based intergroup relations within organizations. In Chapter 12 they argue that organizational practices, such as performance evaluation, salary gradients, and job titles, can instantiate consensually legitimated status hierarchies. Drawing on system justification theory (e.g., Jost & Banaji, 1994), Jost and Elsbach explain how groups at the bottom of the organizational pecking order are unable to be creative in constructing a positive image of their group, but instead internalize their status position and show a range of consequent behaviors including outgroup preferences and bias. Jost and Elsbach review evidence for their own research program that supports their analysis.

Chapters 13 and 14 focus specifically on leadership, which is a high-profile focus of contemporary organizational research. Michael Hogg, in Chapter 13, describes a social identity theory of leadership and sketches out ways in which this new perspective may be able to address leadership phenomena in organizational contexts. Hogg's core argument is that in some circumstances, specifically when group membership is a highly salient basis for self-conceptualization, leadership processes may be strongly influenced by how group-prototypical the leader is and relatively less strongly influenced by generic or specific leader schemes or by specific status characteristics. In Chapter 14, Alex Haslam and Michael Platow focus more specifically on charisma and leadership in organizations. From a social identity perspective, they argue that charisma is not a cause of leadership effectiveness but more probably a correlate or consequence. For Haslam and Platow, the key question about leadership is how an individual gets others to exert effort on behalf of his or her vision of the group. They argue that this can only happen when social processes fuse leader and followers as partners in a common group that is defined by shared membership-defining goals.

Chapters 15, 16, and 17 focus on mergers and acquisitions, which are a particularly problematic aspect of organizational life because they so often backfire and cause human distress and economic setbacks. Deborah Terry in Chapter 15, and Daan van Knippenberg and Esther van Leeuwen, in Chapter 16, together give a solid theoretical overview of the role of social identity and self-categorization processes in the dynamics of mergers and acquisitions. Terry provides a conceptual overview of her own research program, which emphasizes the intergroup context of mergers and acquisitions, and illustrates her analysis with three recent studies. Van Knippenberg and van Leeuwen focus on the impact on merger outcomes of people's perceptions of the extent of continuity between the old organization and the new merged organization and of people's perceptions of the relative entitativity of the old and the new organization. In Chapter 17, Samuel Gaertner, Betty Bachman, Jack Dovidio, and Brenda Banker provide an analysis of mergers that rests on an intriguing parallel between corporate mergers and step-families. A merger is characterized as the marriage of two organizations—an intergroup marriage.

## CLOSING COMMENTS

The chapters in this book are diverse. Nevertheless, they reflect some common themes that may identify directions for future research. Some of these overlapping themes might include (a) recognition and management of diversity in organizations; (b) clarification of the relationship among terms such as organizational identification, organizational commitment, social identification, and so forth; (c) recognition that organizations are multifaceted regarding the provision of identities for members and of the need to understand processes that render different identities contextually salient; (d) study of new organizational structures that rely on virtual groups, distributed groups, CMC groups, and, generally, the new virtual world of work; (e) analysis of hierarchical relationships of power and leadership within groups; (f) mergers and acquisitions; (g) the role of work groups in organizational socialization and commitment and the tension between different levels of nested categorizations within an organization; (h) the mediational role of organizational identification between organizational culture and norms and the extent to which relations within the group are cooperative and trusting or not; (i) the question of what makes people remain in an organization and exert effort on its behalf.

The chapters in this book point, we feel, to a promising future for closer research ties between social and organizational psychology around social identity issues. This articulation will identify conceptual and empirical lacunae and thus highlight new directions for research and theory. Our understanding of basic social identity and identity processes will advance, as will our understanding of social identity and identity dimensions of contemporary organizational life.

*2*

# Social Identity Dynamics in Modern Organizations:
## An Organizational Psychology/ Organizational Behavior Perspective

MICHAEL G. PRATT
*University of Illinois at Urbana-Champaign*

T heories of identity have made a remarkable resurgence in studies of organizational psychology and organizational behavior more generally. Questions of "who are we?" and "with whom (or what) do we identify?" are becoming increasingly important as the nature of organizations, and of work itself, continues to change. For example, what does it mean to identify with an organization or group that is not physically co-located? With what groups do we identify as organizations become increasingly global and more heterogeneous? How does the evaluative component of identification manifest itself in organizations characterized by downsizing and new "psychological contracts"? The purpose of this chapter is to examine these and other questions inherent in modern organizing by using a social identity perspective.

To help narrow this very extensive topic, I take four major points of departure. First, I have limited my review primarily to the application of social identity theory (SIT) and self-categorization theory (SCT) even though more sociological theories, such as identity theory (Hogg, Terry, & White, 1995; Stryker & Serpe, 1982) and organizational identity (Albert & Whetten, 1985; Dutton & Dukerich, 1991), are also being used to examine identity dynamics in organizations. My review, therefore, is mostly concerned with psychological, "microlevel" applications of SIT and SCT. Second, the focus of this chapter is on applications of SIT and SCT in organizational contexts, broadly defined. That is, I examine how these theories have been applied to traditional, bureaucratic, "bricks and mortar" organizations, as well as to more unusual work contexts such as "tainted" occupations (e.g., those with bad reputations) and virtual teams. Third, I have concentrated primarily on two organizational issues that are typically addressed with a SIT or SCT perspective: how the individual relates to the collective (e.g., organizational identification), and how organizational groups interrelate (e.g., managing conflict and diversity). Fourth and finally, I have limited my review to relatively recent research, especially that done within the past decade. There are two reasons for this choice: (a) 1989 is the year in which Ashforth and Mael published *Social Identity Theory and the Organization*, which was extremely influential in "introducing" SIT to organizational scholars; and consequently, (b) much of the extant work on SIT and SCT coming out of business schools has been published in the past 10 to 11 years (Elsbach, 1999). This chapter also attempts to complement recent reviews of identification research in business contexts (Elsbach, 1999; Pratt, 1998) by examining relatively unexplored applications of SIT and SCT.

The bulk of this chapter addresses several key issues in organizational SIT and/or SCT research, which are summarized in Table 2.1. It also discusses how organizational applications of SIT and SCT complement social psychological research and extend the breadth of research in this area.

## KEY ISSUES IN ORGANIZATIONAL SIT/SCT RESEARCH

True to the theories' origins, organizational scholars are primarily interested in using SIT and SCT to better understand (a) how the individual relates to the collective, and (b) intergroup relations. The first issue is most often expressed in the area of *organizational identification*. Organizational identification occurs when "an individual's beliefs about his or her organization become self-referential or self-defining" (Pratt, 1998, p. 172). Organizational identification is a specific type of social identification.

Organizational scholars are particularly concerned with understanding how and why individuals choose to identify with some organizations or work-related groups (e.g., occupations, departments) and not others. Understanding the nature of identification is critical as strong identification has been linked to lower employee turnover, lower levels of burnout due to emotional labor, and increases in employee motivation, job satisfaction, and compliance with organizational dictates (e.g., Ashforth & Humphrey, 1993; Cheney, 1983; Dutton et al., 1994; Mael & Ashforth, 1995). Moreover, organizational members who identify with their organizations are more likely to make decisions and engage in sense making in ways that favor the organization (Cheney, 1983; Pratt, 2000a). Individuals, by contrast, may use a strong identification with organizations to satisfy a variety of needs, including safety, affiliation, self-enhancement, and more holistic needs, such as being part of something greater than themselves (Deaux, Reid, Micrahi, & Cotting, 1999; Pratt, 1998).

Identification with one's organization needs to be managed carefully, however, because there are a number of possible negative outcomes from mem-

TABLE 2.1. An overview of recent SIT/SCT research from an organizational psychology/organizational behavior perspective

| Topics | Theoretical Foundations | Psychological Processes | Contexts | Representative Research |
|---|---|---|---|---|
| | Primary SIT | Identification | "Traditional" | Ashforth & Mael (1989); Dutton, Dukerich, & Harquail (1994); Mael & Ashforth (1992); Pratt (1998) |
| | | Disidentification, ambivalent identification, & deidentification | "Traditional" organizations | Dukerich, Kramer, & Parks (1998); Elsbach (1999); Elsbach & Bhattacharya (2000); Pratt (2000a) |
| Organizational identification | | Identification | "Dirty work" or unpopular organizations | Ashforth & Kreiner (1999) |
| | SIT / SCT | Identification / intergroup behavior | Dispersed groups (e.g., virtual teams) | Brandon & Pratt (1999); Bouas & Arrow (1996); Wiesenfeld, Raghuram, & Garud (2000) SIDE model: Lea & Spears (1992); Postmes, Spears, & Lea (1998); Reicher, Spears, & Postmes (1995); Spears & Lea (1994) |
| | | | Multiple organizational identity environments | Golden-Biddle & Rao (1997); Pratt & Foreman (2000); Pratt & Rafaeli (1997); Scott (1997); van Kippenberg et al. (forthcoming); van Leeuwen, van Kippenberg, & Ellemers (2000) |
| Managing conflict & diversity | SIT / SCT | Identification intergroup behavior | "Traditional" organizations | Brewer & Kramer (1985); Chattopadhyay (1999); R. M. Kramer (1993); Nkomo & Cox (1999); Philips (2000); S. K. Schneider & Northcraft (1999); Tsui, Egan, & O'Reilly (1992); Tsui & O'Reilly (1989) |
| | | | Virtual organizations | Bhappu, Griffith, & Northcraft (1997); Pratt, Fuller, & Northcraft (2000) |

**15**

bers' identifying "too much." As Tajfel and others have noted (Brewer & Kramer, 1985; Hogg, Terry, & White, 1995; Kramer, 1993; Tajfel, 1981, 1982), high identification with a particular ingroup may lead to stereotyping and degrading outgroup members and to more intergroup conflict. Organizational scholars have also noted that "overidentification" can lead to a lack of organizational flexibility, individual vulnerability (especially if the organization's reputation fails); distrust and paranoia, overdependence on and overconformity to organizational dictates; antisocial, unethical, immoral, and even tyrannical behaviors by both leaders and followers; decreased creativity and risk taking; and the loss of an independent sense of self (e.g., Ashforth & Mael, 1996; Dukerich et al., 1998; Dutton & Dukerich, 1991; R. M. Kramer and Wei, 1999; Mael & Ashforth, 1992).

The second issue—intergroup relations—most often takes the form of *conflict and diversity management*. Here, researchers want to know how groups in organizations interact with each other, especially when the groups differ in some demographic characteristic. Again, understanding diversity management is critical because diverse organizations can suffer from individual members who are psychologically alienated and physically unhealthy, groups that are characterized by lower incidents of altruistic behavior and intentions to stay, and elevated levels of intergroup conflict (Chattopadhyay, 1999; K. James, Lovato, & Khoo, 1994; Nkomo & Cox, 1996; Tsui et al., 1992). By contrast, organizations where diversity is managed well can benefit from high degrees of creativity, improved decision making, effective information processing, access to external networks, and higher system flexibility (Cox & Blake, 1991; S. K. Schneider & Northcraft, 1999; Williams & O'Reilly, 1998).

Although I treat organizational identification and conflict and diversity management separately, they are related. Specifically, underlying many of these treatments of identification and diversity management is the assumption *that managers need to ensure that their members are choosing the "right" identity, among many, to act upon*. The notion of multiple identities is inherent in both SIT and SCT. SIT, for example, reminds us that individuals may have as many social identities as they have group memberships. SCT goes further in developing the distinctions among identities existing at different levels of abstraction, from individual or personal, through social, to "self as human being." As I will touch upon, one of the main concerns in both organizational identification and diversity research is that members identify with a social identity *associated with organizational membership* rather than identifying exclusively with a nonorganizational, subgroup identity.[1]

---

1. This distinction between an overarching organizationally related identity and a subgroup identity have been referred to using many terms. The former has been called "group" or "goal group" (Bouas & Arrow, 1996; Brandon & Pratt, 1999; Pratt et al., 2000) or "macroidentities" (Nkomo & Cox, 1996), while the latter have been referred to as "social category groups" (Pratt et al., 2000) or "microidentities" (Nkomo & Cox, 1996).

# ORGANIZATIONAL IDENTIFICATION

As I have argued elsewhere, perhaps the majority of organizational research that applies SIT and SCT has focused on organizational identification (Pratt, 1998). Moreover, because many organizational scholars are concerned with the managerial implications of theories, the focus of much SIT- and SCT-driven research has concerned identifying the organizational characteristics most likely to trigger organizational identification processes in members. I begin this overview of organizational identification by discussing how it has been applied in "traditional" organizations. I then discuss how many of the assumptions underlying this research have been challenged and extended in recent years.

## Organizational Identification in Traditional Organizations

**SIT and Identification Dynamics: An Overview.**    Much of the extant work on organizational identification involves the application of SIT rather than SCT (e.g., Ashforth & Mael, 1989). This research seeks identification-inducing characteristics that build directly from the two processes that underlie identification: *categorization* and *self-enhancement*. Because categorization involves clarifying ingroup-outgroup boundaries, researchers have posited at least three sets of conditions that are likely to make the target or "ingroup" organization perceptually different from outgroup organizations. Specifically, they have argued that identification with an organization is enhanced when: (a) the target organization is distinctive (Ashforth & Mael, 1989; Dutton et al., 1994; Mael & Ashforth, 1992); (b) organizational "outgroups" are salient (Ashforth & Mael, 1989; Mael & Ashforth, 1992); and (c) there is interorganizational competition between ingroup and outgroup organizations (Mael & Ashforth, 1992). The first condition, organizational distinctiveness, allows an organization to be more easily separated from other organizations (or outgroups), thus facilitating categorization, and ultimately, identification. A similar effect is achieved in the second condition in which organizational outgroups are salient, thus exacerbating the perceived differences between one's organization and those in the external environment. The third condition reminds us that intraorganizational competition enhances ingroup differences and diminishes the potential for identification. Alternatively, as noted, interorganizational competition minimizes ingroup differences and maximizes ingroup-outgroup differences, which can result in seeing outgroup members in stereotypical or derogatory ways.

Self-enhancement involves making comparisons with outgroups that increase a member's sense of self-worth. Consequently, organizational scholars predict that identification is more likely under the following conditions: when organizations are (a) highly prestigious (Ashforth & Mael, 1989; Mael & Ashforth, 1992); (b) have attractive images; and (c) have a perceived organizational identity that increases members' self-esteem (Dutton et al., 1994). All three conditions suggest that organizations that are viewed favorably by members are more likely to induce identification than those viewed unfavorably.

**SCT and Identification Dynamics: An Overview.**   SCT explores the cognitive process by which individuals classify themselves as members of social groups by maximizing intracategory similarity and intercategory differences (Hogg, 1996a; Hogg, Terry, & White, 1995; Turner et al., 1987; J. C. Turner, Oakes, Haslam, & McGarty, 1994). As noted, a major tenet of SCT is that individuals can categorize themselves (and others) at various levels of abstraction (individual, social, or member of the human race) depending on which categories are evoked by the social field (J. C. Turner et al., 1987). As individuals move from a personal to a social identity, self-perceptions become *depersonalized* whereby "individuals tend to define and see themselves less as differing individual persons and more as interchangeable representatives of some shared social category membership" (J. C. Turner et al., 1994, p. 455).

SCT (and SIT) also posit that identification is dynamic: whether one invokes a personal or a social identity will depend on the *conditions of the social context* (e.g., which ingroup or outgroup categories are salient) and which *categories seem to best make sense of that social context* (i.e., best explain similarities and differences among social stimuli). More specifically, individuals choose social categories based, in part, on the metacontrast principle that states:

> [A] collection of stimuli is more likely to be categorized as an entity to the degree that the average differences between those stimuli are less than the average differences perceived between them and the remaining stimuli that make up the frame of reference (J. C. Turner et al., 1994, p. 455).

Organizations manage identification via SCT-related processes, therefore, by altering environmental conditions so that organizational identities are evoked rather than identities at some other level of abstraction (e.g., individual or institutional). Put another way, organizations manage identification so that organizational categories are those that best maximize the similarities within, and differences between (or among) stimuli in a social field.

There are at least three contextual conditions that would favor the adoption of an organizational category in order to differentiate among individuals in a social field. First, SCT argues that social identities are more likely to be salient in intergroup contexts, while personal identities are more likely to be evoked in intragroup contexts (J. C. Turner et al., 1994). By extension, organizational identification is more likely to occur in contexts where *interorganizational comparisons* are salient, rather than in conditions where the organization alone (i.e., the ingroup) is salient. When the organization alone is salient, personal identities are more likely to be evoked (Pratt, 1998).

Second, it might be difficult to evoke an organizational category in organizations that are highly heterogeneous (e.g., in terms of race, gender, age, and so on). In these conditions, intragroup differences may make it difficult to find an organizational category that maximizes ingroup similarity in relation to other groups (Ashforth & Mael, 1996). As a result, identification with an organization may be facilitated when there is *intraorganizational homogeneity*. When organizational members are perceived as being too dissimilar, then a personal identity is likely to be evoked (Lau & Murninghan, 1998; Pratt, 1998).

Third, when the target organization is perceived as too similar to organizational outgroups, then interorganizational categories may not best account for similarities and differences in the social context. Thus, if McDonald's employees' see themselves as nearly identical to Burger King employees, then it will be difficult for them to form a "McDonald's" identity in relation to this organization. Rather, members may look at different types of restaurants (fast-food vs. formal restaurants) or look between institutions (food service vs. automotive service) in order to find categories that minimize intracategory similarities and maximize intercategory differences. Thus, organizational identification may also be difficult when members of the organization are perceived as too similar to members of outgroup organizations. Such contexts may evoke more abstract (e.g., institutional) identities (Pratt, 1998). In short, organizational identification is most likely when there is *interorganizational heterogeneity*.

**Identification in Traditional Organizational Contexts: Assumptions and New Directions.** Underlying much of this research on organizational identification has been a number of implicit or explicit assumptions about (a) the nature of identification, (b) the organizational context, and (c) the number of social identities competing for identification. First, the research mentioned thus far has examined "positive" identification. Here, the members view themselves in relation to the social group and have a positive evaluation of that group membership. As noted in Table 2.1, however, more recent research has examined other forms of identification, including disidentification, deidentification, and ambivalent identification.

Second, much of the existing organizational research has examined how identification occurs in high status, traditional organizations where members are physically co-located. However, current research also examines identity dynamics in other contexts, such as low-status organizations (or occupational groups) and organizations where members may not be co-located (i.e., virtual teams and organizations).

Third, emerging research is also examining identification in situations where the work environment is characterized by multiple identities. It has long been known that individuals have multiple social identities as a function of multiple group memberships. Some have assumed, however, that each social group is characterized by a single group-level identity. Recently, organizational scholars have begun to examine identification dynamics in groups that have multiple, and sometimes competing, social identities in a single social context.

### Beyond Positive Identification: Disidentification, Ambivalent Identification, and Deidentification

Tajfel and Turner (1979, p. 44) made a passing reference in their influential work, "An Integrative Theory of Intergroup Conflict," to the possibility that individuals may *disidentify* with their group. The notion of disidentification, as well as other forms of identification, has begun to receive more attention by organizational scholars. This research discusses more fully the evaluative and emotional components of social identity. As Tajfel notes, a social identity is "that *part* of the individuals' self-concept which derives from their knowledge of a social group (or groups) together with the value and emotional significance of that membership" (Tajfel, 1981, p. 255). Thus, scholars are examining the antecedents and outcomes of identifications characterized by negative or ambivalent evaluations and emotions of ingroup membership (see Harquail, 1998, for a discussion of identification and emotion).

In their studies of the National Rifle Association, Elsbach and Bhattacharya (2000, p. 3) define disidentification as occurring when individuals "maintain a sense of self-distinctiveness through perceptions and feelings of disconnection" from an organization. Thus, disidentification is not simply the breaking of an identification (i.e., deidentification, see Ashforth, 1998); rather, it is identification with a set of values and beliefs that are antithetical to those of a group. In addition, unlike positive identification, which involves identifying oneself based on what a group *is*, disidentification is based on identifying oneself based on what a group is *not*. Concurrent with this research are other works that have addressed disidentification. Dukerich et al. (1998), for example, discussed the negative individual and organizational consequences of disidentification, and Anat Rafaeli and I have shown how individuals enact disidentification through symbols (Pratt & Rafaeli, 2000). The concept of disidentification has also been further elaborated by Elsbach (1999) in her expanded model of organizational identification.

In addition to disidentification, researchers have also explored conflicted or ambivalent identifications (e.g., Dukerich et al., 1998; Elsbach, 1999), where individuals are both attracted to and repulsed by their organizations. As with disidentification, research has focused on the individual and organizational causes (e.g., traits and competing ideologies) and consequences (e.g., member burnout) of such a "mixed" identification (Dukerich et al., 1998; Elsbach, 1999; Pratt & Doucet, 2000).

In my own work, I have created a model that attempts to explain how the same organizational practices can cause all three types of identification (positive identification, disidentification, and ambivalent identification) as well as breaks in identification (deidentification). Drawing upon SIT and SCT, as well as other theories, I explain identification as a sensemaking process (Pratt, 2000a). When organizations can both create and fill the need for meaning within members, positive identification occurs. However, when organizations cannot create the need for meaning in members, or when they create the need for meaning but these needs are partially or fully met by nonmembers, then deidentification, ambivalent identification, and disidentification occurs, respectively. In SIT and SCT terms, this model suggests that identification occurs when an organizational identity is salient and when an organization creates strong ingroup-outgroup dynamics. When an organizational identity is not salient, no identification occurs. When the identity is salient, but members' evaluations of the identity are based on the opinions of negative outgroup members, then disidentification occurs. Finally, when the identity is salient, but members' evaluations are based on positive ingroup and negative outgroup members, then ambivalent identification occurs.

## Organizational Identification in Low-Status Organizations and Occupations

As mentioned, most organizational applications of SIT have looked at why individuals are more likely to identify with attractive or highly prestigious organizations than with nonprestigious ones. However, this work does not explain how or why individuals identify with low-status organizations or with social groups that are not prestigious. Such work, however, is critical, as changes in job practices are leading to a greater dichotomy between those with high-status professional jobs and those with low-status (e.g., low-skill service) jobs.

The topic of identification in low-status groups has recently been addressed. Ashforth and Kreiner (1999) have examined how individuals engaged in "dirty work"—work that is physically, socially, or morally tainted (Hughes, 1951)—are able to identify with their work groups or professions. In SIT terms, they suggest that identification occurs as members strengthen ingroup cohesion through the use of two primary strategies. First, they can create a strong occupational ideology that buffers members from negative perceptions by outgroup members (Pratt, 2000b). Here, members may develop rationalizations that reframe, recalibrate, or refocus certain features of the work so that it is less "dirty." Second, groups can change the nature of ingroup-outgroup comparisons. Such tactics, an elaboration of Tajfel and Turner's (1979, pp. 43–44) conceptualization of "social creativity," involve creating new dimensions for comparing ingroups and outgroups and engaging in downward comparisons (e.g., comparing one's self or group to even less fortunate individuals or groups; see also Terry, Chapter 15 of this volume).

## Social Identity Dynamics in Dispersed Groups

In addition to examining identification in "bricks and mortar" organizations, there has been rapidly increasing interest in identification dynamics in dispersed groups that are connected via technology (e.g., telephone, computer, video). Such groups include computer-mediated communication (CMC) groups, virtual or on-line teams (and organizations), Internet groups, and the like. Because these groups can be dispersed *spatially* (e.g., geographically dispersed organizations; see Scott, 1997), *temporally* (e.g., asynchronous groups), or both, I refer to all of them using the general label of *distributed groups* (DGs). The use of DGs as a means of "doing business" is increasing in modern organizations (Lipnack & Stamps, 1997). Given the newfound importance of DGs, Wiesenfeld et al. (2000, p. 7) argue that understanding the role of identification in DGs is critical because, "organizational identification which provides a psychological link between the organization and a dispersed workforce, may facilitate coordination by promoting convergent expectations." That is, identification may provide the psychological "glue" that holds a DG together and allows its members to act as a coordinated unit (DeSanctis & Poole, 1997). For instance, Moore, Kurtzberg, Thomson, and Morris (1999) found that when participants are negotiating over e-mail, ingroup identification facilitated negotiation outcomes (e.g., fewer impasses).

Because of the potential for organizational/group identification to facilitate functioning, and because social identities may be slow to develop in virtual environments where traditional social cues are lacking (Lipnack & Stamps, 1997), research on identity formation and identity salience in such contexts has come to the fore. Bouas and Arrow (1996) utilized SIT and other psychological theories to predict the development and strength of group identity in co-located and dispersed groups. Specifically, they examined behavioral, cognitive, and affective elements of group identity and how they change, over time, in face-to-face and CMC groups where membership changes are occurring. Similarly, Brandon and Pratt (1999) used both SIT and SCT to posit managerial practices that should increase the speed of identity development in on-line groups. Specifically, they suggested that management of identity formation in on-line groups involves the management of information—especially information relevant to building group categories and prototypes. Such findings are congruent with those of Wiesenfeld et al. (2000) who suggest that the quality of communication among members of virtual teams is integral to their identification. Perhaps the bulk of research on identity dynamics in DGs, however, is that which incorporates tenets from the SIDE (Social Identity DEindividuation) model.

**The SIDE Model.** One specific application of social identity (especially SCT) to identification-related issues that has gained increasing popularity is the SIDE model. Although mentioned in previous studies (e.g., Lea & Spears, 1992; Spears & Lea, 1994), the SIDE model seems to have been most fully developed in an article by Reicher, Spears, and Postmes (1995). In essence, the SIDE model explains the process of deindividuation—traditionally associated with a loss of self within a group or group consciousness—as a form of depersonalization in which individuals shift from their personal to social selves (J. C. Turner et al., 1987).

The SIDE model consists of both a cognitive element and a strategic one. Cognitively, the SIDE model predicts that deindividuating circumstances, such as being immersed in a group or being in a highly anonymous situation, affects individuals by changing the salience of a social identity. Specifically, individuals may tend to favor group norms in deindividuating circumstances because the group's social identity becomes more salient to an individual than his or her personal identity, and consequently, individuals tend to identify with the group identity.

Strategically, the SIDE model predicts that in order to enact a salient social identity, ingroup members must have the power to do so. Thus, the SIDE model argues that, "Group members will express those behaviors that are consonant with their social identity but which are disapproved of by the outgroup, only to the extent that they have the power to overcome any anticipated or actual resistance and/or retaliation by that outgroup" (Reicher et al., 1995, p. 186). Specifically, Reicher and colleagues (1995) suggested that when ingroup members become more identifiable *to outgroup members* (especially powerful ones), the ingroup loses power and, therefore, is less likely to engage in behaviors in opposition to the outgroup. By contrast, an ingroup can gain power relative to an outgroup by making other ingroup members more identifiable *to each other* (rather than to the outgroup) because such identification allows ingroup members the opportunity to support each other in the face of opposition.

Just as SIT has been applied to virtual teams, the SIDE model has been applied to groups linked via e-mail and other forms of CMC. In a recent review of SIDE's effects, Postmes et al. (1998) used the SIDE model to reinterpret inconsistent findings in deindividuation theory (LeBon, 1895/1947; Zimbardo, 1969) and in communication theory (Dubrovsky, Kiesler, & Sethna, 1991; Kiesler & Sproull, 1992) regarding why individuals behave as they do in computer-mediated interactions. Their review suggests several findings. First, individuals in visually anonymous CMC groups will tend to favor group norms if their group identity is salient. Such salience is enhanced when members identify with the social (group) identity and when there is an absence of individuating cues or information. Second, they suggest that anonymity may increase intergroup tensions and animosity. Again, salient social identities may transform Internet communications from interpersonal to intergroup among individuals belonging to different groups. In other words, deindividuation helps shift identification from personal to more abstract social identities.

They also note, however, that it is not necessarily anonymity, per se, that is the important factor in explaining their results. Rather, it is the degree to which "members of the ingroup and outgroup are individuated or depersonalized" (Postmes et al., 1998). While anonymity and degree of depersonalization often co-vary, there are situations where they may not. Hence, additional research is needed to explore anonymity effects on deindividuation.

Additional research is also needed to explore the strategic implications of the SIDE model in CMC groups. Although the theoretical implications of such an application has been proposed (Spears & Lea, 1994), and there has been some limited empirical support for the strategic applications of the SIDE model in non-CMC teams (Reicher & Levine, 1994; Reicher, Levine, & Gordijn, 1998), empirical support for the model in traditional and virtual organizational settings remains scant (Postmes et al., 1998).

## Identification in Multiple Organizational Identity Environments

A final trend in organizational identification involves looking at identification processes under conditions where there are multiple work-related social identities (e.g., professional versus organizational) in the organization or where the organization itself consists of multiple identities (Albert & Whetten, 1985; Pratt & Foreman, 2000). An example would be physicians in U.S. health maintenance organizations (HMOs) who are increasingly asked to identify with organizations that have both strong "patient-advocacy" and "business" identities. In this context, they are asked to identify with two legitimate, but often competing, social identities that characterize the HMO. Another context that elicits similar identification dilemmas are in organizations that have recently merged with other organizations (see D. van Knippenberg et al., forthcoming, and van Leeuwen, van Knippenberg, & Ellemers, 2000a for emerging work applying SIT and SCT in the context of organizational mergers; see also van Knippenberg & van Leeuwen, Chapter 16 of this volume, and Terry, this volume).

The dilemma of identification in multiple organizational identity environments (MOIEs) is different from the one posited by the SIDE model, where an individual chooses between a personal and a social identity. It is also different than the dilemma posed in the diversity management research (detailed below) where an organizational identity is competing with a nonorganizational social identity. In MOIEs, identities are at the same level of abstraction (social) and are each organizationally related. Thus, the issue of "identifying with the 'right' social identity" becomes even more problematic due to the fact that each of these multiple identities are often important for organizational survival and are often not entirely complimentary (see Pratt & Foreman, 2000, for a review).

Organizational research in this area has often blended SIT and SCT perspectives with other, often more sociological, theoretical perspectives. Work done in *holographic* (multiple work-related identities embedded in roles throughout the organization) and *idiographic* (multiple work-related identities embedded in distinct units within the organization) multiple identity organizations have combined SIT with theories of organizational identity (Albert & Whetten, 1985). Golden-Biddle and Rao's (1997) study of a nonprofit organization called "Medlay," for example, discussed the difficulties in trying to manage competing holographic identities. Here, both the board of directors and the management team perceived their organization as having two identities: Medlay was a "family of friends," where members treated each other as "colleagues" and "buddies," as well as a "guardian" of the public trust. Golden-Biddle and Rao (1997) documented the significant internal distress that board members felt when faced with the dilemma of which identity to evoke when forced to confront their colleagues about their questionable organizational expenditures.

Similarly, Rafaeli and I have shown how members in a MOIE (a rehabilitation hospital) advocated support for particular work-related social identities via the use of dress symbols (Pratt & Rafaeli, 1997). In this idiographic organization, different social identities were salient for different work groups in different situations. For example, the traditional "rehabilitation identity," in which nurses treat patients as if they are well, was salient with day-shift nurses, while a more traditional "acute care" identity, in which nursed treated patients as if they are sick, was more salient on evening and night shifts. In addition, a "nurse as public servant" professional identity was more salient among nurse managers than it was among floor nurses. In this study, we showed how one individual can identify with multiple work-related identities, but use the same symbols to express these different identifications. We also showed how identity conflicts could be managed symbolically.

Finally, Scott (1997) used SIT and theories of rhetoric (e.g., Cheney, 1983, 1991) to examine member identification in a geographically dispersed organization. Specifically, he examined multiple identification dynamics in members of one state's Cooperative Extension Service (CES), which acts like an "off-campus educational arm of each state's land grant university," to organizational identities existing at the national, state, county, and area levels. He found that individuals working in area and county offices identified more strongly with their corresponding geographic identities (e.g., the county CES organization) than those working in state offices. Moreover, individuals with longer tenure in an organization tended to identify more strongly with the organization.

While this research is intriguing, it is still in its infancy. Thus, SIT and other perspectives are currently being developed to answer questions of identification in MOIE's (see Pratt & Foremans, 2000, and Ashforth and Johnson, Chapter 3 in this volume for continuing efforts in this regard).

## MANAGING CONFLICT AND DIVERSITY

In addition to the management of organizational identification, organizational researchers have also applied SIT and SCT perspectives to issues of intergroup relations. Research on intergroup relations has drawn most heavily from SCT and has shown the conditions that may lead organizational subgroups into conflict (see Brewer & Kramer, 1985, and Kramer, 1993, for review). The logic of such research has been incorporated into a variety of studies examining diversity management from a SIT and SCT perspective.

Although diversity can refer to differences in members' knowledge bases (informational diversity) and in their beliefs about the central mission of the group or organization (value diversity), much of the extant research in applying SIT and SCT to diversity management has to do with differences in demographic characteristics (social category diversity), such as gender and race (see Jehn, Northcraft, & Neale, 1999, for a review of different types of diversity). Such an emphasis on visible characteristics may be due to the fact that individual characteristics that are easier to assess, such as race and gender, are more likely to form the basis for categorization than characteristics that are more difficult to assess, such as personality and abilities (Moreland, Levine, & Wingert, 1996). Moreover, as Lau and Murnighan (1998, p. 328) noted, "Although group members can categorize themselves in many different ways, they typically have a harder time denying their demographic attributes."

As noted in Table 2.1, researchers in diversity management have applied social identity theories in both traditional and nontraditional organizations. In the former, this is exemplified by research on group "fault lines" (Lau & Murninghan, 1998), diversity dilemmas (Philips, 1999; Schneider & Northcraft, 1999), and relational demography (Farh, Tsui, Xin, & Cheng, 1998; Tsui, Egan, & O'Reilly, 1992). In the latter, it often examines diversity issues in the context of virtual organizations (Bhappu, Griffith, & Northcraft, 1997; Pratt, Fuller, & Northcraft, 2000).

## Diversity Dynamics in Traditional Organizations

There have been several emerging streams of research that apply SIT and SCT to the study of diversity in traditional organizations. Much of this research posits the conditions under which demographic differences will be salient or problematic for organizations. I review some of these conditions here. This list is meant to be illustrative, not exhaustive.

1. *Amount of Diversity in the Work Group.* Lau and Murnighan (1998) suggested that "fault lines"—the presence of certain demographic characteristics that have the potential to "split apart" a work group—are more likely to become chronically salient in work groups where there is a moderate amount of demographic diversity rather than extremely high or low levels of such diversity. This prediction fits SCT in that too much heterogeneity (e.g., everyone is different from everyone else) would likely evoke individual identities, and too little (e.g., members are different on only one demographic characteristic) would likely lead to the formation of categories based on demographic rather than work-related characteristics.

2. *The Degree of Overlap between Demographic Characteristics and Functional Areas.* The salience of demographic identities may also be influenced by how they relate to work-related identities. Kawakami and Dion (1995), for example, suggested that memberships in social categories become more apparent when they co-vary with memberships in other groups. Similarly, Lau and Murnighan (1998) suggest that demographic fault lines are most likely to be problematic when member tasks evoke demographic differences. This suggests that when there is an overlap between demographic characteristics and functional areas (e.g., all upper level managers are male and all middle level managers are female), demographic differences will become more salient. For this reason, N. Miller and Harrington (1992) posit the cross-cutting of categories (e.g., varying demographic and functional characteristics) as a means of reducing the impact of demographic memberships.

3. *Age of the Work Group.* Organizational researchers also suggest that demographic differences may be the most problematic for new groups (Lau & Murnighan, 1998; Pratt et al., 2000). New work group members may self-categorize around demographic characteristics because work-related similarities may not yet be salient given the lack of shared expe-

riences in performing work-related tasks. Moreover, new groups may not have formed strong group-related prototypes[2] that define themselves as work groups.

4. *Size and Status of Demographic Subgroups.* Once demographic subgroups are salient, different group dynamics will occur depending on the size of the subgroups. When one subgroup is large in comparison to others, it will tend to dominate other subgroups. These conditions favor the *covert* enactment of dangerous *latent* group conflicts and *persistent* disagreements among members. By contrast, when subgroups are of roughly equal power, conflict will tend to be *intense, overt,* and relatively *short-lived* (Lau & Murninghan, 1998).

5. *Whether Members Are in the Numerical Majority or Minority.* Relational demography, which examines demographic dissimilarity among superiors and subordinates, suggests that high-status and low-status workers experience demographic diversity in different ways. Tsui and O'Reilly (1989), for example, suggest that high-status (e.g., groups in the numerical majority) groups tend to react to diversity with lower levels of perceived effectiveness of, and lower levels of personal attraction to low-status workers. Low-status workers (e.g., groups in the numerical minority), by contrast, are more likely to feel role ambiguity in demographically diverse organizations.

Work in relational demography further suggests that the size and status of the demographic group will affect group and organizational processes differentially depending on which demographic characteristic divides the groups. To illustrate: In *racially diverse* organizations, White members (the majority) have been found to feel less organization-based self-esteem and organizational attachment, to experience poorer peer relations, and to engage in fewer organizational citizenship behaviors than their non-White counterparts (Tsui et al., 1992; Chattopadhyay, 1999). Such asymmetrical effects have also been found for *gender.* For example, the presence of females in male-dominated firms can lead to a variety of negative organizational outcomes for males (Tsui et al., 1992). Findings for gender, however, have not been consistent (see Chattopadhyay, 1999).

*Age* has also been found to influence intergroup behavior. However, Chattopadhyay (1999) found that age dissimilarity was related to positive organization-based self-esteem, altruism, and peer relations among lower status younger workers. To explain these somewhat counterintuitive findings, he suggested that these effects may be due, in part, to the fact that age barriers are more permeable than race or gender barriers for young workers (all young work-

---

2. From a social identity perspective, prototypes are "fuzzy sets that capture the context-dependent features of a group membership often in the form of exemplary group members (actual group members who best embody the group) or ideal types (an abstraction of group features)" (Hogg, 1996a, p. 231).

ers expect to grow old), thus leading young workers to make more interpersonal comparisons than intergroup comparisons (Tajfel & Turner, 1986).

## Diversity Dynamics in DGs: The Role of Technology

The study of diversity management in DGs (especially virtual teams and CMC groups) suggests an additional factor that influences how demographic differences affect member behavior: technology. Since as early as the 1930s, researchers have noticed that technology can either worsen or improve relationships between or among members of demographically diverse groups.

On the one hand, technology is believed to make relations among individuals of different demographic groups more difficult. La Piere (1934), for example, noticed that workers at several American hotels and restaurants were likely to deny a Chinese patron's request for admission to their establishments if an inquiry was made over the phone. However, when workers confronted a Chinese patron face-to-face, admission was almost always granted. This suggests that technology may relax "politeness rituals" that would normally pressure individuals of different groups to behave in a friendly, civilized manner. More recently, effects such as "flaming" and other "uninhibited" behavior on the Internet suggest that the more anonymous the interaction, the more likely one is to act in an extreme manner (Dubrovksy et al., 1991; Kiesler & Sproull, 1992; see Walther, Anderson, & Park, 1994 for a critique of these findings). This suggests that, to the degree that demographic differences are noticeable in DGs, the lack of physical co-presence may make it easier for members to act upon these differences.

On the other hand, the technological mediation of communication may also serve to mask demographic differences. Under these conditions, work- or task-related identities may be more salient and, as a result, improve relations within demographically heterogeneous groups (as suggested by the SIDE model studies). To illustrate, Bhappu et al. (1997) showed that gender-based communication bias is lower in CMC groups than in face-to-face groups.

Clearly, additional research is necessary to help disentangle group identification effects (demographic versus organizational) from technology. Towards this end, Pratt et al. (2000) suggested that whether or not demographic or other "fault line" identities are salient and influence groups varies with technology in a curvilinear fashion. Conditions highest and lowest in their ability to convey social context cues (i.e., "media richness")—face-to-face groups and groups connected via the Internet, respectively—may be the *most* likely to lead to behavior that reflects work-group identities. Such behavior in Internet groups may occur for reasons espoused in the SIDE model (deindividuation leading to conformity to group norms), while strong "politeness rituals" may explain the enactment of group norms in the face-to-face groups. By contrast, technology that lies between these two extremes (e.g., telephone and video-conferencing) may maximize intergroup conflict caused by demographic differences. Specifically, such technology may make demographic differences salient, while at the same time relaxing "politeness rituals."

# CONCLUSIONS

In this chapter, I have provided an overview of some of the most recent applications of SIT and SCT to organizational contexts. Specifically, I show that research in organizational psychology and organizational behavior is currently using SIT and SCT frameworks to explain work behavior in modern organizations. This research sheds new light on "classic" issues such as how individuals relate to their collectives and how different subgroups within the collective interact.

To illustrate, modern organizations are characterized by multiple and competing memberships—especially as organizations are becoming more demographically diverse. Thus, researchers are using SIT and SCT to examine issues of diversity management and identification in multiple identity environments. Organizations are also using more groups that are spatially and temporally dispersed. As a result, researchers have begun to examine social identity dynamics in virtual teams. Finally, changes in the psychological contracts that once bound individuals to organizations have brought to the fore additional identification issues. For example, downsizing has eliminated middle management positions and has widened the gap between high-status and low-status jobs. This trend suggests the need to examine identification in low-status positions. Moreover, the lack of job security has caused different types of identification, such as disidentification and ambivalent identification, to become more salient. These trends, and others like them, are captured in the research summarized in Table 2.1.

This review also suggests how work from the "organizational side of the fence" has contributed to our understanding of social identity dynamics. Specifically, it suggests that its contribution to SIT and SCT research has more to do with breadth than with depth. That is, although social psychologists have done considerable work refining SIT and SCT (adding *depth*), such refinements have yet to appear in many organizational applications of these theories (see Hogg & Terry, 2000). However, organizational theorists do contribute to the *breadth* of SIT and SCT in two fundamental ways. First, they build our understanding of SIT and SCT dynamics by applying these theories to a variety of new contexts. Second, they extend theory by combining insights from SIT and SCT with other theories of social identity (e.g., identity theory), as well as with other theories of organizational behavior (e.g., diversity management).

It is my hope that this review facilitates an appreciation of SIT and SCT from an organizational psychology and organizational behavior perspective. Moreover, like the editors of this volume, I hope that this and other chapters facilitate dialogue between those primarily interested in the development of SIT and SCT for their own sake, and those most interested in their application.

In social identity terms, perhaps the discovery of "inter(disciplinary)-group" similarities will cause researchers to identify themselves as "social identity scholars" rather than to identify with other subgroups, such as psychologists or business school professors. While such distinctive approaches certainly cause the accumulation of social identity knowledge to increase more rapidly, we also know where such ingroup-outgroup distinctions might lead!

# 3

# Which Hat to Wear?

## The Relative Salience of Multiple Identities in Organizational Contexts

BLAKE E. ASHFORTH
*Arizona State University*
SCOTT A. JOHNSON
*San Jose State University*

*B*efore individuals can act in a given organizational context, they need to situate themselves and others—to define the respective social identities of the players. But organizations, particularly large ones, are complex phenomena, and a given context may suggest multiple potential identities. Take the example of a manager in a task force charged with revamping her company's vacation policy. Is she there as a manager, a department head, an organizational representative, a minority employee, all or some combination of these, or as something else? There are, in short, many hats of organizational membership (see also Bartel & Dutton, Chapter 8 of this volume).

In this chapter, we explore what makes various hats more salient or less salient to individuals. Our exploration is divided into four sections. First, we briefly discuss what we mean by salience. Second, we consider the relative salience of "nested" or embedded identities, such as manager → department head → organizational representative. Third, we consider the relative salience of "cross-cutting" identities, such as committees and demographic clusters. Fourth, we offer some speculations on the role of personal identities (i.e., idiosyncratic attributes) in the context of social identities and on the possibility of simultaneously salient identities and even holistic identities. As we will see, the metaphor of "which hat to wear" may be too limiting.

## IDENTITY SALIENCE

Following identity theory (e.g., Stryker, 1980), salience is defined as the probability that a given identity will be invoked, and multiple identities can be ranked in a "salience hierarchy" according to their relative salience. Drawing on identity theory as well as social identity theory (e.g., Tajfel & Turner, 1986), Ashforth (2001) argued that the salience of an identity to an individual in an organizational context is determined by the identity's *subjective importance* and *situational relevance* (cf. context-independent, chronic variation, and context-dependent, momentary variation [Higgins & King, 1981] and accessibility and fit [Oakes, 1987]). A subjectively important identity is one that is highly central to an individual's global or core sense of self or is otherwise highly relevant to his or her goals, values, or other key attributes (cf. Miller, Urban, & Vanman, 1998; Sherman, Hamilton, & Lewis, 1999). The more subjectively important the identity, the more likely one is to seek opportunities to enact the identity, to define a situation as identity-relevant, and to retain and recall identity-related information (especially identity-consistent information; e.g., Swann, 1990).

A situationally relevant identity is one that is socially appropriate to a given context. Whereas subjective importance is defined by internal preferences, situational relevance is defined by external norms. Thus, a person who, to the annoyance of his coworkers, persistently talks shop during a company baseball game is displaying the subjective importance of the work identity, but is defying norms about the identity's low situational relevance. As this example suggests, the situational relevance of a given identity may fluctuate greatly over the course of a day, whereas the subjective importance tends to remain more stable.

## NESTED IDENTITIES

As Figure 3.1 shows, certain identities are nested or embedded within others (Ashforth & Mael, 1989; Brewer, 1995; Dukerich, Golden, & Jacobson, 1996; S. D. Feldman, 1979; Mueller & Lawler, 1999). We will refer to identities toward the bottom as lower order identities (e.g., job, workgroup) and those toward the top as higher order identities (e.g., division, organization).[1] Nested identities form a means-ends chain (March & Simon, 1958) in that a given identity is both the means to a higher order identity and the end of a lower order identity.

It should be noted that identities vary in their organization-specificity. For example, a particular job or division may be relatively unique to a particular organization, whereas another job or division may be found in many organizations. The more organization-specific the identity, the more fully nested within the organization it is said to be.

---

1. Although our focus is restricted to the organization, the notion of higher order identities can be extended to industries, strategic alliances, geographic clusters of organizations, and so on (e.g., Lant, Hewlin, & Rindova, 2000).

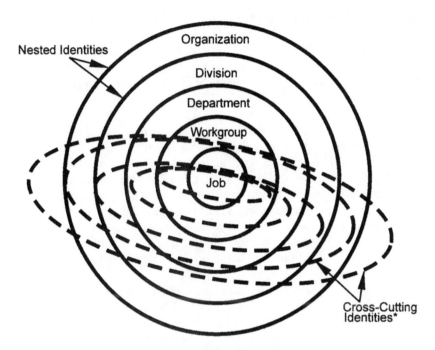

*Cross-Cutting Identities include *formal* (e.g., committees) and *informal* (e.g., friendship cliques) collectives. The larger rings depict identities that cross-cut multiple nested identities, including identities that extend beyond the organization's boundaries (e.g., demographic clusters). Although the rings converge on the job identity for ease of exposition, cross-cutting identities may converge on any nested level (e.g., a task force of departmental representatives).

FIGURE 3.1. Nested identities and cross-cutting identities.

## Identity Dimensions

Nested identities vary on at least three key dimensions: (a) inclusive/exclusive, (b) abstract/concrete, and (c) distal/proximal.

**Inclusive/exclusive.** Higher-order identities are relatively inclusive because they encompass all lower order identities (R. M. Kramer, 1993). Thus, the identity of a large organization encompasses whatever divisions, departments, work groups, and jobs comprise the organization. Similarly, the organizational identity may be claimed by any organizational member regardless of his or her specific job. Further, as Brewer (1991, p. 476) noted, a given identity provides "the frame of reference for differentiation and social comparison" of identities lodged at the next lower level. Members of the cookware department of a Sears store may look to other departments in the store for information about their department's relative performance and what makes the department unique: the store provides a common and inclusive context for the mutually exclusive departments within the store. Lower order identities are more exclusive because they do not include higher order identities and membership is restricted to individuals who meet certain criteria. Thus, the identity of cookware department sales clerk can be claimed only by individuals performing sales tasks in that department.

**Abstract/concrete.**   Higher order identities are relatively abstract because they must include a potentially diverse array of lower order identities, from secretary to senior manager, and accounting department to marketing department (M. E. Brown, 1969). The larger and more diverse the organization, the more abstract the identity. Thus, organizational identities are often defined in relatively general and succinct terms (and perhaps only implicitly), such as organizational mission and performance goals, key values and operating principles, major strategies, and favored traditions (e.g., Albert & Whetten, 1985; Ashforth & Mael, 1996). Organizational identities provide a psychological framework for individual members.

Conversely, lower order identities are relatively concrete because they represent the local means or action levers by which higher order identities are put into play. An organizational identity may espouse the importance of customer service, but it is the front-line service agents who must translate that value into specific behavior. Consequently, job descriptions and operating procedures may be considerably more detailed than the organization's mission statement. Further, S. D. Feldman (1979, p. 403) noted that "As one devotes more and more time, interest, and attention to an activity, one can make finer and finer gradations and see significant distinctions that an 'outsider' may not see." For example, the identity of accountant may be subdivided by specialty, job tenure, clients, productivity, and so on. Thus, a given identity may be subdivided into a network of lower order identities and thereby become increasingly exclusive and concrete.

**Distal-proximal.**   Higher order identities are relatively distal in the Lewinian sense that their impact on the individual tends to be indirect and delayed rather than direct and immediate (Lewin, 1943; Mueller & Lawler, 1999). Higher order identities, as psychological frameworks, set the basic parameters within which organizational members operate. The organization's mission, goals, performance targets, key values, and so on help foster a certain culture(s) and climate(s) that in turn shape individuals' thoughts, feelings, and actions.

In contrast, lower order identities are relatively proximal in the sense that their impact is more direct and immediate. This occurs because lower order identities provide a more localized and concrete rendering of the higher-order identities. In effect, lower order identities largely mediate the impact of higher order identities on the individual. For instance, a key organizational value such as respect for the individual may be instantiated at the work-group level through norms of openness and empowerment.

Clearly, then, the three dimensions of inclusive/exclusive, abstract/concrete, and distal/proximal are mutually reinforcing. It is precisely because higher order identities are necessarily inclusive that they also tend to be abstract, and it is because they are abstract that they tend to be distal. In contrast, because lower order identities are more exclusive, they can be rendered in more concrete terms and exert a proximal impact on individuals.

## The Salience of Lower Order Identities

It seems likely that *lower order identities will generally be more subjectively important and situationally relevant, that is more salient, than higher order identities* (Brewer, 1995; M. E. Brown, 1969; R. M. Kramer, 1991; Lawler, 1992; Scott, 1997). D. van Knippenberg and van Schie (2000) suggest several reasons. First, in the course of performing his or her duties, a typical organizational member is more likely to encounter members of other jobs and work groups *within* the organization than members of *other* organizations and to be approached in terms of his or her job or work group membership than organizational membership. Further, because organizational members have the organizational identity in common, it becomes the water within which they all swim, and therefore less salient than more localized identities (Ashforth & Mael, 1996). In short, lower order social categories are more likely to be one's *primary group*— "the group with which an individual most frequently interacts and . . . [through] which other members of the organization interact with him or her" (R. M. Kramer, 1991, pp. 204–205).

Second, given the greater exclusiveness and concreteness of lower order identities, individuals will tend to perceive that they have more in common with those who share the identities. The principle of "metacontrast" holds that individuals in a given context will tend to be categorized into subgroups to the extent that intragroup differences are perceived to be smaller than intergroup differences (J. C. Turner et al., 1987). Because the members of lower order groups tend to be more homogeneous than the members of higher order groups, the lower order groups become more salient. Further, given task interdependencies at the local level, individuals will tend to interact more with others sharing their local identities and to perceive common goals. In turn, perceived similarity, interaction, and task and goal interdependence may facilitate a perception of *entitativity* (Brewer & Harasty, 1996; Sherman et al., 1999)—of being group-like—and a sense of shared identity and a commitment to the shared identity.

Third, Brewer's (1991, p. 475) optimal distinctiveness theory holds that individuals attempt to balance conflicting needs for assimilation with others and differentiation from others, for "being the same and different at the same time." Thus, individuals may find that the inclusiveness and abstractness of the organization's identity make it difficult for them to discern their uniqueness within the organization. Higher order identities, after all, imply sameness.

Conversely, a more exclusive identity, such as job or work group, enables individuals to share an identity with others and yet attain some distinctiveness within the organization. Consequently, individuals may gravitate toward more localized and therefore differentiating social identities. At the same time, a lower order identity can be *too* exclusive and thus threaten one's desire for inclusiveness (Brewer, 1991). For example, a store's lone security guard may feel somewhat isolated by the guard identity and may therefore prefer to invoke the higher order identity of store worker. However, because we are focusing on *social* rather than personal identities, even a relatively exclusive social category such as security guard will encompass other people (although one may have to imagine them as a generalized ideal).

We can add a fourth reason to D. van Knippenberg and van Schie's (2000) argument that lower-order identities tend to be more salient. As the world has become more dynamic and complex, and competition, globalization, technological development, and customer demands explode, organizations have evolved from ponderous bureaucracies to more organic structures. Top-down command and control systems are giving way to lateral communication and teamwork, decentralized decision making, employee empowerment, and flexible work arrangements. Virtual work environments, where individuals are linked electronically, have even eradicated some traditional office facilities. Thus, individuals are increasingly vesting their sense of workplace self at the job and work group levels (Stroh, Brett, & Reilly, 1994).

Although no study, to our knowledge, has contrasted the salience of nested identities in organizational contexts, work group identification was found to be stronger than organizational identification among samples of local government and university employees (van Knippenberg & van Schie, 2000), military supply company employees (Becker, 1992, Table 1), and a computer manufacturer's telemarketing sales and service employees (Johnson, 2001; however, *occupational* identification was not stronger than organizational identification). Similarly, Barker and Tompkins (1994) found that workers in a manufacturing firm identified more highly with their self-managing teams than with their organization (at $p = .07$), and Scott (1999) found that students in a small group communication course identified more strongly with their project groups and major than with their university. Finally, Russo (1998) found that newspaper journalists identified more strongly with their profession than with their newspaper, although Scott (1997) did not find that occupational identification was stronger than subunit identification in a geographically dispersed government organization.[2] (Each of these studies measured identification by using parallel items across foci to ensure comparability.)

Conversely, we speculate that an organization's identity is likely to remain more subjectively important (although not necessarily more situationally relevant) than lower order identities if, all else being equal, the organization ap-

---

2. The terms "occupation" and "profession" are somewhat more abstract than "job." A job is a bundle of tasks institutionalized in the organization's structure, whereas an occupation or profession may also include collectives that exist beyond the organization's boundaries. Accordingly, an occupation or profession may not be seen as "lower order" per se.

pears to be: (a) more or less *uniquely* associated with particular values and goals (e.g., religious, military, and public service organizations; D. T. Hall, Schneider, & Nygren, 1970); (b) of very high status; (c) *holographic* rather than *ideographic* (Albert & Whetten, 1985), that is, where subunits have a common identity rather than differentiated identities (e.g., a clan organization versus a diversified firm; Ouchi, 1980); (d) highly centralized such that individuals must "look up to" the organization for direction and resources (Lawler, 1992); and/or (e) chronically and severely threatened by external forces (e.g., tobacco companies, abortion clinics; Korn, 1996).

## The Salience of Higher Order Identities

Although higher order identities tend to be less salient than lower order ones, higher order identities are nonetheless extremely important. The more salient a higher order identity, the more likely that an organizational member will think, feel, and act in ways consistent with that identity. For example, a salient organizational identity may encourage one to pursue organizational goals ahead of narrow lower order goals, to interpret issues and events from a higher order perspective, to enact organizational values in ways consistent with organizational norms, to cooperate with other organization members (even though they may have different and possibly conflicting lower order identities), and to engage in organizational citizenship behaviors (Ashforth & Mael, 1996; Dutton et al., 1994; Kramer, 1993; Pratt, 1998).

Additionally, immersion in a higher-order identity allows one to "lose oneself" at least temporarily in something greater than the individual, to become part of a powerful and edifying collective. As Zurcher (1982) documented, occasional deindividuation may be experienced as liberating and empowering. We emphasize "occasional" because the imposition of a superordinate identity may threaten subjectively important subgroup identities and provoke a backlash (Ashforth & Mael, 1998; Hornsey & Hogg, 2000a).

**Substantive and symbolic management.** How are higher order identities made at least temporarily salient in the face of the gravitational tug toward lower order identities? The answer lies in *substantive management* and *symbolic management* (Ashforth & Mael, 1996; Bullis & Tompkins, 1989; Cheney, 1991; Czarniawska, 1997; Elsbach & Glynn, 1996; Gaertner, Dovidio, Anastasio, Bachman, & Rust, 1993; R. M. Kramer, 1991; Pfeffer, 1981; Pratt, 1998; Stern, 1988). Indeed, it could be argued that a major function of senior management is to make higher order identities more salient and thereby unite disparate members in a common cause. Substantive management refers to real, material change in organizational practices. A variety of tactics may induce individuals to view themselves as being in the same boat and regard one another and higher order identities more positively: keeping the organization relatively small and focused, formulating overarching goals and strategies, creating innovative and high-quality products, picking fights with external "enemies," acting in a socially responsible manner, creating task interdependencies and communication channels and minimizing physical proximity between lower order groups, creating dispute resolution mechanisms for intergroup conflicts, providing full-time and permanent employment, socializing newcomers collectively with an emphasis on higher order identities, rotating members through various departments, tying rewards to higher order goals, creating internal labor markets, sponsoring an organization newsletter and organization-wide social events, and so on.

Symbolic management refers to the ways that management portrays the organization to members, and tends to focus on what is (or is presumed or hoped to be) central, distinctive, and relatively enduring about the organization (Albert & Whetten, 1985). Like the levers of substantive management, the levers of symbolic management are legion: articulating a mission statement, celebrating organizational achievements, attributing negative developments to external sources, championing individuals whose actions exemplify the organization's identity, framing lower order goals and accomplishments in terms of the organization's mission, extolling the organization in advertisements and public relations activities, minimizing the trappings of rank and hierarchy, wearing organizational uniforms or formulating a dress code, using the pronouns "we" and "us" rather than "you" and "I," emphasizing member commonalities (although it is no longer socially acceptable to emphasize certain demographic commonalities), creating an organizational logo and a unique argot, relating stories and myths and crafting traditions and rituals that glorify the organization's history and identity, invoking metaphors and labels such as "family" to characterize the organization, housing employees in distinctive and prestigious settings, and so forth. Substantive and symbolic practices tend to blur over time as the substantive takes on symbolic overtones and the symbolic becomes institutionalized in substantive practices.

In sum, substantive and symbolic management are largely intended to counter parochial and insular identifications, creating subjective importance and situational awareness—salience—for the organization as a whole. Thus, although lower order identities tend to have ongoing salience, higher order identities may be rendered at least temporarily salient by various practices that draw attention to the larger entity (cf. Pratt & Foreman, 2000).

## Salience Shifts

Assuming that the subjective importance of identities to an individual is fairly stable in the short term, shifts in the relative salience of the identities are most likely to be caused by their situational relevance. A doctor may focus on her occupational identity when treating a sick patient but may focus on her higher order hospital identity when interviewing prospective interns. However, if an identity is seen to be extremely subjectively important, then it will likely remain chronically salient such that salience shifts are infrequent. One is more likely to invoke the identity at socially inappropriate times, as illustrated by the earlier example of the employee talking shop at the company baseball game.

We speculate that salience shifts between nested identities tend to be quite easy for most organizational members. First, because higher order identities are a more inclusive, abstract, and distal version of lower order identities, there tends to be at least some overlap in the content of nested identities. As Scott, Corman, and Cheney (1998, p. 315) noted: "An engineer, for example, may feel that his or her work is personally rewarding, central to the project group's goals, consistent with the organization's mission, and very much aligned with what the engineering profession is all about." A given act, such as designing a prototype, may be consistent with all of the engineer's nested identities. Thus, it may be relatively easy for the engineer to shift from one identity to another as circumstances warrant.

However, nested identities are not always consistent and may even conflict (M. E. Brown, 1969; R. J. Fisher, Maltz, & Jaworski, 1997; Hornsey & Hogg, 2000a; Rotondi, 1975). Higher order identities, by definition, take a broader and often longer term purview of the organization and may need to counter parochial subunit tendencies and to reconcile conflicts between subunit identities (e.g., marketing's emphasis on sales versus production's emphasis on efficiency; cf. social dilemmas, Polzer, Stewart, & Simmons, 1999). Indeed, an identity lodged at one level may serve as a *foil* for an identity lodged at another level. For instance, Collinson (1992) found that shopfloor workers defined themselves partly in opposition to the organizational identity propounded by management (e.g., militant vs. cooperative, independent vs. interdependent, crude vs. genteel). The degree of inconsistency and conflict between nested identities likely fluctuates over time as new issues arise. Ironically, however, such flashpoints may *facilitate* salience shifts by rendering multiple identities at least momentarily important and situationally relevant, although such shifts are likely to trigger heightened anxiety.

A second reason that salience shifts between nested identities tend to be relatively easy is that identification with a given level tends to *generalize* to other levels such that the subjective importance and therefore the salience of the implicated identities tends to generalize as well. Because the organization provides the context within which local identities may flourish (whether by design or default), the organization may come to be seen as one's "home" or the "vehicle" (Russo, 1998, p. 102) for expressing one's local identities. Thus, identification with a lower order entity, such as one's job, may generalize to higher order entities, such as one's department and organization. Conversely, identification with a higher order entity may predispose one to perceive lower order identities in positive terms and to internalize them as more specific and localized definitions of self.[3]

---

3. Identification with an individual, such as a charismatic manager, high-status peer, or favored client, may similarly generalize to other organization-based entities. For example, Stern (1988) describes how identification with Clifford Garrett, the charismatic founder of Garrett Corporation, generalized to the company as a whole. However, because an individual is not, by definition, a social category (although a group

Combining these two arguments, that nested identities tend to overlap and that identification tends to generalize, it seems likely that a positive correlation would exist between identification at one level and identification at other levels. Research generally supports this contention. Becker (1992) found that identification with one's work group and one's organization correlated at $r = .45$ in a military supply company. Barker and Tompkins (1994) reported that identification with one's self-managing team and one's organization correlated at $r = .68$ in a manufacturing firm (personal communication from the authors, February/March, 1995). D. van Knippenberg and van Schie (2000) report that identification with one's work group and one's organization correlated at $r = .41$ for a sample of university employees, but at $r = .07$ for a sample of local government employees. Johnson (2001) found correlations among telemarketing sales and service employees of $r = .62$ between work team and organizational identification, $r = .60$ between team and occupational identification, and $r = .47$ between occupational and organizational identification. Scott (1997, Table 2) found that bivariate correlations among identification with four foci (occupation and three levels of offices: county, area, state) of a geographically dispersed government organization ranged from $r = .39$ to $r = .68$. And Russo (1998) found that journalists' identification with their profession correlated at $r = .60$ with identification with their newspaper. (However, because these studies measured multiple identifications by using parallel items in a cross-sectional design, the correlations are likely inflated by common method variance.)

However, although the different foci for identification may be conceptually clear and distinct, the foci may blur in practice for organizational members. The same principles of overlap and generalization that facilitate salience shifts may render any given entity less distinct. For instance, Russo (1998) also interviewed the journalists and found that the foci of identification tended to blur, partly because the subordinates, coworkers, and clients with whom the journalists felt a kinship were themselves allied with multiple groupings (journalist, department, newspaper). Thus, it may make little difference to an organizational member if he or she is said to be identified with, for example, the organization or the division, or the job or the work group.

A third reason that salience shifts may be relatively easy is that individuals tend to develop *transition scripts* (Ashforth, Kreiner, Fugate, & Johnson, 2001) over time. As individuals gain experience in shifting between identities, they develop psychological routines for rapidly switching cognitive gears and adopting the necessary affective tone (e.g., getting "psyched up" for a group meeting). Transition scripts may be triggered by external cues (e.g., a reporter phones, cuing the organization identity) or internal cues (e.g., one decides to work, cu-

---

of similar individuals or of followers is), this kind of identification is beyond the scope of the paper. Identification with an individual is commonly referred to as "classical identification" (Kelman, 1961) and follows somewhat different social psychological dynamics than social identification (Ashforth & Mael, 1989).

ing the job identity). With repeated enactments of the transition script, both the cuing and enactment of the transition process are likely to become relatively automatic. Consequently, individuals tend to become adept at shifting identities.

In sum, because lower order identities are more exclusive, concrete, and proximal than higher order identities, they tend to be more salient. However, substantive and symbolic management may render higher order identities at least temporarily salient, and transition scripts, generalization of identification, and overlap in the content of identities typically facilitate salience shifts between nested identities.

# CROSS-CUTTING IDENTITIES

Nested identities are attached to *formal* social categories in the sense that the categories are institutionalized in the organization's structure. A typical organizational chart, for example, depicts the hierarchy of nested categories. In contrast, cross-cutting identities are attached to social categories that are either *formal or informal*. Formal cross-cutting social categories may include committees, task forces, union locals, and so on, whereas informal categories may include friendship cliques, common interest social groups (e.g., a prayer group), family ties (as in a family-run company), demographic clusters, and so on. As Brewer (1995, p. 51) noted, informal categories may be "*external* to the organization and overlap only partially with membership in the organization itself."

## The Salience of Cross-Cutting Identities

Cross-cutting identities are analogous to lower order identities in that they tend to be relatively exclusive, concrete, and proximal. Consequently, such identities tend to be relatively salient. Compared to lower order identities, cross-cutting identities may be more salient or less salient, depending of course on their relative situational relevance and subjective importance. The situational relevance of cross-cutting identities, like nested identities, is determined by external norms and therefore tends to be cued by the local environment. Thus, the situational relevance of a given identity is likely to fluctuate greatly over time. The subjective importance of cross-cutting identities likely varies widely, from a very important friendship clique to an unimportant committee charged with a trivial task. It is unclear whether informal cross-cutting identities will tend to be seen as more subjectively important than formal ones. On one hand, informal identities may be more important because, with the exception of family ties and demographic categories, individuals tend to have more latitude in selecting them. On the other hand, formal identities tend to carry more status, reward, and career growth opportunities because they are more likely to be linked to the organization's mission.

**Demographic identities.**    Demographic clusters represent a special case of cross-cutting social categories. Unlike other categories, the members may seldom interact as members *per se* (although members of *minority* categories often coalesce for mutual support, and demographic similarities do facilitate attraction and interaction; see, e.g., Mehra, Kilduff, & Brass, 1998). For instance, a White male may not seek out other Whites or males to talk about issues related to race or gender. Thus, a given demographic category may be what J. C. Turner (1984) called a "psychological group," that is, "a collection of people that . . . define themselves in terms of the same social category membership" (p. 530) but who do not necessarily interact with other members *qua* members. Turner's psychological group can be distinguished from a "social group" where a relatively clear social structure exists (e.g., roles, norms), and members *do* have interpersonal interdependencies and interactions centered on collective goals—in short, where entitativity is relatively high.

Although demographic categories in the workplace often remain psychological rather than social groups, demographic identities may nonetheless remain fairly salient (Wharton, 1992). First, many demographic attributes are universal (everyone has them) and/or highly visible, thus providing ready stimuli for categorization. For example, gender and race are said to be "primary categories" (Brewer, 1988) because they are perceived automatically and given precedence over other possible categorizations. Potent social stereotypes are often attached to demographic categories and may be invoked to provide a shorthand (and usually flawed) understanding of category members (Oakes et al., 1994). Thus, individuals are routinely perceived through the prism of their demographic attributes, although the salience of these attributes may wane with increased interpersonal familiarity (Ashforth & Humphrey, 1995).

Second, demographic attributes are often correlated with nested identities (e.g., male senior executives) and with each other (e.g., female and ethnic minority maids, young and male bouncers), thus reinforcing the salience of the attributes (Hogg & Terry, 2000; cf. "faultlines," Lau & Murnighan, 1998). Moreover, if demographic categories are correlated with access to resources, the categories may become a salient indicator of status in their own right (Ridgeway, 1991).

Third, given social stereotypes and the historical inequities that have resulted, members of stigmatized demographic categories may feel threatened. The sense of threat may sensitize category members to perceive events and issues through the lens of their demographic category and cause them to band together for mutual support, as alluded to above. In such cases, the psychological group becomes a social group.

Fourth, affirmative action and diversity programs call attention to various demographic attributes, institutionalizing them as surely as the nested identities or formal cross-cutting identities. Affirmative action programs have the laudable goal of righting historic wrongs and various diversity programs are designed to enhance the perceived value and synergy of demographic and other differences. Ironically, however, such programs and the banding together noted above may compound the historic wrongs by rendering the targeted demographic categories more salient to all concerned such that individuals are labeled (by themselves and by others) in terms of their categories and are more likely to be seen as different—as "them" rather than part of "us." Further, to the extent that hiring, promotion, and other important human resource decisions are attributed to the salient categories rather than to merit, the programs may foster resentment and a backlash against the category members (e.g., Day, Cross, Ringseis, & Williams, 1999). Finally, as labeling theory indicates, labels tend to become self-fulfilling as the salient categories color subsequent interaction and reinforce perceived differences (Ashforth & Humphrey, 1995).

### Salience Shifts

**Formal cross-cutting identities.** Salience shifts between formal cross-cutting identities and between these identities and nested identities are likely to be quite easy because of overlapping content (e.g., one is assigned to a task force to represent one's department or to draw on the expertise associated with one's job). Also, given this overlap, identification with other formal categories may generalize to the cross-cutting identities.

A potential exception to this overlap and generalization argument may involve professions, professional associations, and unions vis-a-vis other formal identities. Gouldner's (1957) distinction between cosmopolitans and locals suggests that professional values are antithetical to bureaucratic values such that one identifies with either the profession (cosmopolitan) or the organization (local). However, research suggests that professional and organizational identities are only loosely coupled such that one may identify with one, both, or neither (e.g., Greene, 1978). Similarly, reviews of research on "dual allegiance" to union and company (Gordon & Ladd, 1990) and on "multiple commitments" to profession and company (Wallace, 1993) indicate positive rather than negative associations. Thus, identity overlap and identification generalization may indeed occur between professional/union attachments and other formal identities.

Further, any conflict that *is* experienced between identities may, as noted, actually facilitate salience shifts. Moreover, Meyer and Allen (1997) speculated that many conflicts between identification objects focus on specific and infrequent issues rather than on general and ongoing issues such that the conflicts are *acute* rather than *chronic*. If so, the positive regard that one generally has toward different identification objects may give way to temporary disidentification with one object or another during those times of acute conflict, just as a person can argue with a spouse about specific issues and yet retain an abiding love for him or her.

**Informal cross-cutting identities.** The more that informal cross-cutting identities correlate with formal identities (e.g., male senior executives, coworker friendships), the more likely that the informal and formal identities will blur and shape one another. The result, once again, is identity overlap, identification generalization, and transition scripts, such that salience shifts between the informal and formal will tend to become relatively easy.

In contrast, the less that informal and formal identities correlate (e.g., a prayer group drawn from all corners of an organization), the less overlap and generalization, and the more difficult the salience shifts, although transition scripts may nonetheless emerge over time to regulate such shifts. However, as noted, if conflict emerges between otherwise segmented identities, the identities may become at least temporarily important and situationally relevant such that they are both salient. For instance, a supervisor may be ordered to perform acts that contravene the precepts of her prayer group. Indeed, the more subjectively important an identity, the more likely one is to perceive conflicts involving that identity, and the more one perceives such conflicts, the more acutely important the identity becomes.

In sum, because cross-cutting identities are analogous to lower order identities, they tend to be relatively salient. Due to identity overlap and identification generalization, salience shifts between formal (but not necessarily informal) cross-cutting identities and nested identities tend to be quite easy.

## SPECULATIONS ON CONNECTIONS BETWEEN MULTIPLE IDENTITIES

### The Importance of Personal Identities

We have thus far focused on social identities. However, personal identities likely play a critical role in the dynamics discussed above. First, individuals tend to *personalize* the enactment of their social identities; that is, individuals interpret and execute the identities in more or less idiosyncratic ways. Personalization occurs because no two individuals are alike and the behavioral norms associated with a given identity usually allow some latitude in the way an identity is expressed. Further, because higher order identities are relatively inclusive, abstract, and distal, they are often only loosely coupled with behavioral norms, allowing additional latitude. Thus, once a social identity is cued, one's personal identities tend to inform the social identity, often strongly affecting the way it's enacted. For example, for one police officer the organizational value of public service may mean helping a commuter change his flat tire, whereas for another officer it may mean simply calling a tow truck. Personal identities, in short, become more salient in intragroup contexts (J. C. Turner et al., 1994). Moreover, personal identities may *shape* social identities, particularly lower order and cross-cutting identities because there tend to be fewer individuals comprising the social category. A police officer's behavior is more likely to change the way her squad, rather than her precinct, thinks of itself.

Second, because formal cross-cutting groups often include people from various jobs, work groups, and departments, they tend to be more heterogeneous than a typical lower order nested group. Accordingly, the various nested identities of the cross-cutting group members tend to be relatively salient. For example, a new product development team typically contains individuals from diverse functional departments. Thus, optimal distinctiveness may be attained by invoking one's unique departmental identity in the context of the more inclusive team identity. Conversely, because lower order nested groups tend to be more homogeneous, optimal distinctiveness may be attained by invoking one's *personal* identities. In short, personal identities tend to be more salient in lower order nested groups than in formal cross-cutting groups. (In contrast, *informal* cross-cutting groups, such as a friendship clique or demographic cluster, tend to be more homogeneous than formal cross-cutting groups because they tend to coalesce around perceived commonalities.)

Third, perhaps personal identities rather than the job identity occupy the lowest rung on the nested hierarchy (see Figure 3.1). The rise of employee empowerment and flexible work arrangements, noted earlier, is placing a premium on the qualities of the individual—the values, knowledge, skills, abilities, and so forth—that necessarily undergird job performance. Moreover, employees are increasingly viewed as contingent workers, laboring with a series of employers on specific assignments for limited time periods (Barnett & Miner, 1992). For instance, it has been estimated that individuals change employers every 4.5 years (Sullivan, 1999), whether voluntarily or involuntarily. Consequently, many individuals are adopting a free agent identity, where they strive to continually develop skill sets that are no longer tied to a specific organization, that is, that are *portable* (Arthur & Rousseau, 1996b). As individuals thus become more self-centered and self-directed in their careers, the social identities (nested and cross-cutting) become less salient relative to their personal identities, their portable self.

## Simultaneous Salience

Each lower order, higher order, and cross-cutting identity needs to be salient at certain times. However, there may be times when multiple identities need to be *simultaneously* salient (cf. Gaertner, Dovidio, & Bachman, 1996; Huo, Smith, Tyler, & Lind, 1996). First, following Brewer's (1991) contention that individuals seek similarity and dissimilarity at the same time, cuing a given social identity may activate a counterdesire for a lower order (more exclusive) social identity or a personal identity (cf. Deschamps & Devos, 1998). In short, *ambivalence* may be a cause (and consequence) of simultaneous salience.

Second, bringing multiple identities to bear on a situation may facilitate rich and circumspect actions. For example, a finance executive representing the finance department at a strategic retreat for top managers needs to think in terms of the organization as a whole as well as his department, and a marketing task force may be comprised of demographically diverse individuals precisely because the individuals are expected to bring their demographic identities to bear on the task force's mission. Further, Hogg and Terry (2000) argued that harmonious relations between subgroups may be enhanced by making both subgroup and organizational identities salient.

However, as S. R. Marks and MacDermid (1996) document, the literature on multiple identities and roles indicates that identities tend to be cognitively segmented and buffered, suggesting that individuals are capable of invoking only one identity at a time. For instance, the notions of a salience hierarchy (identity theory) and self- and social categorization processes (self-categorization theory) imply that social identities are discrete psychological phenomena such that as one identity becomes salient, others necessarily become less so.

A provocative question, then, is whether multiple identities can in fact be simultaneously salient. We speculate that simultaneity is indeed possible (cf. Thoits & Virshup, 1997). It seems unlikely that individuals would routinely park their various social identities outside—in a real sense, would forget who they are—when a particular identity is salient. Four factors may affect simultaneity. First, the greater the overlap between identities and the generalization of identification, the more likely that the salience of the identities will in turn be positively correlated. Cuing one identity would make similar identities more cognitively accessible (Higgins, 1996). Second, the more relevant multiple identities are to a given context, the more likely that those identities will be explicitly or implicitly cued via substantive and symbolic management. For example, in the marketing task force mentioned above, a team member may be asked to respond to an issue from the perspective of her gender or ethnicity. Third, the more often that multiple identities are invoked either simultaneously or sequentially, the more likely that a cognitive association will form between them such that invoking one at least primes the other (Higgins, 1996). Finally, the more cognitively complex the individual, the more likely it is that he or she can cognitively attend to the demands of multiple identities (cf. Slugoski, Marcia, & Koopman, 1984). Indeed, consistent with Nippert-Eng's (1996) finding that individuals differ in the degree to which they prefer to integrate their home and work roles, perhaps "preference/tolerance for simultaneity" can be cast as a more or less stable individual difference variable.

Ultimately, salience is not an all-or-none phenomenon; it is a matter of degree. The notion of a salience hierarchy reminds us that identities can be arrayed according to their *relative* salience (Stryker, 1980). Thus, the fact that one identity is highly salient does not necessarily mean that another is not at all salient.

## Holistic Identities

The notion of simultaneous salience still preserves the notion that identities are independent and bounded. Returning to Figure 3.1, each identity is depicted as a discrete part of the whole, and individuals often must invoke transition scripts to move from one identity to another.

Thus, a broader question is whether multiple identities can form a *holistic gestalt* where the boundaries around each identity fade and the contents flow into a rich melange. The notion of holism is reminiscent of the debate regarding whether individuals have a single, unified self or a multiplicity of selves (e.g., Baumeister, 1998, vs. Gergen, 1991).

Personal identities would appear more amenable to holism than social identities because the latter are attached to discrete social categories that are generally deemed meaningful by one's culture (e.g., gender) and may be institutionalized in organizational contexts (e.g., department). Nonetheless, social identities may also have holistic qualities. As noted, nested identities tend to be at least somewhat overlapping and spark generalized identification. Further, the complexity of many organizational issues and the interdependence of nested identities (recall March & Simon's [1958] means-ends chain) often require that one instantiate multiple identities simultaneously, such as manager (lower order identity) of the marketing department (higher order identity). Just as expertise is gained by gradually forming dense connections between data points (a holistic grasp), repeated instantiation of multiple identities may lead to dense connections between the identities. As Thoits and Virshup (1997, p. 128) put it, "When multiple identities are conjoined (e.g., student activist) . . . their meaning and behavioral consequences may reside in the amalgamation itself." Moreover, Dietz and Ritchey (1996, p. 6) argue that identities that accumulate as a set "may have a content and a meaning . . . beyond the sum of [the] parts," a kind of *identity synergy* (cf. Pratt & Foreman, 2000).

Cross-cutting identities may have even more potential for holism than nested identities. The growth of empowerment and teamwork implies that individuals need to marshal their internal resources and be aware of the self as a gestalt whose knowledge, skills, and abilities draw on and transcend categorical identities derived from gender, race, ethnicity, religion, and so on. The atomistic self was better suited to more stable and simple times. Thus, employees in contemporary organizations are less likely to put stock in gender, race, or other categories per se, and more likely to put stock in their holistic capacity to get the work done (although the diversity issues mentioned earlier create a countervailing tendency).

## SUMMARY

Identity salience is a critical construct because individuals have a multiplicity of social identities to choose from in situating themselves and others in a given organizational context. Identities are generally either nested or cross-cutting. Because lower order nested identities are more exclusive, concrete, and proximal than higher order ones, they tend to be more salient. However, organizations often utilize substantive and symbolic management to boost awareness of higher order identities, at least temporarily. Cross-cutting identities are similar to lower order identities and are therefore relatively salient. Shifts in salience between social identities, whether nested or cross-cutting, are facilitated by overlap in identity content, generalization of identification, and transition scripts.

However, as organizations become increasingly organic, salience shifts may give way to simultaneous salience and even holistic identities. Instead of asking which hat to wear, perhaps we should switch metaphors and ask, say, how a diamond is revealed through its facets.

## ACKNOWLEDGMENTS

We thank Mike Hogg and Glen Kreiner for their helpful comments.

# 4

# Identity Orientation and Intergroup Relations in Organizations

SHELLEY BRICKSON
*Harvard University*
MARILYNN BREWER
*Ohio State University*

Within large, complex organizations, many potential social identities—and associated ingroup-outgroup distinctions—arise from the structural and functional differentiation of the organization into departments, roles, work groups, etc. At the same time, prejudices and discrimination based on extraorganizational social categories such as sex and ethnicity also play themselves out in organizational settings, particularly as the workplace becomes more and more sociodemographically diverse (see Milliken & Martins, 1996; Pelled, 1996; see also Pratt, Chapter 2 of this volume). The two major research traditions within social psychology that have addressed the reduction of intergroup prejudice are the contact hypothesis and social identity theory (see Brewer & Brown, 1998; Brewer & Gaertner, 2000, for reviews). More than most areas of social psychology, these two approaches have been used to prescribe policy interventions in schools (see D. N. Johnson, Johnson, & Maruyama, 1984; N. Miller & Davidson-Podgorny, 1987, for reviews) and in organizations more generally (e.g., Ashforth & Mael, 1989; Chatman, Polzer, Barsade, & Neale, 1999; Kramer, 1991).

While interventions derived from research on the contact hypothesis and social identity theory have enjoyed some degree of success, they also suffer significant challenges that limit the practicality and effectiveness of their implementation. The present chapter seeks to address some of these limitations and problems from a new theoretical perspective. It presents a recently developed framework (Brewer & Gardner, 1996; Brickson, 2000) of identification processes that distinguishes among three fundamental forms of identification—personal, relational, and collective. Each form has different implications for social information processing in organizational contact situations with potentially important consequences for the outcomes of intergroup interaction.

The first two sections of this chapter focus on theory. In the first, we present the "identity orientation" framework and argue that identity orientation, because of its effect on social motivation, shapes social cognition of outgroup members. Next, the identity orientation framework is applied to theories underlying interventions designed to improve intergroup relations in organizations. We suggest that a relational identity orientation may underlie successful interventions and that challenges facing interventions may be related to their failure to consistently promote a relational orientation. In the final section, we present some preliminary research findings supporting the arguments presented in the theory sections.

## IDENTITY ORIENTATION, MOTIVATION, AND SOCIAL COGNITION OF OUTGROUP MEMBERS

### The Identity Orientation Framework

A new model of identification processes (Brewer & Gardner, 1996; Brickson, 2000) provides a fresh look at the contact hypothesis and social identity theory that may resolve some dilemmas in applying theory to intergroup contact situations. Brewer and Gardner (1996) recently challenged a long-held assumption, implicit in the contact hypothesis and explicit in social identity theory, that there are only two basic loci of self-definition: the self as an individual or the self as a group member. They argue that there are, in fact, three loci of self-definition. In addition to the two previous conceptions, they propose that a third locus is the self as an interpersonal relationship partner.

Based largely on Brewer and Gardner's work, Brickson (2000) outlined a theoretical framework in which the three loci of self-definition represent distinct *identity orientations*. Individual, interpersonal, and group loci of self-definition correspond with personal, relational, and collective identity orientations, respectively. Each identity orientation is associated with its own social motivation, type of significant self-knowledge, and basis of self-evaluation (see Brewer & Gardner, 1996). While there may be individual differences in terms of inclination toward a given identity orientation, all of us experience each orientation at different times as a function of situational influences. Table 4.1 depicts the major differences between identity orientations.

When a *personal* identity orientation is primed, individuals are motivated by self-interest ("I want to win the Professor of the Year Award to gain personal recognition"), conceive of themselves in terms of their individual traits (e.g., "I

TABLE 4.1. Fundamental aspects of identity orientation.

| Identity orientation | Locus of self-definition | Basic social motivation | Relevant elements of self-knowledge | Self-evaluation frame of reference |
|---|---|---|---|---|
| Personal | Individual | Self-interest | Traits | Interpersonal comparison |
| Relational | Interpersonal | Other's benefit | Roles | Comparison to role standard |
| Collective | Group | Collective welfare | Group prototype | Intergroup comparison |

*Note:* Derived from "Who Is This 'We'? Levels of Collective Identity and Self-Respresentations," by M. B. Brewer and W. Gardner, 1996, *Journal of Personality and Social Psychology, 71,* p. 84. Reprinted from "The Impact of Identity Orientation on Individual and Organizational Outcomes in Demographically Diverse Settings," by S. L. Brickson, 2000, *Academy of Managment Review, 25,* p. 85.

am a good professor"), and utilize comparisons with other individuals as a frame of reference for self-evaluation ("How good of a professor am I compared to Sandra?"). When a *relational* identity orientation is activated, individuals are primarily motivated to procure the other's welfare ("I want to make Sandra happy"). Their most relevant elements of self-knowledge consist of roles vis a vis significant others ("I am Sandra's colleague"). They evaluate themselves in terms of the adeptness with which they perform those interpersonal roles (e.g., "How good of a colleague am I to Sandra?"), which they determine by comparing their performance to their own or to their relationship partner's role standard. Finally, when a *collective* identity orientation is made salient, people are largely motivated to ensure the group's welfare, generally relative to other groups ("If I work hard as a professor this year, maybe I can help ensure that my college is ranked higher than our rival"). They may conceive of themselves in terms of the group prototype (e.g., "What is the prototypical professor like at this college?"), and they are likely to judge their worth by how their group compares to other groups ("How does society view the prototypical professor at this college compared to the prototypical professor at another college?").

## The Impact of Identity Orientation on Motivation and Social Cognition

Social cognition is driven by both automatic and more controlled processing mechanisms (see Brewer, 1988; Brewer & Feinstein, 1999; Fiske & Neuberg, 1990). Automatic processing is effortless, but controlled processing can be more or less effortful and elaborated depending on perceiver motivations and attentional capacity. Impressions based on social categorization and well-learned category stereotypes are generally assumed to represent a low-effort, shallow processing strategy that requires little attention to new information about a specific individual. Brewer's dual processing model of impression formation (Brewer, 1988; Brewer & Feinstein, 1999) distinguishes between two different modes of controlled processing, individuation and personalization, that go beyond this simple categorization strategy. The two differ in that *individuation* is a top-down processing mode in which information about a target is processed in terms of category membership (e.g., a target may be seen as a woman who is somewhat differentiated from other women), while *personalization* is a bottom-up information processing mode in which the target's characteristics are integrated into a unique impression that is person based rather than category based.

The extent to which more effortful individuated or personalized processing is engaged depends upon the perceiver's motivational state in a given situation (Brewer, 1988; Fiske & Neuberg, 1990; Fiske, 1998). Interpersonal interdependence, which exists when individuals' outcomes are linked (Fiske & Neuberg, 1990), affective investment (Brewer, 1988), and trust (Fiske, 1998) appear to increase one's motivation to perceive others in increasingly effortful and complex terms.

Brewer and Miller (1984; N. Miller & Brewer, 1986) suggested that the mode of social information processing that is engaged when members of different social groups interact is a critical factor in determining how that interaction influences subsequent intergroup attitudes and beliefs. Based on Brewer's (1988) model, impressions of specific outgroup members can be the product of simple categorization, category-based individuation, or personalization. Type of processing, in turn, determines what is learned and remembered about the individual outgroup member and the group as a whole. We argue here that the identity orientation that is activated in the interaction context provides the motivational component that determines which processing mode will be engaged.

Differences in identity orientation may be particularly important when contact in the workplace involves interactions between members of majority and minority groups. Elsewhere (Brickson, 2000), a detailed model outlines the way in which identity orientation may mediate majority and minority members' affective, cognitive, and behavioral reactions to one another and the outcomes of those reactions at both the individual and organizational levels. Here we summarize the part of that model focusing on the role that identity orientation may play in majority individuals' social cognition of minority individuals. In the present discussion, *minorities* refers to individuals belonging to social groups (based on similar biological traits, historical experience, or vulnerability to social forces: see Alderfer, 1987) traditionally possessing low power or opportunity, while *majorities* refers to individuals belonging to traditionally high-power or high-opportunity social groups.

**Personal identity orientation.**  When their personal identity orientation is activated, majorities may be somewhat motivated to go beyond mere categorization of minorities, taking into account individuating characteristics that are relevant to the interaction goals at hand. Given that the motivational state corresponding to a personal identity orientation is self-interest and that individuals evaluate their own worth through interpersonal comparison, minorities will be individuated to the extent that task interdependence makes them a relevant basis for social comparison. However, the functional nature of such interdependence is not likely to encourage the level of affective investment or trust (see Lanzetta & Englis, 1989) believed to enhance one's motivation for complex social cognition. Further, the salience of interpersonal competition may promote feelings of insecurity or anxiety, factors that further reduce motivation to perceive others in personalized terms (see Fiske, 1998). Given the cognitive accessibility of socially meaningful demographic categories (Fiske, 1998), a high level of motivation is required to perceive outgroup individuals in a manner that is independent of their category membership.

**Collective identity orientation.** When a collective identity orientation is primed, the resultant motivation state is group-promoting, where the ingroup's welfare is compared to that of an outgroup. Any interdependence between the self and outgroup members is perceived at the intergroup rather than the individual level and is likely to be interpreted in zero-sum terms (Fiske & Ruscher, 1993). Affective investment or trust in outgroup members would be minimal, and simple categorization is the likely default processing strategy, particularly for minority outgroupers (see Fiske & Neuberg, 1990).

Although demographic groups are often among the most salient of collective memberships, they need not necessarily be the cognitive focus of collective identity in specific settings. For example, organizational practices and structures can make departments (and departmental social identities) salient. The impact of salient nondemographic categories on the perception of minorities by majorities depends on whether the two types of group boundaries reinforce each other. Outside the laboratory, demographic and nondemographic groups are typically highly correlated (e.g., Alderfer, 1987). When this results in demographic minorities also being outgroupers in terms of another dimension (e.g., department), category-based processing is enhanced (Arcuri, 1982). On the other hand, if minorities and majorities share nondemographic group memberships, increased cooperative interdependence, affective investment, and trust between minority and majority individuals may lead to greater allocation of cognitive resources in the social cognition of minorities (Marcus-Newhall, Miller, Holtz, & Brewer, 1993). However, because all group members, including the self, are viewed from the perspective of the group when a collective identity orientation is primed, minorities may be individuated (e.g., J. C. Turner & Oakes, 1989) but are not likely to be fully personalized (see Brewer, 1988, 2000; Fiske & Neuberg, 1990).

**Relational identity orientation.** The critical difference between personal and relational identity orientations is that the latter is more other-directed rather than self-focused. The motivation to promote the other's welfare emerges when a relational orientation is made salient. This may take the form of caring and concern (as in close relationships) or obligation and responsibility (as in role relationships). In either case, because self-evaluation depends on one's ability to succor another individual's welfare through one's role performance, it implies a form of cooperative interdependence between individuals whereby the other's well-being enhances one's own.

Promoting another's welfare requires deep-level perspective taking on the other's own terms. Such perspective taking may be particularly important to valuing individuals who are different from oneself (Batson, Turk, Shaw, & Klein, 1995). In addition, knowing that each individual is invested in the other's welfare will also likely lead to greater affective investment and trust between minorities and majorities than would occur under the other identity orientations. Therefore, majority individuals whose relational orientation is activated may be more likely to experience factors underlying the motivation to allocate sufficient cognitive resources to truly personalize minorities. A relational identity orientation provides the conditions that Brewer (1988) proposed as critical to determining whether personalized information processing will occur.

## IDENTITY ORIENTATION AND THEORIES OF INTERGROUP RELATIONS

Breaking from the assumption that there are two loci of self-definition (the self as either an individual or a group member) by adding an interpersonal locus of self-definition provides a new perspective on the main techniques for reducing intergroup prejudice and discrimination that have emerged in social psychology. We argue here that the success of these interventions in promoting positive intergroup relations within organizational settings may hinge on whether a relational identity orientation is activated as an integral part of intervention strategy implementation.

### Interventions Based on the Contact Hypothesis

The contact hypothesis (e.g., Allport, 1954) proposes that negative intergroup attitudes can be reduced through contact between individuals from different groups, provided that the context meets certain preconditions. While theorists have proposed a large number of preconditions (Allport alone proposed 30), the following have received particular attention: acquaintance potential (or intimacy), cooperative interdependence, equal status, and social and institutional sanction (Amir, 1976; Brewer & Brown, 1998; Brewer & Gaertner, 2000). Although contact hypothesis theorists were cognizant of the importance of interpersonal interaction, interventions have implicitly focused on personal and collective identity orientations. They emphasize the role of individuals perceiving themselves and each other at the *individual* level of analysis (e.g., in terms of their individual traits) in reducing the salience of the *collective* identities such as ethnicity.

Perhaps the reason that each of the four major preconditions mentioned above has been associated with improved relations between individuals from different demographic groups is that each may in fact promote a relational identity orientation. Regarding the first, *acquaintance potential* "refers to the opportunity provided by a situation for participants to get to know and understand each other" (Cook, 1962, p. 75). Acquaintance potential, as well as social acceptance, one's willingness to accept the other as a social equal and at least a potential friend, constitute two subconditions necessary for intimacy to emerge. "[Both] concepts were introduced to take account of one of the most frequently reported findings with regard to intergroup contact—the more intimate and neighborly the association, the more favorable the attitude" (Cook, 1962, p. 75). Intimacy may well be the single most influential factor in determining the favorability of intergroup attitudes (Amir, 1976; Pettigrew, 1997) because it alters individuals' motivation state, resulting in greater openness to new types of information (Ashmore, 1970). These various associated terms, acquaintance potential, social acceptance, and intimacy, are all arguably subsumed under the notion of a relational identity orientation. Each would promote a concern for the other's welfare, a motivation state that is more conducive to complex social cognition of minorities than are self- or group promotion.

Just as a relational identity orientation may underlie the precondition of acquaintance potential or intimacy, so too might it deserve credit for the effectiveness of *cooperative interdependence*. Although he maintained it as a separate precondition, Cook (1962) argued that this condition promotes "intimate and neighborly contact" (p. 75) that "induces cooperative, friendly behavior and develops liking and respect . . . " (1984, p. 183). While the specific processes underlying the effectiveness of cooperative interdependence remain elusive (D. W. Johnson et al., 1984), they depend upon the existence of give-and-take interactions based on mutual concern (see Amir, 1976) as well as interpersonal support and acceptance (Johnson, Johnson, & Maruyama, 1984). As a relational identity orientation elicits these interaction qualities, it may be that the hitherto mysterious processes are related to identity orientation.

A meta-analysis of cooperative learning interventions (D. W. Johnson et al., 1984) provided empirical evidence suggesting that a relational orientation is more conducive than personal or collective orientations in eliciting the type of interdependence capable of improving intergroup relations in contact settings. The analysis compared the effectiveness of contact under conditions of interpersonal competition (personal identity orientation), intergroup competition where minorities are part of the ingroup (collective orientation), or interpersonal cooperation within a group whose boundary is not made salient (arguably promoting a relational orientation). Results indicated not only that cooperative interdependence resulted in more favorable attitudes toward demographic outgroup members than interpersonal competition (personal orientation), but also that making one's group boundary salient (collective orientation) reduces the benefit of interpersonal cooperation. The most beneficial type of intervention was that which was most conducive to a relational identity orientation.

Some research suggests that the third major precondition mentioned above, *equal status*, may be less essential than acquaintance potential and cooperative interdependence (see Amir, 1976). In some cases, equal status yields negative results while unequal status elicits positive outcomes. Attempts to eradicate status differences in contact situations can actually make demographic categorizations more salient by provoking a sense of threat and competition (Brewer & Miller, 1984). *Perceiving* the other as an equal, which is promoted by creating relationally oriented contact and minimizing the salience of demographic collective identities, may be more crucial than completely equal status between groups as a precondition of effective contact.

Finally, because *institutional support* (e.g., norms, policies) influences the motivations and goals of participants (Brewer & Miller, 1984), it can increase or decrease the effectiveness of the intergroup contact (Amir, 1976). Clearly, even if the situation fosters meaningful contact and cooperative interdependence, strong norms of interpersonal or intergroup competition would elicit motivation states corresponding to personal and collective identity orientations, thereby inhibiting the emergence of a relational orientation. Institutional support may be necessary to ensure that, first, meaningful and cooperative contact occurs and, second, norms reinforce rather than undermine the other-oriented nature of such contact.

In summary, a relational identity orientation may underlie the effectiveness of various preconditions specified by the contact hypothesis to improve intergroup relations. Meaningful rather than fleeting contact is central to the notion of a relational identity orientation. Conditions encouraging interpersonal cooperation and perspective taking (relational identity orientation) and those discouraging an emphasis on individual gains (personal identity orientation) or group boundaries and intergroup competition (collective identity orientation) are the most likely to elicit such contact.

## Interventions Based on Social Categorization and Social Identity Theories

Almost from its inception, social identity theory (and social categorization theory, on which it is based) has been applied to the development of strategies for reducing intergroup discrimination (see Brewer & Gaertner, 2000; Hewstone, 1996, for reviews.) Interventions derived from social identity theory vary according to whether they advocate enhancing the salience of personal or social identity in the intergroup contact situation. The *mutual differentiation* strategy (Hewstone & Brown, 1986) is based on the premise that generalized improvement in intergroup relations can be achieved if existing social identities are preserved and respected.

Alternative intervention strategies are based on reducing, rather than maintaining, social category distinctions in the contact situation. The *decategorization* approach specifically recommends replacing social identities with personal identities, on the assumption that personal and collective identities are functionally opposed so that priming an individual-level identity inhibits group-level processes such as ingroup bias (Brewer & Miller, 1984).

Two other intervention strategies derived from social identity theory seek to dilute the salience of majority/minority category distinctions by making alternative collective identities salient. *Recategorization* invokes a superordinate group identity on the assumption that subgroup distinctions will be replaced by a common ingroup collective identity (e.g., Gaertner, Mann, Dovidio, Murrell, & Pomare, 1990). *Cross-categorization* invokes multiple social identities that are at least partially nonoverlapping. The argument is that salient cross-cutting categories reduce ingroup/outgroup differentiation along any particular category distinction (e.g., Marcus-Newhall et al., 1993).

A core assumption of social identity theory (e.g., Tajfel, 1969; Tajfel & Turner, 1986; J. C. Turner, 1975) is the distinction between personal identity and social (collective) identity as separate levels of self-definition. The theory does not provide for interpersonal identity. Yet viewed through the lens of the identity orientation framework, relational orientation may play a critical role in the effectiveness of interventions based on social identity theory concepts. In the case of decategorization, for instance, most studies that have found this strategy to be effective involve situations where a relational identity rather than a personal identity would be activated. Manipulations designed to "personalize" intergroup interactions (e.g., Bettencourt, Brewer, Croak, & Miller, 1992; N. Miller, Brewer, & Edwards, 1985) typically involve collaborative projects and the sharing of personal information, conditions that are likely to promote the development of interpersonal relationships between self and others. In fact, the activation of a personal identity orientation (rather than a relational orientation) may undermine the intended effect. For reasons stated earlier, individuals focused on their own selves would not likely seek out, attend to, or process personalizing information about the other.

Under some circumstances, recategorization and cross-categorization may also elicit a relational identity orientation. Recategorization induces cooperative interdependence among individuals from different subgroups by introducing superordinate goals. The effectiveness of cooperative interaction in reducing intergroup discrimination is attributed to the development of a common ingroup identity (e.g., Gaertner et al., 1990), but it is likely that the same interventions also promote the formation of strong interpersonal ties between (former) ingroup and outgroup members. Brewer and Gaertner (2000) have suggested, in fact, that the effects of recategorization may typically proceed sequentially from common collective identity to friendly interpersonal relations. This was demonstrated in a laboratory experiment (Dovidio, Gaertner, Validzic, Matoka, Johnson, & Frazier, 1997) in which the members of two groups were induced to conceive of themselves as one group or two groups and then given the opportunity to self-disclose or to offer assistance to an ingroup or outgroup member. As expected, the degree of both self-disclosure and prosocial behavior toward outgroup members was greater among participants in the one-group relative to the two-groups condition. Self-disclosure and prosocial behaviors are particularly interesting because they elicit reciprocity, which can further accelerate the development of positive interpersonal relationships across group lines.

Finally, a relational identity orientation may also underlie successful cross-categorization interventions. Cross-cutting categories often leads to increased ego-involving interaction between individuals from different groups along one dimension due to shared memberships along another. An example often used to support the efficacy of cross-categorization is that societies are less prone to war when kinship groups cross-cut tribal groups (see R. A. LeVine & Campbell, 1972). However, interpersonal relationships may better explain this result than two competing collective memberships. Kinship bonds, perhaps the strongest relational ties that exist, are characterized by an intense concern for, and identification with, the other. Therefore, it is not at all surprising that one tribe will be reluctant to wage war on a neighboring tribe where many of its family members live.

## Identity Orientation and Challenges of Intergroup Relations Interventions

While all of the intervention strategies derived from the contact hypothesis and social identity theory described above have experienced varying degrees of success, they have also suffered some significant challenges. These challenges can be understood in terms of the activation of personal and collective identity orientations. Strategies focused on the direct activation of a relational orientation would seem to evade some of these challenges.

**The contact hypothesis.** Contact hypothesis–derived interventions are typically criticized on the grounds that (a) there are too many preconditions and (b) positive results often do not generalize beyond minority individuals to entire outgroups. Regarding the first criticism, numerous preconditions may have been necessary because none directly and consistently induces a relational identity orientation. While contact hypothesis theorists have long recognized the importance of interpersonal interaction as a condition of successful contact, the dichotomous conceptualization of identity as personal versus collective generally produced interventions focused on promoting individuation of outgroup members, rather than directly on relationship building.

The second significant concern with the contact hypothesis is that positive results (i.e., improved attitudes toward outgroup members in the contact setting) often do not generalize beyond the immediate interactants. Generalization requires perceiving, but not focusing on, the other's outgroup membership. If this membership is not sufficiently salient, outgroupers with whom one has contact are apt to be individuated and viewed as "exceptions to the rule" rather than as typical outgroup representatives (Wilder, 1984), hence precluding generalization from the individual case to perceptions of the outgroup as a whole.

We contend that interventions designed to promote a relational identity orientation would fare better in terms of positive attitude generalization. As an information-processing mode, individuation involves *separating* the individual outgroup member from the social category, encoding specifically what makes this particular individual different or exceptional relative to the category stereotype. Personalization, on the other hand, is not based on category comparison. During the course of interpersonal interaction, the other's social category identities become an integral part of what is known about the relationship partner and is incorporated into the relational self (Aron & McLaughlin-Volpe, in press). In a sense, then, having an involving relationship with an outgroup member inevitably changes affect toward the group as a whole.

A review of the contact hypothesis research literature supports the idea that close intergroup relationships play a special role in mediating the positive effect of contact on improved intergroup attitudes (Pettigrew, 1998; Pettigrew & Tropp, 2000). For instance, possessing an outgroup friend, not merely a co-worker or neighbor, is associated with lower levels of subtle and blatant prejudice, greater support for pro-outgroup policies, and generalized positive attitudes toward a number of outgroups (Pettigrew, 1997). Similar results have been found regarding relationships between gay and straight individuals (Herek & Capitanio, 1997). Positive consequences of meaningful relationships may be related to empathy with the other (Pettigrew, 1997) or to the fact that minorities may feel sufficiently safe to reveal information about themselves related to their minority group membership (Herek & Capitanio, 1996). Interactions based on a relational orientation may be critical to this degree of self-disclosure comfort. In an interpersonal relationship with a majority group member, minorities will be in a position to express identities that they would otherwise be apt to minimize or hide due to a fear of categorization.

Also encouraging is evidence suggesting that when individuals interact in terms of a relational orientation, positive results may generalize not only to other members of the outgroup but also to other ingroup members who have had no direct contact with outgroup individuals. Even indirect outgroup relationships, if they are sufficiently ego-involving, can improve attitudes toward outgroup members. S. Wright, Aron, McLaughlin-Volpe, and Ropp (1997) documented what they call an "extended contact effect," whereby the mere knowledge that some ingroup members have close relationships with outgroup individuals enhances positive attitudes toward members of that outgroup. Brickson (in press) found that the effect even results in improved attitudes toward members of entirely different outgroups.

**Social identity theory.** While contact hypothesis interventions have influenced policy in schools, social identity–based interventions have generally been more influential in organizational theory (e.g., Ashforth & Mael, 1989; Chatman et al., 1999; R. M. Kramer, 1991). Unfortunately, significant concerns surround what appear to be the two favorite interventions, recategorization and cross-categorization. In organizational contexts, both cross-categorization and recategorization can actually reinforce the very collective identities they are meant to minimize. Because of the real-world correlation between demographic and nondemographic groups, making nondemographic social identities salient may have the effect of increasing the number of category distinctions separating individuals. This will almost ensure that intergroup contact will take place under a collective identity orientation focused on group differences (see Diehl, 1990; Pepels, 1999).

Second, results from cross-categorization and recategorization can be inconsistent, especially in the field. One reason is that reducing the salience of demographic social categorization by emphasizing other group memberships has proven extremely difficult to achieve in the field. For example, since categorizations outside the laboratory have unequal significance, cross-cutting categories will often not cancel each other out (see Brewer & Brown, 1998; Pepels, 1999). In terms of recategorization, very specific conditions (e.g., especially strong unifying goals, relatively small group size) are necessary to ensure a continual emphasis on the superordinate collectivity (Brewer & Brown, 1998). Another reason for inconsistent results is that reducing the salience of one social identity does not necessarily promote significant interpersonal ties across group lines. If cross-categorization successfully inhibits a collective identity orientation, either a personal or relational orientation could emerge. While a personal orientation may be preferable to an emphasis on demographic or ethnic differences, personalization of outgroup members is unlikely. If recategorization within a common group identity is achieved, individuals will be collectively oriented, perceiving demographically different individuals as generic members of the superordinate ingroup. This, too, may preclude personalization of minorities.

A third concern with recategorization as an intervention is assimilation pressure. Because minority individuals may not be truly personalized under recategorization, they may be less willing to express their own unique views. When a superordinate collective social identity is emphasized, minority group members may feel particularly pressured to conform to the collective group prototype at the cost of both their own social identity and organizational diversity.

In summary, then, while successful interventions derived from the contact hypothesis and social identity theory may share an ability to activate a relational identity orientation, this has not typically, if ever, been the direct intent. As a result, personal and collective identity orientations have sometimes been primed, which may underlie the various challenges encountered by interventions from both paradigms.

## AN ANALOG EXPERIMENT

Our analysis thus far has been largely post hoc, using the identity orientation framework to reassess previous work on intergroup contact in organizations. At this point, we introduce a preliminary experiment conducted to test directly the proposition that an intervention explicitly focused on activating a relational orientation will improve intergroup attitudes (Brickson, 1999). The experiment was a laboratory analog of an organizational team in which a relationally oriented intervention was compared to the collectively oriented intervention of recategorization. The hypothesis being tested was that individuals who interact with a demographic outgroup member will demonstrate more positive attitudes toward both that individual and other outgroup members when a relational identity orientation is activated than when a collective identity orientation is activated.

## Method and Design

Participants in the experimental study were 82 undergraduate Caucasian males. Two Caucasian male and two Caucasian female undergraduates served as confederate "teammates." Confederates were trained to behave in either a relationally or a collectively oriented fashion. Two male Caucasian undergraduates were hired as experimenters, who read directions for the teams from a prepared script. Confederates and experimenters were blind to the hypotheses and served for half of the experimental sessions for each condition.

Prior to the experiment, participants had been given a questionnaire to ostensibly measure their "business orientation." Items in this questionnaire elicited both relational and collective responses. In the experimental conditions, two (male) participants and two confederates, one of each gender, constituted a "team." Teams met in a conference room equipped with a video camera in one corner as well as a TV and a VCR.

The manipulation of identity orientation during team interaction consisted of two interventions. First, teams were told that their questionnaire results indicated that they possessed either a relational or collective business orientation. The questionnaire feedback consisted of one of the following formats:

> Your questionnaires indicate that your business orientation is what is called relational. A relational orientation focuses on interpersonal relations. You believe it is important that each individual does his or her part to ensure that other members' needs are being met. You believe that when everyone makes an effort to support each other, teams are not only better environments in which to work, but they also have a better chance to prosper. Research does indicate that such an orientation is enormously beneficial.

> Your questionnaires indicate that you share a collective orientation. A collective orientation emphasizes the importance of group solidarity. You believe it is important for group members to feel loyalty toward their groups and for all individuals to perform to their maximum capacity for the sake of the group. Unless there is group solidarity, teams may not perform well. They also may not obtain sufficient recognition from the larger organization. Research does indicate that such an orientation is enormously beneficial. Groups like yours that possess a collective orientation will be compared with groups with other orientations.

The second manipulation was the kind of role play performed. Two role plays were performed with one confederate and two with the other participant.

(Only data from the 41 participants who interacted with the female confederate are presented here.) While the *content* of the role plays was identical for the two conditions, the *context* was either interpersonally oriented or intergroup in the relational and collective manipulations, respectively. Furthermore, instructions were varied, so that participants in the relational condition were asked to take turns giving and seeking advice and told that the important thing was to take the other's perspective, to listen empathetically to his or her concerns, and to provide the type of feedback that the other seeks. Meanwhile, participants in the collective condition were instructed to jointly problem-solve and told that the important thing was their ability to assess the current threat to team integrity and to generate concrete solutions for solving the problems. Therefore, relational role plays encouraged interpersonal relationship formation, while collective role plays encouraged group boundary formation.

Following the four role-playing experiences, participants completed several different response measures. Dependent measures included both behavioral and implicit measures of attitudes toward the female with whom participants had interacted as well as toward females more generally. In the first task, participants allocated up to 100 *credit points* to each of their fellow team members. Credit points allotted to the female confederate provided a behavioral measure of attitudes toward the female with whom participants had interacted directly.

Second, the *teammate selection task* assessed participants' willingness to "hire" a female who they did not know into their team, which provided a behavioral measure of their attitudes toward another demographic outgroup member. Participants believed that the purpose of the study was to assess whether a team's business orientation impacted its ability to incorporate a new group member. Supposedly, if they passed this "screening test," they would be asked to select a new member and then the team plus the new member would return at a future date for the "real" study. After the role plays, groups were informed that they passed the screening test. Each individual was asked to watch videos of four individuals, including one Caucasian female, and rank-order them according to personal preference. (While participants believed that the individuals had generated responses to the question of how to induce organizational innovation, the responses were actually generated by Harvard Business School faculty.) All scripts were rated as equally competent and all actors as equally desirable on a number of dimensions. Both the order of actor presentation as well as the answer read by each actor were varied systematically.

A *projective test* was used as a measure of implicit attitudes toward female workers in general. Each participant was given a photograph of a man and woman in business attire discussing the content of some papers and was asked to write a short vignette about their interaction. Answers were coded for the number of times the man or the woman was given the initiating role in the conversation.

Finally, an *implicit stereotype test* (see Banaji & Hardin, 1996) was also designed and used to assess implicit attitudes toward female workers in general. On laptop computers equipped with Super Lab, participants were presented with occupational titles that were either stereotypically male or female. These titles quickly disappeared and either a male or female name appeared. The task was to categorize ten names as either male or female. Response latencies were measured for name categorization on all trials. Difference scores were taken between stereotypically male occupations paired with female names as compared to stereotypically congruent occupation-name pairings (e.g., doctor, Liz vs. doctor, Ted). Male and female name and occupation lists were matched in terms of number of letters, syllables, and perceived familiarity. (Occupations used were heavily occupied by either males or females, according to 1990 census statistics.)

## Results

Overall, the results of the analog experiment provided some degree of support for the hypothesis that participants interacting with a female team member under a relational identity orientation would respond more favorably to her, as well as to other women, than those interacting with a female teammate under a collective orientation. On three of the four measures, participants in the relational condition demonstrated more positive attitudes toward women than those in the collective condition, though the results were not always statistically significant given the small $n$ in this preliminary study.

On the behavioral measure assessing attitudes toward the female teammate with whom participants had interacted, participants in the relational condition allotted the female team member marginally more credit points ($M = 88.75$) than those in the collective condition ($M = 88.14$) ($F(1,25) = 1.755$. $p < .10$).[1] Results from two of the three measures assessing attitudes toward other women also supported the hypothesis. Relational condition participants were much more likely to give the female in the projective test the initiating role in the vignettes that they wrote (12/20) than were those in the collective condition (4/19) ($\chi2 (1) = 6.11, p = .01$). This is a particularly interesting finding because it indicates that identity condition affected the likelihood that participants would attribute agency to a female. It is highly unlikely that the result is due to greater self-presentation concerns among participants in the relational condition. While some participants in both conditions mentioned actively trying to make the conversations between the male and female egalitarian, none suggested that they thought about who should begin the conversation itself.

Participants in the relational condition also showed marginally significantly less sex stereotyping on the reaction time task, as demonstrated by lower difference scores between "male" jobs paired with female names as opposed to "male" or "female" jobs paired with stereotypically congruent names ($z$ scored $M$ for

---

1. Experimenter and confederate were included as blocking variables in all analyses comparing condition effects because initial analyses indicated that which experimenter or which male/female confederate was involved in a session had significant effects on some of the dependent variables.

composite of two comparisons $= -.263$ versus $M = .238$, respectively) $(F(1,36) = 2.978$, p $< .10)$.[2] The only measure of the four that did not support the hypothesis was the teammate selection measure, on which individuals from neither condition showed any discrimination against a woman as a potential future teammate (mean ranking $= 2.30$).

# CONCLUSION

This study provides some preliminary evidence regarding the impact of identity orientation on attitudes toward members of demographic outgroups. Results indicate that interventions promoting a relational orientation among team members may be more beneficial in improving attitudes toward outgroup members than those promoting a collective orientation. When compared to individuals exposed to the collective identity orientation manipulation, those introduced to the relational manipulation tended to display more positive attitudes toward demographically different others as evidenced by both behavioral and implicit attitude measures. While these results are preliminary and by no means offer a definitive conclusion that all organizations should hasten to implement relational identity interventions, there is reason to believe that results should probably be viewed as presenting a very conservative estimate of the potential benefits of relational interventions.

From a theoretical perspective, the relational intervention was pitted against what is arguably the front-running intervention approach in the field at this point. Furthermore, the potential benefits of relational interventions as well as potential drawbacks of recategorization were constrained in the experiment. Because no pre-existing friendships existed and no personal information was shared at any time, the identity orientation effects on mechanisms underlying complex social cognition—interdependence, affective investment, and trust—were minimal. As a result, the potential advantages of a relational orientation were almost certainly lower than they would be if individuals actually knew and cared about each others' well-being. At the same time, potential disadvantages of a collective orientation due to recategorization were minimized through experimental control. The common ingroup (team) was continually salient, and attitudes toward demographic outgroup members on other teams were not measured.

In light of this conservatism, results are encouraging in the sense that they indicate that promoting an interpersonal relational orientation within the organization may be a promising approach to managing a diverse workforce. While the present study did not directly address the preconditions of contact hypoth-

---

2. The analysis for the stereotype test included a blocking variable indicating whether participants were exposed to a gender or race (presented in Brickson, in press) stereotype test first. Experimenter and confederate variables were not included in this analysis due to limited $df$.

esis interventions, it does suggest that the long list of preconditions may perhaps be reducible to one general principle. In the intervention here, there was little or no acquaintance potential since individuals never shared real personal information about themselves. While a *willingness* to cooperate and *perceived* equal status with the other are probably inherent in a relational orientation, individuals can certainly be invested in the other without actively cooperating on a concrete task and without sharing equal rank (mentoring relationships being a good example of the latter). Further studies would need to address whether these two preconditions can also be subsumed by the presence of a relational identity orientation in the contact situation.

The evidence presented here also indicates that there is generalization of positive attitudes derived from the relational manipulation. The relational intervention promoted the extension of positive attitudes toward other members of the demographic outgroup as a whole. This finding indicates that personalization of an outgroup member is not incompatible with generalization at the group level. Interpersonal interaction with an outgroup member leads to attitude and stereotype change that is extended from the particular interaction partner to other members of his or her group.

The social identity approach has taken us a long way in understanding the dynamic relationship between identity and social cognition. Recognizing that individuals can organize their perceptions of self and others in terms of personal identities or group identities helped make sense of many confusing findings from the research literature on intergroup contact and cooperation. But limiting the set of alternative orientations to only two processing modes—individuation and categorization—may have been unnecessarily restrictive and not fully representative of the range of orientations that persons may bring to social interactions. An interpersonal, relational orientation (and associated personalized social cognition) may provide a key element for creating an organizational environment that fosters positive intergroup relations.

# 5

# Majority-Minority Relations in Organizations:
## Challenges and Opportunities

**MILES HEWSTONE**
*Cardiff University*
**ROBIN MARTIN**
*University of Queensland*
**CLAUDIA HAMMER-HEWSTONE**
*Fischer-Gaertner Gruppe Management Consultants*
**RICHARD J. CRISP**
*University of Birmingham*
**ALBERTO VOCI**
*Università Degli Studi di Padova*

*I*n the course of a lifetime women have made great strides in their quest towards equal opportunities in the workplace. Indeed, we see many more women in charge of large organizations like Hewlett Packard and the Body Shop. At a closer look, however, women (and members of other minorities) are still severely underrepresented in professional and managerial jobs and disproportionately overrepresented in special staff jobs that have no line responsibility as well as in job categories that fit the stereotypically female domains of helping others (e.g., human resources and customer services; see Henderson, 1994) .

In this chapter we begin by exploring some of the negative effects that being in groups of different sizes can have for both individuals and organizations (see B. Simon, Aufderheide, & Kampmeier, 2001). We then consider some possible social psychological remedies for problems generated by group size effects, with a focus on improving intergroup relations within organizations and managing diversity rather than eliminating it. We wish to emphasize, however, that numerical minorities can be sources of dissent, influence, and creativity within organizations. For example, Allmendinger and Hackman (1995) acknowledged that gender-homogeneous groups often have "smoother" processes. There is less conflict, other members of the organization are more predictable, and there is less anxiety about interacting with other colleagues. However, as Allmendinger and Hackman also pointed out, "smooth processes are not necessarily advantageous" (p. 424). The norms characteristic of gender-homogeneous groups can restrict opportunities for personal learning and development as well as collective task performance (P. Y. Martin, 1985). Moreover, within limits, the conflict generated by diversity can challenge and change norms that are out of date, conservative, restrictive, or inappropriate and can enhance group creativity (see Nemeth & Staw, 1989).

Throughout this chapter our theoretical focus is on the contribution of ideas provided by, and extrapolated from, social identity theory (Tajfel, 1978a; Tajfel & Turner, 1986). As we shall see, this theory helps to explain why minorities act as they do and are perceived as they are, it provides a compelling basis for models of intergroup relations that allows for the provision of distinct group identities and overarching, superordinate identities, and it contributes to our understanding of the conditions under which minorities can make positive contributions to group creativity and productivity.

# SOME EFFECTS OF GROUP PROPORTIONS WITHIN ORGANIZATIONS

What do women in the U.S. Senate and House of Representatives, the academic senate of every British University, the Marylebone Cricket Club (the governing body of English Cricket), and the Vienna Philharmonic have in common? They are all members of a tiny minority. Kanter (1977a, 1977b) was the first to argue that such differences in group proportions, or relative group size, can lead to qualitatively different "perceptual phenomena" and "interaction dynamics." She carried out a qualitative case study of 20 saleswomen in the 300-person sales force of a multinational corporation and concluded that, "The life of women in the corporation was influenced by the proportions in which they find themselves" (Kanter, 1977a, p. 207). Although she focused on imbalanced sex ratios, she made clear that the phenomena she identified also applied to other groups characterized by cultural or status differences.

## Kanter's Theory of Group Proportions

Kanter (1977a, 1977b) distinguished the following four group types, based on the proportions of the larger and the smaller subgroups within a particular setting (her examples of the proportions of each group are given in parentheses).

1. *Uniform groups* (100:0) contain only one kind of person or significant social type, such as groups that are completely homogeneous with respect to gender (e.g., the membership of the Oxford and Cambridge Club in London) or racial-ethnic categories (e.g., a WASP golf club).
2. *Skewed groups* (85:15) entail a large preponderance of one type (Kanter called them *dominants*) who control the group and its culture. Kanter labelled the smaller group *tokens*, because they are often treated as representatives of their category. In extreme cases, tokens are termed *solos*, but this term does not refer exclusively to solitary individuals (e.g., the only woman in an engineering firm), but rather to cases where the absolute size of the smaller group is extremely small (Pettigrew & Martin, 1987).
3. *Tilted groups* (65:35) are less extreme in size (Kanter refers to the subgroups here simply as *majority* and *minority*), and the minority is large enough to form coalitions and affect the culture of the group.
4. *Balanced groups* (60:40–50:50) contain two groups more similar in size, which may be further subdivided based on, for example, roles and abilities.[1]

Kanter was especially interested in the kinds of interactions found in face-to-face groups with highly skewed sex ratios, since so many women (especially in organizations) encounter such unequal numerical distributions of gender in their workplace. She proposed that these women's proportional rarity (or token status) was associated with three *perceptual phenomena* (visibility, polarization, and assimilation) and three parallel *interaction dynamics* (performance pressures, group-boundary heightening, and role entrapment).

*Visibility and performance pressures* refer to the fact that tokens are highly visible, receive more attention than dominants, and hence feel "different" (cf. Milliken & Martins, 1996; S. E. Taylor, 1981). This awareness of difference leads to performance pressures for tokens, who must both act for themselves and represent their category. It can adversely affect their performance in work groups (e.g., C. G. Lord & Saenz, 1985), increase their perceptions of vulnerability (Niemann & Dovidio, 1998), and decrease feelings of comfort (Bourhis, 1994) and job satisfaction (Mellor, 1996; Milliken & Martins, 1996; Yoder, 1994). which may increase turnover rates of such employees. The increased feelings of distinctiveness can themselves increase the salience of negative stereotypic expectancies (Milliken & Martins, 1996; Niemann & Dovidio, 1998) and have significant detrimental effects on both feelings and performance (see Steele, 1997). Ironically, even though distinct minorities may, in fact, receive dispro-

---

1. There are 9 women among the 100 U.S. senators and 56 women in the 435-member House of Representatives (*New York Times*, 2000); only 5.6% of full professors in the U.K. are women (statistics compiled by the Association of University Teachers, reported in *The Guardian*, 1997); the MCC and the Vienna Philharmonic have only recently admitted their first women members.

portionately more attention, they may also be seen as "whiners" and "social losers," who are less trusting or even paranoid members of the organization (R. M. Kramer, 1998).

*Polarization and group-boundary heightening* refer to the contrast drawn between tokens and dominants, which might be reflected in negative perceptions of the relations between the two groups. The presence of the tokens can lead to dominants' exaggerating both their within-group commonalities and differences between the two gender groups (cf. Tajfel & Wilkes, 1963). This overgeneralization leads to a tightening of group boundaries, as dominants emphasize their culture (e.g., by talking about the need to be tough at senior levels in an organization) and remind tokens of their difference (e.g., by referring to women's split loyalties between work and family life). It can also lead to more insidious, but no less powerful, exclusion whereby tokens are isolated from informal social and professional networks (Meyerson & Fletcher, 2000).

Finally, *assimilation and role entrapment* refer to the fact that tokens' personal characteristics tend to be distorted to fit the generalization, and the target of these processes is forced to confirm the perceiver's stereotype. These processes are evident when a token woman is mistaken for another member of her category, treated as though she resembles women on average, and forced to play a gender-stereotypical role (trapped in her gender role). According to Henderson (1994), at its most extreme women find themselves in a "catch-22": they are devalued if they display "feminine" behaviors (nurturing, cooperative, passive) and disliked when they exhibit "masculine" behaviors (assertiveness, independence, aggressiveness). This experience can reduce job satisfaction and be a source of stress (Kanter, 1977a, pp. 283–284; see also Gutek, 1993).

### Evidence Relating to Kanter's Theory

Kanter's ideas have great intuitive appeal and there is extensive evidence that token women suffer in some of the ways she predicted, whether as the first policewomen on patrol (e.g., Ott, 1989), women academics (Young, Mackenzie, & Sherif, 1980), women enlisted in the armed forces (e.g., Rustad, 1982), or women physicians (Floge & Merrill, 1986). Token women are especially likely to report being the target of stereotyping and discrimination (e.g., Beaton & Tougas, 1997; Floge & Merrill, 1986), being perceived as physically weak (Yoder, Adams, & Prince, 1983), and being seen to lack leadership qualities (Ott, 1989).

In short, compared with women in more balanced settings, minority women in male domains experience greater prejudice and discrimination (Nieva & Gutek, 1981; see also Eagly, Makhijani, & Klonsky, 1992; Eagly & Mladinic, 1994). These negative effects are typically magnified in the case of solos, who are especially likely to suffer from being perceptually distinct and the source of attention (see Heilman, 1980; S. E. Taylor, 1981). Critics have, however, identified a number of key limitations to Kanter's theory and associated research (see Yoder, 1991, 1994). The most damaging critiques refer to Kanter's confounding of numerical proportions with three other factors: (gender) status, occupational inappropriateness, and intrusiveness.

Status is typically confounded with gender (see, e.g., Eagly, 1987; Geis, 1993; Ridgeway & Diekema, 1992). Relatedly, several studies have shown that token men (e.g., male nurses; Floge & Merrill, 1986) avoid the negative consequences of numerical imbalance (e.g., Fairhurst & Snavely, 1983a, 1983b). In fact, visibility may have no effect on men (e.g., Sackett, DuBois, & Noe, 1991) or may even confer advantages such as enhanced promotional opportunities (e.g., Heikes, 1991; Ott, 1989; Yoder & Sinnett, 1985). Thus the phenomena Kanter outlined are best seen not specifically as gender effects, but as consequences of membership in numerically small groups with low status (see Alexander & Thoits, 1985; Frable, 1993). In fact, the negative effects of distinctiveness may be restricted to token or solo members of culturally stigmatized groups in a given context (Crocker & Major, 1989; Frable, Blackstone, & Scherbaum, 1990; B. Major & Crocker, 1993; see also Niemann & Dovidio, 1998).

The occupational inappropriateness of a profession refers to its gender stereotyping or the extent to which women or men stand out as members of that profession. As Yoder (1991) noted, the gender stereotyping of an occupation has a strong normative component that includes two types of sex ratio (for the occupation as a whole, and for the organization as a whole) which should be considered alongside Kanter's (1977a, 1977b) focus on the sex ratio in the work group. Yoder pointed out that all of the studies on women and men tokens involved gender-inappropriate occupations. From these studies Yoder concluded that distinctive women in gender-inappropriate occupations do tend to experience performance pressures, isolation, and role encapsulation, but men do not.

Intrusiveness refers to those pioneer members of the minority group who are the first, or the first significant cohort, to break into a new occupation or organization (Laws, 1975; Yoder, 1991, 1994). If women are seen as "intruders," the benefits of decreased distinctiveness that Kanter envisaged may be gained at the cost of one or more types of 'backlash' reaction from the majority. Increasing proportions of the minority might worsen the situation for tokens if the majority view them as a threat to their status and then react with increased discrimination (see Blalock, 1967; South, Bonjean, Markham, & Corder, 1982), which does not level off until the minority proportion of the whole group reaches about 30% to 40% (Allmendinger & Hackman, 1995; P. Y. Martin, 1985; Pfeffer & Davis-Blake, 1987). Men in male-dominated occupations may react especially strongly to women's intruding, because jobs dominated by men are accorded higher prestige (e.g., Jacobs & Powell, 1985; but cf. Glick, 1991) and pay better wages (Glick, 1991), benefits which are likely to be eroded with the intrusion of women in significant numbers (Pfeffer & Davis-Blake, 1987; Reskin & Roos, 1990; Shaffer, Gresham, Clary, & Theilman, 1986; Toren, 1990). In contrast, women may believe, or at least hope, that the intrusion of men into their less prestigious, female-dominated occupations will increase their pay and prestige.

Based on this review of the literature, we can conclude that group proportions can be associated with the negative perceptual processes and interaction dynamics outlined by Kanter (1977a, 1977b). However, these effects will occur primarily, and be strongest, when the token group has low status and/or is stigmatized and is attempting to pass for the first time into a traditionally gender-inappropriate occupation or role (e.g., women entering the mostly homogeneous male White domain of senior management). To track such processes, Allmendinger and Hackman (1995) emphasized that future work must take a more dynamic approach. Their extensive, cross-cultural study of women entering the traditionally male-dominated domain of concert orchestras concluded that gender dynamics differ qualitatively at three successive temporal stages, and they argued that research should study *changes* in organizations. Their three stages were: (a) when an organization has only a few token women (e.g., 10% or less); (b) when it is in transition (e.g., 10% to 40%); and (c) when it has become relatively gender balanced (e.g., 40% to 60%). These minority proportions are, of course, very similar to Kanter's (1977a, 1977b) three group types—skewed, tilted, and balanced—but Allmendinger and Hackman's findings paint a more complex picture.

According to Allmendinger and Hackman (1995), at token levels of representation women may have to keep a low profile and be nonintrusive; they are less satisfied than men, but both they and men are more satisfied than they are at the transitional stage. Allmendinger and Hackman reported a qualitative worsening of organizational life (e.g., decreased satisfaction and motivation) for all members as the proportion of women rose to 40%. This stage can include the phenomena of group boundary tightening, outgroup stereotyping, and decreased social support across gender boundaries, all of which tend to heighten tension for all members of the organization (Kanter, 1977a, 1977b; South et al., 1982). Only when the "tipping point" of 40% is reached (see also P. Y. Martin, 1985; Pfeffer-Davis & Blake, 1987) are gender relations more interdependent and mutually supportive. It is noteworthy, however, that male musicians responded more strongly and negatively to changes in gender composition, whereas women's reactions became more favorable as their representation moved from token to relatively balanced.

As this review of the literature shows, although results are mixed, being in a very small minority with low or stigmatized status can affect several of the most important organizational outcomes. These include job satisfaction, organizational commitment and turnover, and health-related organizational outcomes, such as stress, absenteeism, and job performance (see Meyerson & Fletcher, 2000). It is therefore imperative that we understand better the nature of these effects, and what can be done about them.

## Contributions of Our Own Research

We introduced the concept of perceived variability to this research literature, because it appeared to be a variable that was central to Kanter's theorizing, but one that had not yet been related to it. This construct has its origins in Tajfel's (1978b) discussion of processes leading to the exaggeration of both within-group similarities and between-group differences (see Tajfel & Wilkes, 1963). In particular, we were interested in the finding that group members tend to perceive outgroups as being less variable, or more homogeneous, than ingroups (the "outgroup homogeneity" effect; Jones, Wood, & Quattrone, 1981; for reviews, see Linville, 1998; Ostrom & Sedikides, 1992); but that under some circumstances there is an opposite, "ingroup homogeneity: effect (B. Simon & Brown, 1987; for reviews, see Devos, Comby, & Deschamps, 1996; Voci, 2000). The relevance of perceived variability to Kanter's (1977a, 1977b) theory is most obvious in her discussion of "assimilation." She gives as an example dominants' mistaking one token for another (see Lorenzi-Cioldi, Eagly, & Stewart, 1995; S. E. Taylor, Fiske, Etcoff, & Ruderman 1978) and states that when proportions become less extreme (i.e., from skewed to tilted) the 'minority', as opposed to tokens, "begin to become individuals differentiated from each other" (Kanter, 1977b, p. 966).

Simon's (1992) theoretical account of the ingroup homogeneity effect owes much to social identity theory. He argued that being in a minority, which is often associated with lower status (Farley, 1982), tends to make group membership more salient (see Brewer, 1993b; Mullen, Brown, & Smith, 1992) and may pose a threat to group members' self-esteem. Minority members may respond by perceiving their ingroup as more homogeneous, thus promoting in-group solidarity and accentuating social identity (Tajfel & Turner, 1986; see Ellemers & van Rijswijk, 1997). The effects of gender and group size converge when being in a distinct minority heightens women's consciousness of their stigmatized status and/or gender group. This awareness does indeed increase their perceived similarity to women as a group (Foster & Matheson, 1998; Hogg & Turner, 1987). We therefore sought to compare women's and men's perceptions of group variability under male-skewed and male-tilted settings.

Our most relevant research was carried out using academic staff at universities in the United Kingdom and Italy, whose group size varied as a function of their academic discipline (Hewstone, Crisp, Contarello, Conway, Voci, & Marletta, 2000). Although university women are not necessarily seen as occupationally distinct (Niemann & Dovidio, 1998), they may still be seen as occupationally inappropriate (Laws, 1975) and intrusive, especially in stereotypically male domains, which is where the male majority is likely to be most strongly skewed (Laws, 1975; Yoder, 1991, 1994). We compared perceptions of group variability by men and women academics who were members of male-skewed or male-tilted departments using the "range" measure of perceived group variability (Jones et al., 1981). This measure assesses the "perceived dispersion" component of variability (see Park & Judd, 1990), by asking respondents to mark the central tendency of a group on each one of a set of rating dimensions and then to mark where they think the most extreme group members they know or can imagine would fall, either side of the mean. The distance between the two extremes ("full range") constitutes a robust measure of how respondents perceive members of a group to be dispersed around the mean. We provided a strong replication of R. Brown and Smith's (1989) findings, that men in the majority showed an outgroup homogeneity effect and women in the minority showed an ingroup homogeneity effect. We extended their research by showing, as Kanter's theory would predict, that men's out-group homogeneity effect was stronger in the male-skewed than the male-tilted settings (dominants assimilated token women more to the stereotype than did majority men), and women's ingroup homogeneity effect was stronger when they were a smaller minority (token women in a male-skewed setting felt more distinctive and emphasized ingroup cohesiveness; B. Simon, 1992).

In our first study we were only able to study men in a majority and women in a minority; in our second study, carried out at a university in Italy, there were some academic departments with a balanced sex ratio, and one department with a female-tilted sex ratio (we were unable to find any female-skewed university departments). We found that perceived variability for men and women varied as a linear function of group proportions. The outgroup homogeneity effect for men tended to disappear as they lost their ingroup majority status, and women's tendency to show an ingroup homogeneity effect disappeared as they lost their ingroup minority status. In related research, we have found consistent evidence that group size affects perceived variability for other occupational groups. Both female nurses and policemen (as majorities) showed an outgroup homogeneity effect, but male nurses and policewomen (as minorities) showed an ingroup homogeneity effect (Hewstone & Crisp, 2000). Across four different studies, this evidence provides powerful testimony to the impact of group size and shows that group proportions can affect men and not just women (see Sackett et al., 1991). These results confirm that perceived dispersion is a useful variable for research testing Kanter's (1977a, 1977b) hypotheses regarding the effects of group proportions, because it reflects quite subtle quantitative and qualitative changes in intergroup perception and dynamics across different sex ratios (see also Hewstone, Crisp, Richards, Voci, & Rubin, 2000).

Perceived variability is also a variable that has widespread consequences for stereotyping and intergroup relations. Notably, perceiving an outgroup as relatively homogeneous can increase the impact of categorical versus individuating information (Krueger & Rothbart, 1988), and the likelihood that perceivers judge specific individuals in a stereotypic manner (Ryan, Park, & Judd, 1996). By affecting these and other processes, perceived homogeneity tends to enhance stereotype maintenance and may promote intergroup bias (Hewstone & Hamberger, 2000; Richards & Hewstone, in press). Thus the fact that group proportions appear to have reliable and pervasive effects on perceived group variability is reason alone to study them and be aware of their consequences.

## Summary

Kanter's (1977a, 1977b) theory of group proportions argues that proportional rarity is associated with distinct, negative perceptual processes and interaction dynamics. However, these effects occur primarily, and are strongest, for low-status or stigmatized token groups, which are attempting to pass into a traditionally inappropriate occupation for the first time. Group proportions also consistently affect perceived group variability, a variable that affects many aspects of group perception and intergroup relations. Because group proportions can have negative effects on both intergroup relations and organizational outcomes, we now turn our attention to possible interventions to overcome them.

## IMPROVING RELATIONS BETWEEN MAJORITIES AND MINORITIES WITHIN ORGANIZATIONS

Thus far we have argued that the consequences of group proportions are pervasive and pernicious. How, then, can they be overcome, or at least mitigated? One possibility is some form of structural intervention to bring the proportions of the two groups (e.g., men and women) closer to balance, and this has been done with limited success (see the huge literature on affirmative action, e.g. Crosby, Ferdman, & Wingate, 2001; Crosby & VanDeVeer, 2000). We believe in both the ethics and the effectiveness of this intervention. However, given space considerations and the focus of this volume, we will focus instead here on how various, selected social psychological interventions typically used to improve interethnic relations could be applied in this case.

There are two main types of intervention aimed at changing intergroup perceptions and improving intergroup relations (see Hewstone, 1996). The first is based on bringing about more positive and cooperative contact (see also Brickson & Brewer, Chapter 4 of this volume) and the second attempts to change the structure of social categorizations. Both interventions may be aimed at changing various aspects of intergroup perception, including making attitudes towards the social category as a whole more positive, increasing perceived outgroup variability, and decreasing category use (see Brewer and Miller, 1988).

### Contact Between Members of Different Groups

One source of inaccurate, stereotypical views of the outgroup may be the relative scarcity of contact between groups (see Lee & Duenas, 1997). It is worth noting that even one positive encounter with a member of the other group, although it is unlikely to change the stereotype of an outgroup in general, can sometimes bring about change in perceived group variability, revealing that "they" are not "all alike" (Hamburger, 1994). To be most effective, however, contact should be cooperative, between equal-status members of the two groups, in a situation that allows the individuals to get to know each other on more than a superficial basis, and with the support of superiors (Hewstone, 1996; Pettigrew, 1998; Pettigrew & Tropp, 2000).

Indirect contact may also be effective, in which knowledge that a fellow ingroup member has a close, positive relationship with an outgroup member is used as a catalyst to promote more positive intergroup attitudes (see S. Wright et al., 1997). This form of contact might be particularly useful in cases of extreme group proportions (e.g., just a handful of women engineers in a large firm otherwise made of men) where the probability of outgroup contact is low.

Despite the theoretical and practical limitations to intergroup contact (see Hewstone & Brown, 1986), we believe that efforts should be made to promote contact between majorities and minorities within an organization, because unless proactive attempts are made to bring about contact, many people tend to avoid contact with what is perceived as an outgroup. In addition, an organization may be so segregated that unless we intervene there is almost no opportunity for contact. This is the case in organizations where gender overlaps with function and/or seniority (women still account for less than 4% of the uppermost ranks in Fortune 500 companies; Meyerson & Fletcher, 2000). We acknowledge too that contact between groups within an organization could, and sometimes certainly does, exacerbate conflict, especially when it leads to intergroup comparisons concerning inequalities of salary and working conditions. We still believe that, in principle, some contact, especially where it can be made positive and cooperative, is desirable. The absence of contact is likely to reduce the likelihood of future contact, strengthen the assumption that the two groups have different (even irreconcilable) beliefs, maintain intergroup anxiety, and reinforce the boundary between groups (see Hewstone, 1996).

One of the most serious limitations of the so-called "contact hypothesis" is that participants do not necessarily generalize their positive attitudes and perceptions of the few outgroup members they get to know, either beyond the specific situation in which the positive contact took place or to the group as a whole. Hewstone and Brown (1986) therefore argued that unless contact can be characterized as *intergroup* (i.e., between individuals *as group representatives*), it is unlikely to generalize to the group as a whole. This does not mean that categories should be emphasized at all times, but rather that group affiliations should still be clear in contact situations, and that when members of one group meet members of the other group, they should both be seen as, at least to some extent, *typical* of their groups (R. Brown, Vivian, & Hewstone, 1999; Van Oudenhoven, Groenewoud, & Hewstone, 1996; Wilder, 1984).

Thus, somewhat counterintuitively, stereotype-disconfirming information should be linked to typical outgroup members (Rothbart & John, 1985). Unless this is the case, people tend to react to stereotype-disconfirming information by assigning disconfirming members of the outgroup to a "subtype," consisting of atypical group members, unrepresentative of the group as a whole and thus an ineffective vehicle for changing stereotypes (R. Weber & Crocker, 1983). Thus it is more effective to present a constant amount of stereotype-disconfirming information by "dispersing" it across several members of the outgroup (each of whom will only slightly disconfirm the stereotype, while also appearing somewhat typical of the group in other ways), than by "concentrating" it in one or two members who clearly disconfirm the stereotype, but just as clearly are unrepresentative of the group as a whole and thus can easily be subtyped (see

Hewstone, 1996, for a review). Here again we see that extreme group proportions place serious limitations on change; if the minority in an organization only consists of a handful of tokens, then it is practically impossible to disperse rather than concentrate stereotype-disconfirming information. In discussing the process of assimilation, Kanter (1977a) noted that, "If there are enough people of the token's type to let discrepant examples occur, it is possible that the generalization will change to accommodate accumulated cases. But if individuals of that type are only a small proportion of the group, it is easier to retain the generalization and distort the perception of the token" (pp. 971–972).

## Changing Social Categorizations

The interventions reviewed in this section start from the premise that since social categorization is the cause of discrimination, an improvement in intergroup relations must be brought about by reducing the salience of existing social categories (Brewer & Miller, 1984). These interventions are all inspired theoretically by social identity theory (Tajfel, 1978a) and, more recently, self-categorization theory (e.g., J. C. Turner et al., 1987). These theories emphasize that we all typically belong to several social categories and therefore may have a series of social identifications, one of which is salient at any given time. Self-categorization theory develops the earlier social identity perspective by arguing that self can be conceived on a number of levels of inclusiveness (e.g., me as: a team member, a group member, an employee, a woman, a human being). The level at which the self is defined determines how one relates to others, including members of the same group. Despite their shared theoretical roots, these approaches try to reduce bias by very different means. The first, decategorization, seeks to eliminate categorization; the remaining alternatives—recategorization, subcategorization, and cross-categorization—seek to alter *which* categorizations are used.

**Decategorization.** Brewer and Miller's (1984, 1988) *personalization* model uses a specific form of between-group contact to reduce the salience of category memberships. They argued that when members of the two distinct groups come together, the contact should be "differentiated" (allowing for distinctions to be made among outgroup members) and "personalized" (allowing for perceptions of the uniqueness of outgroup members). The goal then is a more interpersonally oriented and non-category-based form of responding. Studies have confirmed the hypothesized effects of personalized contact (Bettencourt et al., 1992; Bettencourt, Charlton, & Kernahan, 1997). Participants who adopted an interpersonal focus displayed significantly less ingroup favoritism than did either those who focused on the task or those in a control condition. Participants also differentiated among outgroup members more in the interpersonal conditions, and there was a strong correlation between perceived similarity of outgroup members (to each other) and the degree of intergroup bias shown. Personalization aims to, and can, achieve decategorization: individuation of outgroup members results in the category being seen as less useful and, thus, being used less often. This intervention may also succeed in changing perceived group variability, encouraging a more complex and differentiated perception of the outgroup. However, the very conditions that promote personalization impede generalization of attitudes from individual members of the outgroup to the outgroup as a whole (see Scarberry, Ratcliff, Lord, Lanicek, & Desforges, 1997), and the beneficial effects of personalized contact may be restricted to majority groups (Bettencourt et al., 1997).

**Recategorization.**   Gaertner, Dovidio, and colleagues proposed that intergroup bias can be reduced by factors that transform members' perceptions of group boundaries from "us" and "them" to a more inclusive "we" (Gaertner & Dovidio, 2000; Gaertner et al., 1993). They acknowledge that several factors influence intergroup bias and conflict, but their *common ingroup identity* model regards the cognitive representations of the situation as the critical mediating variable (for a review, see Gaertner & Dovidio, 2000). While a representation of the situation as one involving two groups is thought to maintain or enhance intergroup biases, recategorized (i.e., common ingroup identity) representations are expected to reduce tension by increasing the attractiveness of former outgroup members, once they are included within the superordinate group structure. The common ingroup identity model resolves ingroup versus outgroup conflict by changing group boundaries and creating a superordinate identity.

There is extensive support for the common ingroup identity model from sophisticated laboratory experiments, and, more recently, Gaertner and colleagues have shown that their theory can be successfully applied to organizational groups, specifically to formerly distinct groups drawn together in a business merger (see Gaertner et al., 2000). In this business context, corporate banking executives felt more positive towards a new corporation when it "felt like one group." Consideration of such models of intergroup relations could make a significant contribution to countering the poor success rate of corporate mergers and could attack the problem of employees' low levels of commitment to the merged organization (see Terry, Chapter 15 of this volume; Van Knippenberg & Van Leeuwen, Chapter 16; and Gaertner, Bachman, Dovidio, & Banker, Chapter 17).

Despite the impressive empirical support for the common ingroup identity model, it shares a limitation with the decategorization approach; both seek to deemphasize sometimes valued identities. The fundamental truth of social identity theory is that because groups often provide a source of desired social identity (Tajfel, 1978a), their members will therefore often resist alternative categorization. Thus a more successful strategy may involve a superordinate identity *and* distinctive subgroup identities, and research has begun to consider the possibility of maintaining simultaneously dual categorizations at different levels of social categorization.

**Subcategorization.** One risk of bringing groups together, especially when they are similar on an important dimension (such as their status in the work-place), is that their distinctive group identity may be threatened, to which they respond by using various strategies aimed at reestablishing their "positive distinctiveness." Thus a number of different perspectives have suggested that, rather than eliminating preexisting categories and introducing a new, superordinate categorization, former categorizations should still be valued and maintained, but in the context of a superordinate identity (see Gaertner & Dovidio, 2000; Hewstone & Brown, 1986; Hornsey & Hogg, 2000b). A number of studies by Gaertner, Dovidio, and colleagues support this *dual-identity* model (e.g., Dovidio, Gaertner, & Validzic, 1998; Gaertner, Rust, Dovidio, Bachman, & Anastasio, 1994; see also Gaertner & Dovidio, 2000). The goal, they argued, should be to establish a common ingroup (i.e., superordinate) identity, while simultaneously maintaining the salience of subgroup identities (e.g., identities prior to a merger or identities based on function within a superordinate, corporate identity). One supportive study was carried out in an occupational setting, in which actual employees were asked to imagine that their current organization was about to merge with another (Mottola, Bachman, Gaertner, & Dovidio, 1997). Employees were most positive about a hypothetical merged organization in which the two groups had equal status but also positive distinctiveness (e.g., one was higher on sales, the other on profit), compared with other fictional mergers in which their own company was described as either higher status or lower status, respectively. Maintaining dual identities also promotes generalization of positive intergroup contact beyond that with selected members of the other group to more positive views of the group as a whole (see Gaertner & Dovidio, 2000; Gaertner et al., 2000).

**Cross-categorization.** A final model for changing the structure of social categorization begins from the fact that where others can be classified as outgroup members on multiple dimensions, bias is typically high (so-called converging boundaries; Brewer & Campbell, 1976). But where categories can be made to overlap, so that previous "others," "out-groupers," or "opponents" share group membership on one dimension, bias can be reduced (Crisp & Hewstone, 1999; Migdal, Hewstone, & Mullen, 1998; Urban & Miller, 1998). By making perceivers aware that the outgroup consists of different components, some of which share group memberships with sections of the ingroup, this intervention can achieve a more differentiated view of the outgroup, reduce the importance of any one category, force the perceiver to classify other individuals in terms of multiple dimensions, and point to at least some similarities between groups (see Crisp, Hewstone, & Rubin, 2001; Vanbeselaere, 1991).

Although the effects of cross-categorizations are much more complex than had at first been thought (see Vescio, Hewstone, Crisp, & Rubin, 1999), a relatively small number of different patterns of discrimination seem to be most important (see Hewstone, Islam, & Judd, 1993). Overall there is best support for an "additive" pattern of discrimination (i.e., where the two dimensions of categorization are combined additively to influence intergroup bias). In this model, evaluation of a "double ingroup" member (e.g., someone sharing ingroup membership on both available dimensions) is most positive; evaluation of a "partial group" member (e.g., ingroup on one dimension, but outgroup on another) is neutral or intermediate; and evaluation of a "double outgroup" member (e.g., someone who has outgroup status on both available dimensions) is most negative (see Crisp & Hewstone, 1999).

As regards underlying process, both Migdal et al. (1998) and Crisp and Hewstone concluded that, although relatively weak, the best evidence for an underlying process driving the effect was for category differentiation (see Crisp & Hewstone, 2000a, 2000b). The category differentiation model (Doise, 1978) posits that cognitive organizing principles in a two-group context lead to an accentuation of differences between, and an accentuation of similarities within, the categorizations. In a situation of cross-categorizations, however, the normal processes accentuating differences between *and* similarities within categorizations are working against each other when applied to crossed-category composite groups that contain conflicting cues for group membership (e.g., ingroup on one dimension, outgroup on another). Thus the two processes of accentuation cancel each other out. However, although category differentiation processes are important, they have not yet been shown to mediate reduced bias (Crisp et al., 2001). It should also be noted that if the groups involved become so similar that their distinctive social identity is threatened, similarity can *increase* bias (see Jetten, Spears, & Manstead, 1998).

## Summary

There are several promising social psychological interventions to promote harmonious relations between majorities and minorities (or indeed equal-sized groups) within organizations. Optimal intergroup contact can bring about generalized change in outgroup attitudes, and changing the structure of social categorizations can reduce or change the salience of existing categorization in a complementary fashion. Indeed, interventions most likely to succeed will integrate these perspectives, some of which (e.g., the dual-identity model of subcategorization and cross-categorization) have obvious structural similarities.

## MINORITIES AS VALUABLE SOURCES OF DISSENT, INFLUENCE, AND CREATIVITY

Thus far we have outlined some of the negative consequences (for minority members) of extreme group proportions within organizations, and we have reviewed some of the interventions designed to improve majority-minority relations. In the last section we emphasized interventions that do not cleave individuals from their cherished identities, bur rather allow individuals within organizations to have multiple identities and multiple loyalties (Guetzkow, 1955). This preference is based on both ethics and effectiveness; individuals should be free to choose and maintain their own social identifications and interventions that permit them to be more effective at improving intergroup relations. There is another reason to adopt this pluralistic perspective, namely, that diversity can be a resource to be exploited (Adler, 1997), rather than something to be eliminated or avoided, and minority views can offer vitality and creative challenges to organizations, broadening their perspective and actually increasing productivity (De Dreu & De Vries, 1997). A homogenous workforce in which minority dissent is suppressed may reduce creativity, innovation, individuality, and independence (see also Nemeth & Staw, 1989; West, in press), whereas minority dissent can contribute significantly to improving group decision making (Nemeth & Owens, 1996; West, Borrill, & Unsworth, 1998).

## From Majority to Minority Influence

The predominant focus of research on social influence has been on the ability of the majority to influence the minority (e.g., Asch, 1951). However, over 30 years of research on "active" minorities has taught us that the minority, despite lacking size, status, or power, can also influence the majority and that it appears to do so in distinct and subtle ways (for a review, see De Vries & De Dreu, in press). Moscovici (1976) argued that social influence arises from the *conflict* between the established opinions of the majority and the new opinions of the minority. While the impact of minorities on public responses is generally low, probably because individuals wish to avoid publicly agreeing with a deviant group, it is greater on private or indirect dimensions (for a review, see Wood, Lundgren, Ouellette, Busceme, & Blackstone, 1994). Moscovici's (1980, 1985) conversion theory contrasted majority and minority influence in categorical terms. In the face of a discrepant majority, individuals engage in social comparison and, since identification with a majority is desirable, they conform to the majority position without the need for a detailed appraisal of the majority's message. This results in public compliance with the majority position with little or no private or indirect attitude change. Faced with a discrepant minority, however, social comparison is unlikely, as minority membership is often associated with undesirable characteristics. However, through its distinctiveness, Moscovici proposes that the minority can encourage a *validation process* leading individuals to engage in more detailed processing of the message. While minority influence may not lead to public agreement, for fear of being categorized as a minority member (Mugny, 1982), the close examination of the minority's position may bring about attitude conversion on an indirect, latent, or private level.

In the present context, where we are considering the impact of minorities within organizations, we are most interested in three lines of evidence relevant to conversion theory: these concern cognitive activity, attitude change, and creativity (for reviews, see De Vries, De Dreu, Gordijn, & Schuurman 1996; R. Martin & Hewstone, 2001). Regarding cognitive activity, Moscovici predicted that a minority, compared with a majority, will lead to greater cognitive activity aimed at understanding its persuasive message and that people are more likely to generate arguments and counterarguments to a minority than a majority message. Studies on these questions have, however, been inconclusive (R. Martin & Hewstone, in press). Regarding attitude change, Moscovici predicted that minorities will have more private than public influence, whereas majorities will have more public than private influence. Wood et al.'s (1994) meta-analytic review of 97 studies did indeed conclude that the impact of the minority was greater on measures of influence that were private from the source and indirectly related to the content of the appeal, but they found less evidence that majority influence takes the form of greater public than private attitude change.

The research on creativity is more supportive of the thesis that minorities could make a distinctive, positive contribution to organizational life. This research owes most to Nemeth's (1986, 1995) adoption of a broader concept of influence, one that refers to any change in thought processes, opinions, and decisions, independent of the direction of these changes. Like Moscovici, Nemeth believed that minorities induce more cognitive effort than majorities and that the nature of the thought processes itself is also different. Nemeth contended that minorities capture more attention and induce more divergent thinking, leading to the consideration of a multitude of alternatives, including alternatives not proposed explicitly by the minority. As a consequence the presence of a minority viewpoint, even when it is objectively incorrect, can contribute to judgments that are both more original and qualitatively better than those provided in the absence of minority dissent, because more alternatives are weighed against each other. Majorities on the other hand, tend to command less attention and induce convergent thinking, leading to the mere imitation of the alternative proposed.

A diverse body of evidence supports Nemeth's hypotheses. In tasks where performance benefits from divergent thinking, minority influence has been shown to lead to better performance than majority influence (e.g., Martin & Hewstone, 1999; Nemeth & Kwan, 1987; Nemeth & Wachtler, 1983), while on tasks where performance benefits from convergent thinking, majority influence has been found to lead to better performance than minority influence (e.g., Nemeth, Mosier, & Childs, 1992; Peterson & Nemeth, 1996). Further evidence for Nemeth's predictions comes from studies showing that exposure to a minority leads to the generation of more creative and novel judgments compared to exposure to a majority (e.g., Nemeth & Kwan, 1985; Nemeth & Wachtler, 1983; see also R. Martin, 1996). Furthermore, exposure to a minority leads to the use of multiple strategies in solving problems, whereas a majority leads individuals to focus on the majority-endorsed strategy (e.g., Nemeth & Kwan, 1987; Peterson & Nemeth, 1996).

Although the difference between majority and minority influence is not as sharply drawn as Moscovici's provocative theory implies, there is some evidence of both quantitative and qualitative differences in their impact. In organizational contexts, however, the most striking findings emerge from Nemeth's radical perspective, which suggests that minority influence (even when it consists of promoting an objectively incorrect solution to a problem) leads individuals to consider a wider range of alternatives than would have been considered without exposure to the minority, and this can result in improved judgements and performance, and greater creativity. Minority dissent is especially likely to predict innovation when groups have high levels of participation and allow an exchange of ideas (see West, in press).

Notwithstanding some support for Moscovici's conversion theory and Nemeth's convergent-divergent theory, a more recent perspective based on self-categorization theory has also made an important contribution to this literature. Turner and colleagues (J. C. Turner et al., 1987; J. C. Turner, 1991) have argued that the most effective minority is an ingroup minority, that is, a minority source that shares group membership with the influence target on at least one dimension. Similar others provide consensual validation for one's opinions and therefore disagreement with such individuals can result in influence occurring. Dissimilar others do not provide consensual validation and therefore are unlikely to be a source of influence.

Applying self-categorization theory to minority influence suggests that a minority will only have influence if it is defined as a subgroup of the target's ingroup and avoids being categorized as being an outgroup. Evidence for self-categorization comes from research by David and Turner (1996, 1999), who found majority compliance and minority conversion *only* when the source of influence was categorized as similar to the target of influence. More generally, research has shown that ingroup minorities have more public or direct influence than outgroup minorities (for a review, see Pérez & Mugny, 1998). This finding is entirely consistent with the research reviewed above on models for changing social categorization. The perspectives offered by recategorization, subcategorization, and cross-categorization all ensure that members of previously nonoverlapping groups are made to see that they share group membership on at least one dimension. In the terms used by those models, a minority with a "common in-group identity" is likely to be influential, and certainly more so than a minority that can be categorized as a "double outgroup" (e.g., Crisp & Hewstone, 1999; Gaertner & Dovidio, 2000).

## The Impact of Diversity on Group Productivity

The findings on minority influence are consistent with a growing literature showing that diversity is a positive resource for innovation, creativity, problem solving, and overall financial performance in organizations. Moreover, these findings are not limited to *cultural* diversity (see Cox & Finley, 1995). Diversity in terms of gender and function (e.g., marketing vs. engineering) works in similar ways (see Ancona & Caldwell, 1992b; Bantel & Jackson, 1989; Murray, 1989; Wanous & Youtz, 1986). However, this literature is also careful to emphasize that diversity needs to be managed (Hofstede, 1991; Thomas, 1990). Adler (1997) pointed out that culturally diverse teams tend to become the most or the least effective team, whereas single-culture teams tend to be average. Unmanaged diversity (e.g., heterogeneous work teams brought together without adequate support or training) often leads to either no improvement over homogeneity, or even to unfavorable outcomes. Interestingly, Ancona and Caldwell (1992b) highlighted, as has the literature on minority influence, the contribution of diversity to *creativity and problem solving*, but they also acknowledge that it can obstruct *implementation*, because heterogeneous teams may be less capable of coordinated teamwork than are homogeneous teams.

The benefits of diversity emerge clearly from research on group performance. It is a fact of organizational life that much work requires group interaction, perhaps especially creative and scientific work (Dunbar, 1997; Paulus, 2000; West, 2000). As work itself becomes more complex, organizations increasingly have to rely on collaborative work teams (Sutton & Hargadon, 1996), thus posing the question; Which teams work best? (see West, in press; West et al., 1998).

One intriguing answer to this question was provided by Stroebe and Diehl (1994) in their research on "brainstorming" or generating ideas in a group. They point out that practitioners often criticize the fact that the groups used in research on brainstorming tend to be similar in their knowledge, and this overlap in their knowledge about the brainstorming topic could plausibly impede the stimulating impact that group members are supposed to have on one another during brainstorming. Perhaps such interstimulation only occurs when groups are *heterogeneous* with regard to their knowledge.

Stroebe and Diehl (1995) reported on a study that manipulated the homogeneity or heterogeneity of the knowledge structure of the group. They deliberately assigned some participants to brainstorm with homogeneous group members, others to work with heterogeneous members, and a third group was assigned at random. They also used both nominal groups (four individuals whose ideas were pooled, so that the same idea only counted once) and interacting groups (four individuals working under classic brainstorming rules). The impact of these different groups was assessed by calculating both the number of nonredundant ideas produced and the "flexibility of performance" (both the variability and diversity of ideas produced). The results showed that, as usual, real groups were less productive than nominal groups (see Mullen, Johnson, & Salas, 1991; Paulus, Leggett Dugosh, Dzindolet, Putman, & Coskun, in press), but only if the groups were either homogeneous or random. When care was taken to form heterogeneous groups, real groups performed as well as nominal groups in terms of both number and diversity of ideas produced.

More recently, Gruenfeld, Martorana, and Fan (2000) reported on the effects of group members who temporarily leave, then return to, their work groups. They found that "itinerant" members' unique knowledge and experience could be transferred from their original group to a new group, leading to an increase in the production of unique ideas. However, their findings also hinted at the deviant status of minority members. On their return to their original groups, itinerant members were perceived as highly involved in group activity, but also more argumentative, and their ideas were less likely to be used by the group.

The results of these and other studies on heterogeneous groups are consistent with the view that *exchange* of information and ideas among collaborators who are both knowledgeable and diverse is a requirement of intellectual progress and creativity (see Csikszentmihalyi & Sawyer, 1995; Dunbar, 1997) and that social factors play a key role in the development of many creative contributions (see Simonton, 1999). They also fit nicely with the view emerging from organizational research, that organizational effectiveness can be facilitated by a diverse workforce that marshalls its knowledge and ability to confront organizational problems (see Adler 1997; Chemers, Oskamp, & Costanzo, 1995; Henderson, 1994).

## Summary

Minorities can influence majorities, often in subtle and indirect ways. Of perhaps greatest impact on organizational effectiveness, minorities can offer a fresh perspective and a challenge to orthodoxy and can help their organization to boldly go where it has not gone before. Minorities are most likely to have this impact when, consistent with the research reviewed earlier on social categorization, they cannot be categorized, and rejected, as outgroup, but share ingroup membership with the majority on at least one dimension. More generally, diverse work groups have a potential advantage on creative, problem-solving tasks, but diversity is a resource that needs managing, and a diverse work force is one that needs training to achieve its potential.

# CONCLUSION

We began this chapter by acknowledging that organizations with homogeneous work forces might enjoy a smoother ride, but their path might be less interesting and less productive than that of more diverse work groups. One difficulty experienced by diverse work forces arises when one or more minorities is present only in very small numbers and as a result experiences various negative perceptual processes and interaction dynamics (Kanter, 1977a, 1977b). These effects occur primarily for low-status or stigmatized token groups, which are attempting to pass into a traditionally gender-inappropriate occupation for the first time. They appear to have numerous implications for organizational outcomes.

One means to attack the source of these problems is provided by social psychological interventions to improve majority-minority relations, namely, intergroup contact and changing the structure of social categorization. We are most sanguine about approaches that involve categorizing former outgroup members as ingroup members on at least one dimension. The need to deal with the pernicious effects of minority group membership should not, however, lead to either depriving members of valued social identities or avoiding diversity. Numerical minorities can exert subtle and effective influence on majorities, contributing to organizational effectiveness by offering new perspectives. This impact is likely to be greatest when the minority shares ingroup membership with the majority on at least one dimension. Consistent with the impact of minorities on creativity, heterogenous or diverse work groups enjoy an advantage when it comes to creative, problem-solving tasks, although a diverse work force must be educated to achieve its potential.

Throughout this chapter we have sought to underline the heuristic value of social identity theory (Tajfel, 1978a; Tajfel & Turner, 1986). This rich theory deals with the fundamental processes of categorization and perception that guide majority-minority relations, constitutes the foundation for recent models of pluralistic intergroup relations, and helps us to identify when minorities can make positive contributions to group creativity and productivity. This theory certainly does not yield answers to all our questions, but it has already proven remarkably fruitful as a seedbed for ideas on the challenges and opportunities posed by majority-minority relations in organizations.

# ACKNOWLEDGMENTS

This chapter was prepared while Miles Hewstone was a Fellow at the Center for Advanced Study in the Behavioral Sciences, Stanford, CA. He gratefully acknowledges financial support provided by the William and Flora Hewlett Foundation, and he and Robin Martin acknowledge a grant from the Economic and Social Research Council (R000236149).

# 6

# Self-Categorization and Work Group Socialization

RICHARD L. MORELAND
JOHN M. LEVINE
JAMIE G. McMINN
*University of Pittsburgh*

Our goal in writing this chapter is to explore the role that self-categorization processes may play in work group socialization. Socialization has become a popular topic in organizational psychology. Evidence of that popularity can be found in four major reviews, all published recently, of theory and research on organizational socialization (N. Anderson & Thomas, 1996; Bauer, Morrison, & Callister, 1998; Moreland & Levine, 2000; Saks & Ashforth, 1997). Why are organizational psychologists so interested in socialization now? One reason may be the apparent failure of socialization practices in many organizations. Few workers seem to feel much loyalty to their organizations anymore (see S. L. Robinson & Rousseau, 1994). This weakens productivity, makes turnover more likely, and probably contributes to tardiness, absenteeism, theft, and other misbehavior. Improvements in organizational socialization might help to solve some of these problems. Another reason why interest in socialization has increased may be the current trend toward hiring temporary workers, who move constantly in and out of different organizations. Such hiring creates special problems for both temporary and regular workers, which might be ameliorated if socialization in organizations were better understood. Finally, the recent spate of downsizing, restructuring, and mergers and acquisitions may also explain why socialization has become a more interesting topic, because all these practices raise issues involving the reactions of workers who have gained or lost membership in organizations.

Both the quantity and quality of work on organizational socialization have improved because of that topic's popularity. Nevertheless, further improvements are possible, especially in terms of three concerns that we have expressed before (see Moreland & Levine, 1982, 2000). First, much of the work on organizational socialization still reflects a narrow temporal perspective: researchers have focused on newcomers entering organizations, without considering the many other experiences (before and after entry) that socialization entails. Second, much of the work on organizational socialization still reflects a narrow social perspective: perhaps because of their focus on newcomers, researchers have emphasized how workers adapt to organizations, rather than the reverse. Finally, much of the work on organizational socialization has ignored the contexts in which socialization experiences take place. We believe, in particular, that work groups deserve more attention than they have yet received. The importance of work groups for organizational socialization has been noted by others as well (N. Anderson & Thomas, 1996; D. C. Feldman, 1981; Noon & Blyton, 1997).

## ORGANIZATIONAL SOCIALIZATION IN WORK GROUPS

Work groups are important for two related reasons. First, most organizational socialization probably takes place within work groups. Some organizational psychologists seem to believe that every worker is involved in a close, personal relationship with his or her organization (see Eisenberger, Huntington, Hutchison, & Sowa, 1986; Rousseau & Wade-Benzoni, 1995; Tsui, Pearce, Porter, & Hite, 1995). But in most organizations, that is just not possible. Instead, relationships between organizations and workers are usually more distant and impersonal. Such relationships can thus be shaped by various contextual factors. Small work groups, both formal and informal, may be critical in this regard.

Several kinds of evidence suggest that organizational socialization takes place primarily in work groups. Consider, for example, the work of Ancona and her colleagues (Ancona, 1990; Ancona & Caldwell, 1988, 1992a), who found that successful work groups develop special roles and activities to manage the flow of information across their boundaries with other groups or individuals in the same organization. This has implications for organizational socialization. To some extent, a work group can control what an organization learns about its members, and what they learn about the organization, by regulating members' contacts with people outside the group and by restricting the information that each worker and the organization receive about each other (Yan & Louis, 1999). Even when information cannot be controlled in these and other ways, work groups can still influence the *interpretation* of information and thereby affect the socialization process (D. C. Feldman, 1981; Louis, 1980). Messages from organizations to workers, organizational efforts to create new programs or practices, and evaluations of organizations by outsiders can thus vary considerably in their meaning and importance for people working in different groups (Baba, 1995; Rentsch, 1990; Schmitz & Fulk, 1991).

Other evidence comes from studies suggesting that organizational socialization occurs primarily in work groups. Socialization is neglected by some organizations, whose workers are forced to acquire the knowledge they need from other sources, such as coworkers or outsiders (Chao, 1988). And many organizations socialize their workers poorly, providing them with "information" that is not very useful because it is irrelevant, vague, misleading, or erroneous (Comer, 1991; Darrah, 1994; Dirsmith & Covaleski, 1985). The workers in these organizations must also depend on other sources, such as coworkers, for whatever knowledge they need. Of course, organizational socialization *can* provide information that is useful to workers, but that frequently occurs during work group interactions.

Many socialization tactics can be used by organizations and newcomers as they adjust to one another (see Levine & Moreland, 1999; Moreland & Levine, 2000). Organizations, for example, can hold orientation sessions, offer training programs, encourage mentoring, and distribute information through newsletters, memos, e-mail, and so on. But training in most organizations is informal and occurs while newcomers are actually working at their jobs (see Moreland, Argote, & Krishnan, 1998); mentoring involves personal relationships and interactions between particular supervisors and their proteges (Kram, 1988); and the information (gossip) that newcomers receive is often distributed through social networks (Noon & Delbridge, 1993). Of course, newcomers have their own set of socialization tactics: they can monitor the behavior and outcomes of other workers, seek feedback about their own performance, search for mentors, and collaborate with one another. But once again, the settings for such tactics are often work groups. When newcomers are asked to evaluate the helpfulness of their socialization experiences they typically report that experiences involving their supervisors and coworkers were the most helpful (see Burke & Bolf, 1986; Comer, 1991; Louis, Posner, & Powell, 1983; Nelson & Quick, 1991; Ostroff & Kozlowski, 1993). Other research on newcomers also indicates that coworkers play a key role in the socialization process (see Chatman, 1991; Dansky, 1996; George & Bettenhausen, 1990; Kram & Isabella, 1985; M. W. Kramer,1993a, 1993b; Morrison, 1993). These findings all suggest that organizational socialization takes place primarily in work groups.

# WORK GROUP SOCIALIZATION

Aside from providing a context for organizational socialization, work groups are important in another way as well. An organization can be viewed as a set of allied work groups, whose activities and outcomes are interdependent. Organizational socialization thus involves the passage of a worker through *several* groups, from the organization itself to the many work groups (formal and informal) it contains. In a *holographic* organization (Albert & Whetten, 1985), work groups are similar because they embody the organization's central features. A worker can thus relate to different groups (and they can relate to him or her) in similar ways. But in an *ideographic* organization, work groups are less similar, which makes the socialization process more complex. Although one could argue that every work group is unique (see, for example, Levine & Moreland, 1991; Moreland, Argote, & Krishnan, 1998), a more common claim is that work groups can be sorted into clusters or *subcultures*, each with its own unique approach to organizational life. Organizational subcultures have been analyzed by several theorists who focused on why they develop and how they might affect organizations and workers (e.g., Johns & Nicholson, 1982; Louis, 1983; Van Maanen & Barley, 1985). And several studies of organizational subcultures offer evidence for their existence and importance (e.g., Baba, 1995; Fulk, 1993; Gregory, 1983; Rentsch, 1990; Sackman, 1992). This theory and research suggest that for many workers, *organizational socialization and work-group socialization are different processes*. While newcomers and organizations are trying to adjust to one another, analogous adjustments are occurring in work groups. Are these processes equally important, or does one matter more than the other?

In our opinion, work group socialization is more important for two reasons. First, we believe that most workers are more committed to their work groups than they are to their organizations. Much of a worker's time, especially in this era of teamwork, is spent in work groups whose members become familiar and attractive as a result (cf. Moreland & Beach, 1992). And in many organizations, employee compensation systems now take work group performance into account, making outcome dependence among group members a salient issue. Work groups are also more likely than organizations to satisfy workers' psychological needs. These include the need to belong (Baumeister & Leary, 1995), the need to feel distinct (Brewer, 1993a), and the need to exert control (Lawler, 1992). Finally, organizational socialization can be stressful (Katz, 1985; Louis, 1980; Nelson, 1987), and coworkers (especially work group members) are an important source of encouragement, advice, and help for people who seek social support (Nelson, Quick, & Eakin, 1988; see also Nelson, Quick, & Joplin, 1991). Only a few researchers have actually measured both work group and organizational commitment, but their results suggest that (a) these two kinds of commitment are often independent or only weakly related to one another (see Becker & Billings, 1993; S. D. Hunt & Morgan, 1994; Mathieu, 1991; Meyer & Allen, 1988; Randall & Cote, 1991; P. L. Wright, 1990; Yoon, Baker, & Ko, 1994; Zaccaro & Dobbins, 1989) and (b) work group commitment is usually stronger than organizational commitment (Barker & Tompkins, 1994; Becker, 1992; Gregersen, 1993; Zaccaro & Dobbins, 1989).

Another reason why work-group socialization is more important is that groups have more power over workers than do organizations. One obvious source of this power is the greater commitment that work groups apparently command. Moreover, coworkers are especially good socialization agents, because they have more contact with each other than with anyone else in the organization, which makes it easier to monitor behavior and take corrective action when someone's behavior becomes problematic (see Noon & Blyton, 1997). The close relationships that coworkers often build with each other also make their efforts at socialization more likely to succeed. Finally, several theorists believe that adjustment to work groups is an early and critical step in the process of organizational socialization (see Ashforth & Mael, 1989; D. C. Feldman, 1981; C. D. Fisher, 1986; Katz, 1985).

Many studies indicate that work groups indeed have more influence on people than do organizations. Some of these studies show that people from different work groups *in the same organization* often think, feel, and act in distinct ways. The research that we noted earlier on organizational subcultures is relevant here, as is research on differences among work groups in job performance (Ellemers, De Gilder, & Van den Heuvel, 1998; George & Bettenhausen, 1990; Joyce & Slocum, 1984), citizenship behaviors (Becker, Randall, & Riegel, 1995; George, 1990; George & Bettenhausen, 1990; Maslyn & Fedor, 1998; see also Ellemers, Chapter 7 of this volume; Tyler, Chapter 10 of this volume), lateness (Becker, Randall, & Riegel, 1995), and absenteeism (George, 1990; Markham & McKee, 1995). Other studies show that work group norms are good predictors of workers' behaviors, often better than organizational norms or feelings of organizational commitment among workers (see Baratta & McManus, 1992; Blau, 1995; Ellemers, De Gilder, & Van den Heuvel, 1998; Hallier & James, 1999; Lusch, Boyt, & Schuler, 1996; D. A. Major, Kozlowski, Chao, & Gardner, 1995; Martocchio, 1994; Mathieu & Kohler, 1990; Wech, Mossholder, Steel, & Bennett, 1998). More dramatic evidence for the power of work groups can be found in situations where conflicting demands are made by groups and organizations. When people choose to act in ways that please the members of their work groups but displease the organization, the power of work groups becomes quite clear.

## A MODEL OF GROUP SOCIALIZATION

We have argued that organizational socialization occurs largely in work groups and that it is usually less important than work group socialization. If we are correct, then a better understanding of the socialization process requires a familiarity with theory and research on small groups (Feldman, 1989). A model of group socialization, especially one that could be applied to work groups, would be especially helpful.

We have developed just such a model (see Moreland & Levine, 1982, 2000; see also Levine & Moreland, 1994), one that describes and explains the process of group socialization. In our model, the relationship between a group and an individual is assumed to change over time in systematic ways, and both the group and the individual are viewed as potential influence agents. The model was developed for analyzing socialization processes in small, autonomous, voluntary groups whose members interact regularly with one another, are behaviorally interdependent, have feelings for each other, and share a common viewpoint. Groups of many kinds, including work groups, can thus be analyzed using the model.

## Basic Processes

Our model is built around three psychological processes: *evaluation, commitment*, and *role transition*. Evaluation involves attempts by the group and the individual to assess and improve one another's rewardingness. Evaluation produces feelings of commitment, which can rise and fall over time. When commitment reaches a critical level, which we call a *decision criterion*, a role transition occurs. The relationship between the group and the individual is transformed and both parties begin to evaluate one another again, though often in different ways than before. A cycle of socialization activity is thus created, one that moves the individual through the group.

Evaluation by the group involves assessing a person's contributions to the achievement of group goals. This includes identifying the goals to which the person can contribute and the behavioral dimensions on which such contributions will be measured, developing normative expectations for each dimension, and finally comparing the person's expected and actual behavior. If someone fails to meet a group's expectations, attempts may be made to modify his or her behavior. A similar evaluation process is carried out by the individual, who focuses on the group's contributions to the satisfaction of personal needs. Through their mutual evaluations, the group and the individual develop a general sense of the rewardingness of their relationship.

Evaluations are not limited to the present. The group and the individual may also recall how rewarding their relationship was in the past and speculate about how rewarding it will be in the future. Evaluations can extend to alternative relationships (actual or potential) as well—other individuals are evaluated by the group, and other groups are evaluated by the individual. All of these evaluations can influence commitment through three comparisons. For either the group or the individual, commitment is stronger to the extent that (a) their past relationship was more rewarding than other relationships in which they were or could have been involved; (b) their present relationship is more rewarding than other relationships in which they are or could be involved; and (c) their future relationship is expected to be more rewarding than other relationships in which they will or could be involved. A detailed analysis of how these comparisons combine to produce an overall feeling of commitment was offered by Moreland and Levine (1982).

Commitment has important consequences for both the group and the individual. When a group is strongly committed to an individual, it is likely to accept that person's needs, work hard to satisfy them, feel warmly toward the person, and try to gain (or retain) the person as a member. And when an individual is strongly committed to a group, he or she is likely to accept that group's goals, work hard to achieve them, feel warmly toward the group, and try to gain or maintain membership. Problems can arise if commitment levels between the group and the individual diverge, so each party monitors the other's commitment and responds to any divergence by changing its own commitment or trying to change the commitment of its partner.

If changes in commitment are large enough, then the relationship between a group and an individual can be transformed. These transformations are governed by *decision criteria,* or specific levels of commitment that mark the boundaries between different membership roles that the person could play in the group. The group will try to initiate a role transition when its commitment to an individual reaches its decision criterion, and the individual will make a similar effort when his or her commitment to a group reaches a personal decision criterion. Role transitions often involve ceremonies or other activities that signify changes in the relationship between the group and the individual (see Trice & Beyer, 1984).

After a role transition, the group and the individual relabel their relationship with each other, and they may change their expectations for one another as well. Evaluation then continues, producing more changes in commitment and possibly other role transitions. In this way, a person can experience five distinct phases of group membership (investigation, socialization, maintenance, resocialization, remembrance), separated by four different role transitions (entry, acceptance, divergence, and exit). Figure 6.1 offers a typical example of how the relationship between a group and an individual might change over time.

## Passage Through a Group

Group membership begins with a period of investigation, when the group engages in recruitment, searching for individuals who can contribute to the achievement of group goals, and the individual (as a prospective member) engages in reconnaissance, searching for groups that can contribute to the satisfaction of personal needs. If the commitment levels of both parties rise to their respective entry criteria (EC), then entry occurs and the person becomes a new group member.

Entry marks the end of investigation and the beginning of socialization. Throughout this membership phase, the group and the individual try to change one another in ways that make their relationship more rewarding (Moreland & Levine, 1989). The group wants the individual to contribute more to the achievement of its goals, while the individual wants the group to contribute more to the satisfaction of his or her needs. To the extent that these efforts succeed, the individual experiences assimilation and the group experiences accommodation (Levine, Moreland, & Choi, 2001). If the commitment levels of both parties rise to their respective acceptance criteria (AC), then acceptance occurs and the person becomes a full member of the group.

Acceptance marks the end of socialization and the beginning of maintenance. During this phase of membership, the group and the individual negotiate about functional roles (e.g., leader) for the individual that promise to maximize both the achievement of group goals and the satisfaction of personal needs. If role negotiation succeeds, then the commitment levels of both parties rise and maintenance continues, perhaps indefinitely. But if role negotiation fails, commitment levels fall. If they reach the respective divergence criteria (DC) of both parties, then divergence occurs and the individual becomes a marginal member of the group.

Divergence marks the end of maintenance and the beginning of resocialization. During resocialization, the group and the individual try once more to change one another so that the group's goals are more likely to be achieved and the individual's needs are more likely to be satisfied. If enough assimilation and accommodation occur, then the commitment levels of both parties may rise again to their respective divergence criteria. This produces a special role transition (*convergence*) that allows the individual to regain full membership. Convergence is rare, however. Commitment levels usually continue to fall (as in Figure 6.1) until they reach the respective exit criteria (XC) of the group and the individual. Exit then occurs and the individual becomes an ex-member of the group.

Group membership ends with a period of remembrance, when both parties look back at their relationship. The group recalls the individual's contributions to the achievement of its goals, while the individual recalls the group's contributions to the satisfaction of his or her needs. Some of these memories may be incorporated into the group's traditions and/or the individual's reminiscences. If they still have an influence on one another's outcomes, then both parties may also evaluate their current relationship. Over time, commitment between the group and the individual eventually stabilizes, often at a low level.

Figure 6.1 is an idealized representation of how the relationship between a group and an individual might change over time and thus masks several complexities (see Moreland & Levine, 1982). For example, group and individual commitment levels may undergo sudden shifts, rather than gradual changes. Group and individual decision criteria are sometimes unstable, and changes in decision criteria could affect how long people remain in various membership phases. If two adjacent criteria are similar, for example, then the membership phase they demarcate will be short. And if those decision criteria are identical, the membership phase may not occur at all. Some decision criteria can also vary in their relative positions, which would alter the order in which role transitions occur. There are situations, for instance, where exit might occur during the investigation or socialization phase of membership. And finally, the figure suggests that the group and the individual have exactly the same decision criteria and are equally committed to one another throughout their relationship. When decision criteria or commitment levels diverge, conflict is likely to occur.

## SELF-CATEGORIZATION AND SOCIALIZATION

Self-categorization theory (see J. C. Turner, 1985; J. C. Turner et al., 1987; Turner & Oakes, 1989) was originally developed to explain intergroup relations, but has been extended recently to intragroup relations as well, providing insights into such phenomena as group formation, deindividuation, conformity and de-

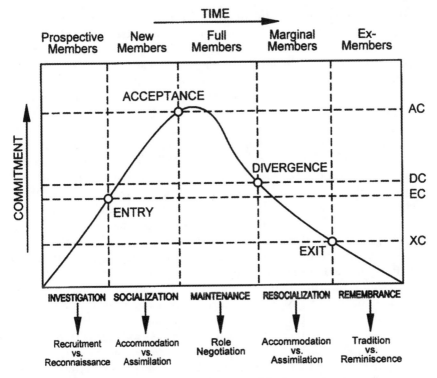

**FIGURE 6.1.** Moreland and Levine's model of group socialization.

viance, cohesion, leadership, and decision making. For our purposes here, a few central ideas from the theory are especially important. First, people are motivated to make sense of the world around them (cf. Abrams & Hogg, 1988; Hogg & Mullin, 1999), so they can cope more effectively with whatever problems occur. Categorization is helpful because it allows people to respond rapidly to stimuli, without evaluating them exhaustively. Second, social as well as nonsocial stimuli can be categorized, and the categorization of social stimuli involves the self as well as others. Self-categorization plays an important role in guiding many forms of social behavior. Finally, self-categorization can be carried out at different levels of abstraction. A sense of *social identity* develops when people categorize themselves as members of one group rather than another. In contrast, a sense of *personal identity* develops when people categorize themselves as unique individuals within a group. Choosing one level of self-categorization over the other depends on the accessibility of the relevant category and how well it "fits" the situation. A categorization scheme that maximizes the *meta-contrast ratio* (the mean difference between social categories divided by the mean difference within categories) provides the best fit for a given situation.

Categorization, which focuses attention on both the similarities within and the differences between groups, promotes the use of *prototypes* to characterize group members. A prototype (in this context) is a mental image of the type of person who best represents the group. Any characteristic (e.g., appearance, background, abilities, opinions, personality traits) that makes a significant contribution to the meta-contrast ratio on which a self-categorization is based will be incorporated into the group's prototype. A prototypical member, whether real or imaginary, is thus someone who embodies whatever characteristics make the group distinctive.

The potential relevance of this theory to socialization in organizations and work groups has been noted (see Ashforth & Mael, 1989; Hogg & Terry, 2000), but has not been discussed in detail. One way to extend self-categorization theory to work group socialization is through the notion of group prototypes. In our socialization model, the evaluation process is analyzed in social exchange terms. The relationship between a group and an individual generates rewards and costs for both parties, who compare the value of their own relationship with the value of any alternative relationships available to them. Feelings of commitment, for both the group and the individual, depend on how much *more* rewarding their relationship is than those other relationships. But suppose evaluations of the group and the individual were made in a different way, using the group prototype as a standard. The group's commitment to the individual and the individual's commitment to the group might then depend on how well that person matched the prototype. A closer match would produce greater commitment, for both the group and the individual. Commitment could rise and fall over time with changes in either the individual or the prototype, which would make the match between them better or worse. If the commitment levels of both the group and the individual reached their decision criteria, then a role transition would occur and new evaluations (prototype matching) would begin. In this way, as in our original model, the individual would pass through the group, experiencing a series of membership phases separated by role transitions.

To put this in another way, suppose that a group's prototype described full members of the group better than other members. Passage into and out of the group would then depend on a person's resemblance to the group's full members. From the group's viewpoint, commitment to prospective and new members would rise as they acquired the special qualities possessed by full group members, whereas commitment to marginal and ex-members would fall as they lost those qualities. From the viewpoint of the individual, commitment to the group as a prospective or new member would rise as a person's self-concept changed to include the special qualities possessed by full group members, whereas commitment to the group as a marginal or ex-member would fall as those qualities were excluded from a person's self-concept. Note that this evaluation process is simpler than the one in our original model: the same criteria are used to evaluate everyone in the group, whatever phase of membership they may be in, assuming that the group's prototype is clear and stable.

There is no research, to our knowledge, on whether or how prototypes actually affect work-group socialization. But indirect evidence for such effects can be found in two other areas of research. First, the influence of *social attraction* on several aspects of intragroup relations has been studied extensively (see Hogg & Terry, 2000; Oakes, Haslam, & Turner, 1998). Unlike personal attraction, which reflects the rewardingness of someone's behavior and his or her physical appearance, perceived similarity, and so on, social attraction reflects a person's perceived prototypicality. Group members who seem more prototypical are more popular, in the special sense that they generate stronger feelings of social attraction in others. Personal and social attraction are likely to be correlated, because group prototypes frequently include qualities that are appealing to everyone, both inside groups and out. But these two forms of attraction are distinct and have different effects on the behavior of group members.

Hogg and his colleagues have investigated the role of social attraction in both group cohesion (see Hogg, Cooper-Shaw, & Holtzman, 1993; Hogg & Hains, 1996; Hogg & Hardie, 1991, 1992; Hogg, Hardie, & Reynolds, 1995) and leadership (see Fielding & Hogg, 1997; Hains, Hogg, & Duck, 1997; Hogg, Hains, & Mason, 1998). Their research on cohesion showed that when social identity is salient, prototype matching becomes important to group members, whose feelings of social attraction for one another produce a special type of group cohesion that can affect a variety of group behaviors, including conformity and decision making. Similarly, their research on leadership showed that when social identity is salient, prototype matching by group members, and the feelings of social attraction that activity produces, become important in decisions about who should lead the group, how much and what kinds of influence that person should have, and how effective the person is as a leader. (Interestingly, it seems to be more important for leaders to match group prototypes, rather than more general stereotypes of leaders, at least in groups where social identity is strong.) All of these studies indicate that prototype matching and social attraction are important aspects of group life, so it would be surprising if group socialization were not affected by them as well.

Another research area that provides indirect evidence for the effects of prototypes on work-group socialization involves studies of the hiring process by organizational psychologists. In some of these studies, researchers have investigated how organizations (represented by their recruiters) decide which job applicants to hire (Dalessio & Imada, 1984; Perry, 1994; see also Chatman, 1991; Rowe, 1984; Schmitt, 1976). The results showed that prototypes of the ideal worker are often used by recruiters to evaluate job applicants; jobs are offered to applicants who match those prototypes most closely. In other studies, researchers have investigated how applicants decide which job offers to accept (Moss & Frieze, 1993; see also Dutton et al., 1994; Van Vianen, 2000). The results suggested that job applicants use prototypes of the typical worker in an organization to determine whether they want to work for that organization themselves. The closer applicants believe they are to such prototypes, the more likely they are to accept job offers. Other research by organizational psychologists, showing that workers who got their jobs through friends or relatives tend to have better job outcomes (less turnover, better performance, more satisfaction) than workers hired in other ways (see Griffeth, Hom, Fink, & Cohen, 1997; Werbel & Landau, 1996) and that work groups are homogeneous for a variety of worker characteristics (see Jackson, Brett, Sessa, Cooper, Jilin, & Peyronnin, 1991; B. Schneider, Goldstein, & Smith, 1995), can also be viewed as indirect evidence for the effects of prototypes.

Taken altogether, these findings suggest that incorporating self-categorization processes into an analysis of work group socialization is possible, justifiable, and potentially useful. But before moving further in that direction, we should pause to consider a few possible complications.

## COMPLICATIONS

Several issues arise when self-categorization processes are examined more closely in the context of socialization in work groups (or elsewhere). One such issue involves the nature of the prototypes group members use to evaluate one another. Suppose that just one prototype is used for all evaluations, as we suggested earlier. Does it describe the ideal group member, the typical group member, or maybe some real person whom the group admires? Such prototypes may arise naturally in a work group, or they may be encouraged or imposed by the organization in which the group is embedded. And what if evaluations are made using more than one prototype? There may be a different prototype for every phase of group membership. Prospective members might be compared to one prototype, for example, while ex-members are compared to another. Finally, whose prototype will be used? Different members of the group might use different prototypes to evaluate the same individual. When multiple prototypes are used for evaluations, socialization is likely to be confusing and problematic.

Another issue worth considering involves the process of matching a person to a prototype. Most of the prototypes found in work groups are probably complex, including several features. Is the matching process somehow wholistic, or does it require the separate matching of every feature? And if features are matched separately, then are some features more important than others, in some cases so important that they must be examined first and can make further comparison unnecessary if a clear match or mismatch occurs? Finally, if several (or all) of the features in a prototype are evaluated, then how close must someone be to qualify as an overall match? Is the final decision simply a "match" or "mismatch," or are different levels of matching possible? And if different levels of matching are possible, then how do they translate into feelings of social attraction? Is the relationship linear or more complex?

A third issue involves the stability of group prototypes. As time passes, the composition of a group will change (see Moreland & Levine, 1992). Newcomers will enter the group and marginal members will depart; every member of the group will develop in some way (e.g., by learning new skills or changing opinions); and through self-disclosure and careful observation, group members will learn more about one another's characteristics. The composition of outgroups will change as well, in similar ways. All of these changes can influence the group's prototype. Even if a group's composition were constant, temporal changes could occur in the categorization process that produces its prototype. Group members might compare their own group to a different set of outgroups, for example, or attach more importance to some outgroups than to others. And even if the same outgroups served as comparison targets, the focus of attention might shift to different characteristics of outgroup members. The point is that prototypes in work groups are probably very *unstable*, complicating socialization even further.

Finally, if social attraction, based on prototype matching, is the key to understanding group socialization, then what about personal attraction? There are many reasons to like or dislike a coworker, reasons that are unrelated to how closely that person matches the group prototype. Should such feelings be ignored, or can they still affect socialization? Self-categorization is such a rapid and flexible process that it may provide an ephemeral basis for evaluation. At a given moment, people may choose to categorize themselves at the individual rather than the group level, making personal rather than social identities more important. Even when people categorize themselves at the group level, their social identities may be quite unstable. As we noted earlier, changes in the ingroup and outgroups can alter which social categories provide the best "fit," as determined by the meta-contrast ratio. Different categories may then become salient, causing a variety of social identities to emerge and recede. When someone belongs to a group but is not currently thinking about himself or herself as a member, does the person feel any commitment to the group? And when a group is not currently thinking about someone as a member, does it still feel any commitment to that person, even though he or she is still in the group? If not, then one can imagine odd situations in which many rewards and costs are being exchanged among group members, yet self-categorizations focus everyone's attention on other social identities, so that neither the group nor the individual experiences any change in their commitment to one another.

These and other issues have two important implications. First, self-categorization in work groups is probably far more complex than one would guess from the theory itself or from the many experiments that have tested the theory in laboratory groups. In practice, it may be difficult for the members of real work groups (especially prospective members and newcomers) to know what a group's prototype is or how to apply it to themselves or others. After thinking about this problem and reading qualitative studies that offer insightful analyses of what group members actually say and do together (see, for example, S. A. Hunt & Benford, 1994; Lyon, 1974), we have come to believe that self-categorization is not always a private activity, carried out cleanly and precisely in the minds of individual group members (consider the meta-contrast ratio!), but often is a messy and public activity carried out by group members who struggle together to identify the qualities that make their group distinctive, preferably in a positive way (Levine, Resnick, & Higgins, 1993). If we are correct, then another implication arises, namely, that self-categorization has a political element that has mostly been ignored by theorists and researchers. Socialization is important for groups and their members—critical decisions are always being made about who can belong to the group, which group members can be trusted (and how far that trust should extend), and what it takes to become a full group member, with the privileges and duties of that role. Because group prototypes are often fuzzy, and people rely on one another to clarify them, it may be possible for people to manipulate prototypes in ways that help them and harm others. For example, someone might change the balance of power in a group by altering the group's prototype to include more of the qualities shared by friends and fewer of the qualities shared by enemies. Such manipulation could be blatant or subtle, but it undoubtedly occurs in many work groups and thus deserves attention.

# CONCLUSIONS

Self-categorization theory has already been extended to many other group phenomena, so extending it further, to group socialization, might persuade more researchers to study the socialization process and build bridges that would link socialization more closely to other aspects of group life. Self-categorization theory is stimulating—it is not difficult to imagine interesting hypotheses about work group socialization that might be derived from that theory. When intergroup comparisons are made more salient, for example, there ought to be more agreement among workers about which prospective members to allow into their group or which marginal members to eject (cf. Abrams, Marques, Bown, & Henson, 2000; Marques, Abrams, Paez, & Martinez-Taboada, 1998). Moreover, personal qualities among prospective and marginal members that are relevant to the group prototype should become more important in admission and expulsion decisions, whereas personal qualities that are irrelevant to that prototype should become less important. Another interesting hypothesis is that general beliefs across work groups about the qualities that make newcomers more desirable, or marginal members less desirable, will have a weaker impact on evaluations of such persons than will local beliefs related to each group's prototype (but see Rush & Russell, 1988).

Although these and other research ideas are intriguing, the conceptual issues we just raised are troubling, and research on prototype matching certainly would not be easy, especially if it involved changes over time in how well work group members matched a prototype. But self-categorization theory has proven to be a powerful, flexible tool for analyzing other group phenomena, and so we expect it to be useful for analyzing group socialization as well.

# 7

# Social Identity, Commitment, and Work Behavior

## NAOMI ELLEMERS
### *Leiden University*

## CURRENT DEVELOPMENTS IN THE WORKPLACE

Various recent societal developments have had important implications for work organizations. Although the scope and specific content of these developments may vary depending on local circumstances, it seems possible to distinguish some general tendencies that have had comparable effects in different national contexts.

A first area in which this is visible refers to *work conditions* (V. Smith, 1997). Even in large multinational firms, lifetime employment, or movement along predetermined career paths is no longer a self-evident prospect. Instead, personnel is more often than not hired on a temporary basis, and even in countries that have always relied on collective arrangements to secure continuity of income (after retirement or illness), this tends to be seen more and more as an area of individual responsibility. Fashionable terms such as "flexibility" or "employability" are sometimes little more than fancy labels to justify the decreasing job security or related developments that signal a gradual withdrawal of organizational responsibility for the careers of individual workers.

At the same time, there seems to be a change in *work content* (Cascio, 1995). Especially in Western Europe, North America, and Australasia, manual labor in large manufacturing industries either is made redundant by technical developments and computerization or is relocated to parts of the world where labor is cheaper and environmental requirements are less strict. As a result, in these so-called knowledge-economies, more and more employment is found in the service sector (Goldstein & Gilliam, 1990), where people tend to collaborate in teams (V. Smith, 1997). Consequently, it is essential for business success that workers are available, take initiative, or are prepared to help their coworkers, in order to foster the achievement of common goals ("contextual performance"; Schaubroeck & Ganster, 1991).

Finally, the *labor force* has changed (Chemers et al., 1995). Demographic developments, along with the tendency to spend more time on education on the one hand and to retire early on the other hand, imply that the pool of potential workers is shrinking, and companies have more difficulty attracting and keeping personnel. Due to ethnic migration and an emphasis on equal rights, the labor force has also become more diverse. Together, these different developments have resulted in more tension than before in the relationship between employer and employee: while employers have more difficulty attracting employees, they offer less security than before. At the same time, business success is more than ever dependent on employee effort. Thus, an important question is how businesses may motivate their employees to exert themselves on behalf of the organization.

Traditionally, work organizations have tended to prevent or resolve conflicts of interest between employee and organization by emphasizing the contingency between business success and employee well-being. For instance, bonuses for superior performance or shareholding are commonly used for such purposes. Furthermore, company policy may be geared toward attracting ambitious people and offering them career opportunities, based on the assumption that the ambition and additional effort that people expend to advance their personal careers will be beneficial in reaching organizational goals.

However, an important implication of the recent developments as outlined above may be that these traditional strategies are less effective than before. That is, it is less easy to specify or reward people for their contextual performance, as this involves rather diffuse activities such as helping one's colleagues, showing initiative, or being a 'good sport' at work (Brief & Motowidlo, 1986). Additionally, an important question may be whether it is beneficial to focus on ambition and individual advancement, when the nature of the tasks at work require that people collaborate with each other in teams. Finally, with the increasing diversity of the labor force, for substantial groups of employees, earning a lot of money or making a career may not constitute a primary motivational force. Working mothers, for instance, are likely to attach value to different work aspects and may for this reason even be less attracted to "career-track" jobs, insofar as this implies that they have to relocate or cannot work on a part-time basis.

In sum, given the changing nature of work content, work relations, and the labor force, it may no longer be suffient to rely on strategies that have traditionally served to connect people's self-interest to the interest of the organization. Therefore, it seems important to gain more insight into the different reasons why and the various circumstances under which individuals are likely to be motivated to exert themselves on behalf of some common goal. In this chapter I will take a social identity approach to examine these processes. I will first review theoretical and empirical work on the causes and consequences of social identity before turning to the question of how this may help us understand people's behavior in a work context.

## THE SOCIAL IDENTITY APPROACH

Theory and research in the area of social identity may help understand what drives people to work toward the achievement of common goals (see also Fielding & Hogg, in press). Although some researchers have mainly used this framework to argue that social identification is just another way to connect individual interests with group interests, the more intriguing implication of this theoretical approach is that it enables us to specify conditions under which people may value the group's well-being as an outcome in itself, that is, even if this comes at the expense of their personal self-interest (see J. C. Turner, 1987a).

Research on social identity processes has so far mainly focused on the effects of certain group features or characteristics of the social structure that are likely to foster or undermine the development of a strong common identity among members of particular groups (see Ellemers, 1993, for an overview). Although empirical work has been done with a variety of groups, ranging from experimentally created laboratory groups to members of natural categories at various levels of inclusiveness, most of these studies have used similar research approaches, in the sense that they have mainly compared how people respond to specific group features (notably the relative size or status position of the group; see Mullen et al., 1992, for an overview). Furthermore, the dependent measures in these studies usually focus on whether social identification elicits ingroup-favoring biases in evaluations of groups or group products or in outcome allocations (Ouwerkerk, Ellemers, & De Gilder, 1999).

Despite this relative invariance in the research methodology that has been used, previous investigations have yielded results that would seem inconsistent at first sight. Below I will argue that this may be due to the fact that different components of identification have all been subsumed under the same label. In a similar vein, research results with respect to various bias measures appear unequivocal. Again, this may be due to a lack of conceptual precision, causing researchers to use bias measures as a proxy for group members' motivation to achieve group advancement, while at least under certain conditions, group evaluations or allocations may just as well reflect how people perceive the current standing of their group (e.g., Ellemers, Van Rijswijk, Roefs, & Simons, 1997).

Thus, in order to generate knowledge that may be applied to problems in organizational settings, it is important to gain more insight into (a) sources of variation of identification within groups of people that share similar features or work under identical conditions, and (b) the *behavioral* consequences of differential levels of identification in terms of people's willingness to exert individual effort on behalf of the group. Recent experimentation has started to address these questions by more closely examining the content and causes of group identification and by expanding the range of dependent measures to include indicators that are modeled after behavioral responses employees may show in work settings.

## CAUSES AND CONSEQUENCES OF SOCIAL IDENTITY

A basic assumption of social identity theory is that membership in groups that compare positively to other relevant groups may yield a positive social identity (e.g. Tajfel, 1978a; Tajfel & Turner, 1979). Accordingly, in various experiments it has been demonstrated that overall levels of ingroup identification are higher as the group's relative standing in a comparative hierarchy is more favorable (see Ellemers, 1993, for an overview). However, as we know from research on relative deprivation and collective action, members of lower status social groups may differ from each other in the extent to which they are likely to perceive their disadvantage either as a result of personal inadequacy or as a common fate they share with other group members (e.g., Kawakami & Dion, 1995). As a result, given identical group status, people may show fundamentally different responses, depending on their tendency to think of themselves and others as separate individuals or in terms of their respective group memberships (Branscombe & Ellemers, 1998).

In a similar vein, it has turned out that other group features, such as relative ingroup size, may either increase or decrease levels of ingroup identification (see Mullen et al., 1992.). One way in which this problem has been addressed in the literature is by pointing out that the relative size of the group may carry different value connotations under different circumstances. For instance, in a societal context, the term *minority group* is commonly used to imply disadvantaged social standing, rather than merely referring to the fact that the group is smaller than the dominant majority. Indeed, there is by now converging empirical evidence showing that, when the relative size and the relative status of a group are considered as orthogonal group features, each contributes independently to the resulting level of ingroup identification (e.g. Ellemers, Doosje, Van Knippenberg, & Wilke, 1992; Ellemers & Van Rijswijk, 1997).

An additional source of confusion in empirical research has been that different aspects of ingroup identification have been subsumed under the same label and have been included in the same measurement scales. Nevertheless, in line with Tajfel's (1978a) original definition, three different components of social identification can be distinguished, namely, a cognitive component (acknowledging inclusion of the self as part of a particular social category), an evaluative component (the value of that group in comparison to other groups), and an affective component (the extent to which one feels committed to that group). Importantly, this distinction is not only valid at a conceptual level, but also in terms of the way different components should be related to group features on the one hand and to group members' behavior on the other hand.

When we consider these three components more closely, it becomes clear that, although they may and often do covary, they do not necessarily do so. For instance, it may well be that membership in a group with inferior status only affects the evaluative component of social identification (resulting in an unfavorable value connotation), while people nevertheless acknowledge their inclusion as members of that group (at a cognitive level) or may even have reason to feel strongly committed to the group and its members (at the affective level). However, to the extent that the three components are considered as constituents of one and the same concept and are assessed with a single identification scale, it may be difficult to disentangle these effects or to determine which component drives an overall reduction or increase in ingroup identification under specific circumstances.

To examine this issue more specifically, Ellemers, Kortekaas, and Ouwerkerk (1999) conducted an experimental study in which they aimed to investigate the separate contribution of each of the three above-mentioned components of social identification to the understanding of group-related behavior. For this purpose, research participants were allegedly categorized as either inductive or deductive thinkers and were asked to work on a group problem-solving task. However, various group features were manipulated experimentally in order to assess how this would affect participants' social identification.

First, the composition of the groups either resulted from participants' own conviction of what their problem-solving style was (*self-selected group membership*) or was made by the experimenter, allegedly on the basis of the results of a test on participants' individual problem-solving styles (*assigned group membership*). Second, the relative size of the ingroup was manipulated by informing participants that the group to which they belonged constituted either 70% of the population (*majority group*) or 30% (*minority group*). Finally, after they had worked on a first group task, either participants were informed that their group had scored above the norm, and had outperformed the other group (*high ingroup status*), or they were led to believe that their group's performance fell below the norm score and was lower than the score of the other group (*low ingroup status*). Furthermore, on the basis of existing scales, in their measure of social identification Ellemers et al. included items referring to cognitive (self-categorization), evaluative (collective self-esteem), and affective (commitment) aspects of the overarching concept.

At the measurement level, Ellemers, Kortekaas, & Ouwerkerk (1999) established that the three sets of items represented three orthogonal factors, although they could all be included in one reliable scale (alpha = 0.82). An investigation of this overall score revealed that all three group features significantly affected reported levels of social identification. That is, social identification was higher in high-status than in low-status groups, it was higher in minority groups than majority groups, and it was higher when group membership was self-selected rather than assigned. However, further analyses revealed that these overall effects were driven by different components in each case. Specifically, it turned out that high ingroup status increased group self-esteem and group commitment, while levels of self-categorization remained unaffected. By contrast, ingroup size only influenced the extent to which people perceived themselves in terms of this group membership (the cognitive component), but did not alter the evaluative connotation of group membership or the level of affective commitment to the group. Finally, whether inclusion in the group membership had been self-selected or assigned only resulted in differential levels of group commitment, while no effects of this manipulation were established on the level of group self-esteem (the evaluative component) or self-categorization (the cognitive component).

Thus, both at the measurement level and in terms of the effects of different group features, it may be important to distinguish between these three aspects of social identification. A final way in which Ellemers, Korkekaas, & Ouwerkerk (1999) examined differences between the three components was by providing group members with the opportunity to favor the ingroup in group ratings and outcome allocations and assessing the extent to which each aspect of social identification could account for any ingroup-favoring biases. Overall, there was a general tendency to favor the ingroup both in evaluative group ratings and in outcome allocations. More importantly, for both indicators of ingroup bias, regresssion analyses revealed that, of the three components of social identification, only *group commitment* reliably mediated displays of intergroup differentiation. That is, the extent to which participants felt affectively committed to their group was the sole factor to determining whether they *behaved* in terms of their group membership, while group self-esteem or self-categorization proved less relevant as behavioral predictors.

## DISPLAYS OF COLLABORATIVE EFFORT

Although the occurrence of ingroup-favoring biases is commonly used as a behavioral indicator in research on social identity and intergroup relations, there is arguably a difference between the expression of such relatively effortless and anonymous ratings or allocation preferences and actual effort expended on behalf of the group (see also Barreto & Ellemers, 2000; Ellemers, Barreto, & Spears, 1999). In order to investigate whether similar effects might emerge when dependent measures would more closely resemble the behavioral options people have in work settings, Bruins, Ellemers, & De Gilder (1999) conducted two studies in which they attempted to simulate behavioral patterns as these might occur in actual organizations.

In these studies, participants were asked to make interactive decisions on a stock-trading task in a simulated investment company. They collaborated with a partner in a power hierarchy, in which the participant always held the subordinate position, and their (alleged) partner had to supervise and if necessary correct their work. However, the frequency with which the supervisor overruled participants' decisions was varied systematically to manipulate the level of power exertion. Furthermore, false feedback was provided about the supervisor's and participant's relative competence at the task in order to render the behavior of the supervisor more or less legitimate. In addition to asking participants about their satisfaction, evaluation of the supervisor, and legitimacy judgments, the dependent measures in the first study assessed participants' willingness to collaborate with this supervisor and their inclination to take over the supervisor's position.

The results of the first study revealed that, overall, participants rated the situation as well as their partner more favorably when the supervisor had granted them relative autonomy than when the supervisor had frequently overruled them. Accordingly, after frequent power use they were relatively unwilling to continue the collaboration with this partner. However, and most relevant to the present argument, it turned out that when frequent power use behavior was consistent with the superior task competence of the supervisor, participants rated the supervisor's behavior as relatively legitimate and were not very keen to take over the supervisor's position. Bruins et al. (1999) explained this finding by arguing that, although in general, frequent overruling of the participants' decisions would likely reduce their level of commitment to the partner (see also Tyler & Lind, 1992), these adverse consequences of power use might be overcome, and commitment might be maintained, if subordinates thought the supervisor's behavior could be justified (see also Fiske & Dépret, 1996).

This post hoc explanation was further examined in the second study, which used the same experimental paradigm but more explicitly focused on commitment as an explanatory variable and included actual collaborative behavior as a central dependent measure. The results of the second study showed that, again, frequent power use resulted in lower satisfaction and evaluation scores than infrequent power use. However, Bruins et al. (1999) also replicated the finding from the first experiment that the legitimacy of frequent power use was considered to be relatively high when this was consistent with the supervisor's superior task ability. To examine the behavioral consequences of these ratings, participants were presented with a second task that allegedly involved the preparation of an annual report. Given his or her position in the organization, the supervisor would be responsible for the completion of this task, however, participants could choose whether or not to help the supervisor by adding up numbers of shares that had been bought and sold for each company. A second behavioral measure presented participants with an alleged job offer from a similar investment company and asked them to indicate whether they wanted to stay with the same company or leave.

An examination of actual collaborative task behavior revealed that participants were relatively reluctant to exert themselves on behalf of the team when a less competent supervisor had engaged in frequent power use, but they were more cooperative when their lack of autonomy seemed justified in view of the greater relative competence of their supervisor. Participants' decisions to stay with or leave the organization showed a similar pattern. That is, subjecting participants to frequent power use caused them to leave the organization unless the supervisor's power use behavior was consistent with his or her greater competence at the task. Most important for the current argument, however, is that different considerations were examined as possible explanatory variables for these findings. These included (individual and collective) instrumental considerations, the desire to "get back at" the supervisor for his or her behavior during the previous task, and feelings of commitment to the supervisor. Further mediational analyses revealed that, for both behavioral indicators, the observed effects could only be explained by the reported level of *commitment*. That is, although frequent power use was considered undesirable, to the extent that this seemed justified by differential competence at the task, participants maintained a sense of commitment to the supervisor. As a result, they opted to stay in the organization and engaged in collaborative effort to help the partner.

The role of commitment in the emergence of cooperative behavior was further examined in a study by Ellemers, Van Rijswijk, Bruins, & De Gilder (1998). This study employed the same basic paradigm that was developed by Bruins et al. (1999), however, its aim was to systematically vary a priori levels of commitment by recruiting students with different majors and assigning participants to either an ingroup supervisor or an outgroup supervisor. In addition to various evaluative ratings, the dependent measures included self-reported levels of commitment and actual collaborative effort on the task developed by Bruins et al. (1999, second study). The results of this study again showed that frequent power use was generally evaluated less favorably than infrequent power use. However, participants displayed more cooperative behavior after frequent power use by an ingroup supervisor than when an outgroup supervisor had frequently overruled their decisions. Further analyses revealed that any cooperative behavior towards an outgroup supervisor was accounted for by instrumental considerations (achieving a good team performance), while commitment to the supervisor was the only consideration that predicted cooperative behavior towards an ingroup supervisor.

Taken together, then, the results of the empirical work by Bruins et al. (1999) and Ellemers and van Rijswijk (1998) on subordinates' responses to power use quite consistently reveal the same pattern. That is, team members' willingness to engage in collaborative effort was only explained by the extent to which they felt *committed* to their supervisor, even though, given variations in the experimental designs that were used, this sense of commitment originated from other aspects of the situation in the different studies. Thus, these results again attest to the importance of group commitment as a precursor of people's willingness to exert themselves in the interest of collective goals. Furthermore, they extend findings obtained in traditional research on consequences of social identification in the sense that in these studies actual collaborative effort was assessed, instead of relying on evaluative ratings or outcome allocations. Nevertheless, some limitations have to be pointed out as well. First, it is important to note that these studies only speak to collaborative behavior in two-person teams, working in an asymmetrical power structure. Second, although these studies consisted of organizational simulations and employed measures of actual behavior in the work group, they were still conducted in an experimental setting. Obviously, only certain work aspects were simulated, and it is quite possible that additional or different considerations come into play in real work settings.

Therefore, it seems crucial to investigate whether similar relations between group commitment and work behavior can be observed in an applied context.

## COMMITMENT AND BEHAVIOR AT WORK

On the basis of social identity theory, Ashforth and Mael (1989) proposed that "organizational identification" should predict the extent to which people are willing to serve the organization's best interest. Accordingly, research has revealed that organizational identification is related to various behavioral indicators, such as the intention to stay with the organization (Wan-Huggins, Riordan, & Griffeth, 1998; see also Abrams, Ando, & Hinkle, 1998). However, in applied research, the general idea that the subjective importance of people's work team or organization should affect their behavior at work has been examined from a variety of theoretical traditions and perspectives. As a consequence, different terms and conceptualizations, such as *identification* (Ashforth & Mael, 1989), *commitment* (Allen & Meyer, 1990), 'cohesion' (Mudrack, 1989), or *collectivism* (Moorman & Blakely, 1995) have all been used to refer to similar processes (see also Abrams & Randsley de Moura, Chapter 9 of this volume, and Pratt, Chapter 2).

For instance, Earley (1989) compared the performance of management trainees working on an in-basket task in the United States or in the People's Republic of China and observed that social loafing only occurred among the U.S. participants. Earley explained this finding by arguing that, in a collectivist culture (i.e., in China) people are more inclined to exert themselves on behalf of the group than in an individualist culture (i.e., in the United States). Nevertheless, a recent study that also compared workers in a collectivist (Japanese) with workers in an individualist (British) cultural setting demonstrated that within each national sample people may also vary in the extent to which they feel committed to their work organization, and that they are likely to behave accordingly. Specifically, the results of this study revealed that, in both cultural contexts, people were less willing to quit as they reported stronger organizational identification (Abrams, Ando, & Hinkle, 1998). Accordingly, other researchers have conceived of the level of individualism/collectivism as an *individual difference* variable, instead of as a dimension of cultural variation. That is, in a financial service organization it turned out that workers with collectivist values were more likely than individualists to report organizational citizenship behavior (Moorman & Blakely, 1995).

In the literature on organizational psychology, the term *organizational commitment* is commonly used to refer to similar processes (see Allen & Meyer, 1990; Meyer & Allen, 1991). Although various forms and foci of commitment have been distinguished, it seems that, compared to more instrumental considerations, *affective* commitment is most relevant in predicting behavior in organizations (Allen & Meyer, 1996; Meyer, Paunonen, Gellatly, Goffin, & Jackson,

1989). Over the years, research has established that affective organizational commitment correlates with a variety of behavioral indicators, such as employee turnover, attendance, tardiness, and absenteeism (Mathieu & Zajac, 1990). As far as performance measures are concerned, affective commitment is most closely related to organizational citizenship behavior (see Organ & Ryan, 1995, for a meta-analysis), which is consistent with the general idea that commitment may motivate workers to "go the extra mile" for the organization.

Because of the proliferation of different concepts and operationalizations to refer to similar psychological processes, various attempts have been made to clarify the distinction between terms that tend to be used interchangeably. For instance, Mael and Ashforth (1992) proposed reserving the term *identification* to cognitive/perceptual processes (as in the self-categorization component discussed above), indicating an awareness that one shares certain characteristics and experiences with others (see also Mael & Tetrick, 1992). By contrast, as we have done in our previous analysis, they used the concept of *commitment* to indicate a sense of affective involvement with the organization and demonstrate that this is the main factor that predicts satisfaction and work involvement, which is consistent with the experimental evidence reviewed in this chapter.

## TEAM-ORIENTED COMMITMENT AND CONTEXTUAL PERFORMANCE

Although meta-analytic reviews (such as that of Mathieu & Zajac, 1990) have revealed that there is an overall relationship between affective organizational commitment on the one hand and various work-related behaviors on the other hand, a number of problems are also associated with applied research in this area to date. First, it has been pointed out that the observed relations are not as strong as might have been expected. In order to account for this, it has been argued (e.g., Reichers, 1985) that organizational commitment is a rather broad concept that may incorporate a variety of goals and values. Furthermore, the relative importance (or indeed even the precise nature or content) of such values may differ depending on the organizational constituency that is most salient for the worker in question. Accordingly, when aiming to predict specific work-related behaviors, more focused commitment measures should be used. Thus, in terms of our current research question, people's willingness to exert individual effort on behalf of one's work team, should depend on their commitment to that work team which is not necessarily related to reported levels of commitment to the organization as a whole (see also Becker, 1992; Becker & Billings, 1993).

In a similar vein, it seems important to specify the nature of the behavioral outcome that should be assessed in order to examine the impact of commitment levels on work-related effort. In view of the fact that we are trying to understand how people collaborate in work teams, it would seem essential to focus on *contextual* performance (or prosocial organizational behavior, see Brief

& Motiwidlo, 1986; Organ, 1988) instead of individual task performance. Previous research has demonstrated that these two types of performance at work are independent of each other (George & Bettenhausen, 1990), while both may be equally important for organizational success (MacKenzie, Podsakoff, & Fetter, 1991). Indeed, given the current developments in the workplace (as outlined at the outset of this chapter) implying an increase of teamwork and work in the service sector, it would seem that contextual performance is more important than before, and in some work settings it may well be more important than individual task performance.

In order to address these issues and more closely examine the relationship between commitment and work behavior, Ellemers, De Gilder, and Van den Heuvel (1998) conducted two field studies in work settings. The primary aim of these studies was to distinguish between different motives for exerting oneself and giving a good performance at work. For this purpose, in addition to overall organizational commitment, Ellemers et al. developed a scale to assess a primarily individualistic form of commitment (career-oriented commitment) as distinct from a commitment to common team goals (team-oriented commitment; see also Podsakoff, MacKenzie, & Ahearne, 1997). Subsequently, they tested the hypothesis that, although career-oriented commitment may predict individual task behavior, the extent to which people are willing to exert themselves on behalf of their work team should depend on their level of team-oriented commitment.

The first study examined a representative sample of the Dutch working population ($N = 690$). They were asked to complete a questionnaire assessing the different forms of commitment and to respond to two work-related dilemmas. Then, the same respondents were approached one year later to provide information about certain work-related behaviors during the past year, referring to their work effort and activities related to job change. A confirmatory factor analysis indicated that it was indeed possible to distinguish between general organizational commitment, team-oriented commitment, and career-oriented commitment. Although organizational commitment was correlated with team-oriented commitment, the three forms of commitment showed different patterns of interrelations with personal (e.g., age, level of education) and work-related (e.g., job-level, tenure) background variables.

Most relevant to the present argument, however, are the observed relations between the three forms of commitment on the one hand and work-related behavior on the other hand. The work-related dilemmas had been presented to tap people's preferred responses in two hypothetical situations. The first dilemma asked respondents to indicate whether, if pressed for time and unable to do both, they would help out a colleague or complete their own work. Responses to this dilemma situation only depended on the level of career-oriented commitment. That is, the more they reported feeling committed to their own careers, the more respondents were inclined to indicate that they would complete their own work instead of helping their colleague. The second scenario depicted a dilemma in which respondents could either help a colleague or engage in some leisure activity for themselves. In this case, only team-oriented commitment emerged as a significant predictor, indicating that with increasing levels of team-oriented commitment, respondents were more likely to indicate that they would sacrifice their leisure time in order to help their colleague.

Although these dilemma choices refer to stated behavioral preferences in hypothetical situations, a similar pattern of results was observed for the concrete behavioral indicators assessed one year after the commitment measures were taken, which referred to the actual work situation of the respondents during the past year. That is, career-oriented commitment predicted the extent to which respondents had focused on the advancement of their own career, while team-oriented commitment was related to respondents' willingness to invest time on behalf of common goals. More specifically, in a logistic regression analysis, only career-oriented commitment emerged as a significant predictor of whether or not respondents had taken the initiative to participate in additional professional training and whether or not they had made a voluntary job change. In a similar vein, only the initially reported level of team-oriented commitment was related to the likelihood that respondents indicated they had worked overtime during the past year.

Thus, these findings provide some initial support for the general argument that people may feel committed to their work for different reasons and that specific forms of commitment are related to particular work-related behaviors. However, although data were collected at different points in time, and respondents were asked to report on concrete behavioral indicators, a weakness of this first study is that it relies entirely on self-reports. Furthermore, while the broad sample of workers that was used provides some reassurance that the distinction between the three forms of commitment is generally valid and not dependent on a specific population of workers or a particular work context, this also implies that it remains unclear to what extent individual task performance and contextual performance would indeed both be important in the work situation of the people that were examined.

To address these weaknesses, Ellemers, De Gilder, & van den Heuvel (1998) conducted a second study, which focused on a specific group of workers in a single organization. These were all (*N* = 287) workers with concrete prospects for career advancement (because they can enter a management-trainee trajectory) in a financial service organization, whose current work requires that they successfully complete common tasks. As a result, for the participants in the second study it was possible to make sure that both individual advancement and successful collaboration with one's team of coworkers constituted relevant and important work goals. Furthermore, these participants were all working under similar conditions, so that a possible variation in work conditions could be ruled out as an alternative explanation for differential commitment or differences in work-related behavior. Finally, in this second study, each worker's self-reported levels of commitment could be related to the way his or her work performance was evaluated by the supervisor. These work evaluations comprised a number of specific performance dimensions referring to individual task performance as well as to contextual performance.

The results of this second study corroborated the previously made distinction between career-oriented commitment on the one hand and team-oriented commitment on the other hand and confirmed that these could be distinguished from general organizational commitment. Furthermore, as in the first study (and after correcting for the effects of possibly relevant background variables), any attempts to change jobs were only related to the level of career-oriented commitment of the workers involved. However, respondents' task performance (as rated by their supervisor) was not reliably related to any of the forms of commitment. By contrast, and in line with the theoretical argument developed above, the level of contextual performance as well as the supervisor's overall performance rating could only be predicted from the extent to which the worker in question had reported feeling committed to his or her team of coworkers. Thus, the results of this study again corroborate the argument that feelings of commitment to one's work team are an important precursor of employees' willingness to exert themselves on behalf of common team goals and to give the performance that is required in modern-day organizations.

## CONCLUSIONS

This chapter set out by outlining various societal developments that have significantly altered the nature of work in organizations in order to explain why it is more important than ever to understand the circumstances under which individual workers are likely to exert themselves on behalf of common organizational goals. Furthermore, as is also illustrated with the findings from the last two studies reviewed in this chapter (Ellemers, De Gilder, & van den Huevel, 1998), it is no longer self-evident that strong instrumental ties between the individual and the organization or the motivation to advance in one's own career elicit the kind of work performance that is required in many modern businesses.

A consideration of relevant research on social identity theory and applied research on behavior in organizational settings revealed that there is considerable conceptual imprecision in both strands of research. Nevertheless, upon closer analysis empirical support from both domains seems to converge in showing that people's sense of *affective commitment* with the group may be the crucial factor that determines whether they are likely to behave in terms of their group membership. Indeed, unlike what is sometimes suggested, other—more instrumental—considerations, such as perceived interdependence with other group members or the evaluative implications of group membership, seem less central in this respect. Thus, while the studies that are reviewed in this chapter encompass experiments with different research designs as well as observations in actual work settings, they consistently support the general notion that the

extent to which individuals feel committed to their group is an important predictor of their willingness to exert themselves in order to achieve common group
goals. In this sense, then, this chapter illustrates the validity of a theoretical
analysis of work-related behavior in social identity terms, and underlines the
usefulness of a social identity approach to behavior in work organizations.

# 8

# Ambiguous Organizational Memberships:
## Constructing Organizational Identities in Interactions With Others

CAROLINE BARTEL
*New York University*
JANE DUTTON
*University of Michigan*

*I*n theory, the process of organizational identification begins simply with knowing that one is a member of an organization. In reality, organizational boundaries that distinguish members from nonmembers are increasingly less transparent and knowable. Membership in modern organizations is based on diverse types of ties to organizations that do not clearly delineate whether an individual is an insider or outsider. As Rafaeli (1997) described, traditional perspectives on organizations tend to view membership as a simple dichotomy and to deny membership status to individuals with nontraditional work relationships. For example, defining membership according to physical or temporal interactions (Pfeffer, 1982) excludes individuals who do not work within an organization's physical structure during standard work hours (e.g., telecommuters, virtual workers, and part-timers). In contrast, defining membership based on contractual relationships (Jensen & Meckling, 1976) fails to include contingent and temporary workers who are paid by employment agencies and volunteers who receive no financial remuneration for their services. Although formal definitions may classify certain individuals as nonmembers, these same individuals may identify psychologically with an organization, having feelings of membership and belonging (Ashforth & Mael, 1989).

Contemporary views emphasize that organizational membership is less a matter of being in or out than knowing when and to what degree one is a member (Rafaeli, 1997; Tyler, 1999). By conceptualizing membership as a matter of degree, this redefinition transforms how one thinks about the processes through which individuals come to identify with their work organization. In this chapter, we examine how the process of organizational identification begins (i.e., perceiving oneself as an organizational member) for individuals whose membership status is ambiguous. We use the term *ambiguous* to describe those situations in which memberships are experienced as vague, problematic, or unstable. We emphasize that membership ambiguity is situation-specific. An individual may perceive his or her organizational membership status as strong in a given setting, yet weak in another context (Hogg & Terry, 2000; see also Ashforth & Johnson, Chapter 3 of this volume). Central to our discussion is the idea that individuals aim to resolve ambiguity about their organizational memberships through social interactions.

Our chapter focuses on the work that individuals do in constructing an organizational identity in interactions with others inside or outside of their work organization. We explore how a sense of membership in an organization is constituted through daily interactions with others in the form of claiming and granting acts. We describe specific interactive strategies that individuals use to construct organizational memberships by word and by deed and how others grant membership status to individuals through their own words and actions. Thus, the identity work through which organizational memberships are created involves a social and interactive process (Snow & Anderson, 1987; Van Maanen, 1998).

Our perspective on the daily work of constructing a sense of organizational membership in interaction with others is consistent with two goals that we have for our chapter. First, we aim to shift the focus in organizational identification processes from a self-in-isolation to a self–in-relation perspective (Gergen & Gergen, 1988; Surrey, 1991). Our perspective emphasizes that organizational membership is sensed through daily encounters with others rather than being solely an intrapsychic act of cognitive categorization that typifies current perspectives on organizational identification (Ashforth & Mael, 1989; Dutton et al., 1994). Our second goal is to highlight the work, effort and resources that individuals expend in these encounters to construct a viable sense of organizational membership. Our chapter aims to elaborate how organizational scholars depict processes underlying identification by acknowledging the degree to which they are more relational and more effortful.

## THE BASIC NEED TO IDENTIFY WITH SOCIAL GROUPS

We assume that individuals are motivated to believe that they are part of the settings in which they work. Researchers in social psychology (Baumeister & Leary, 1995) and evolutionary psychology (Caporael, 1997; Stevens & Fiske, 1995) contend that the need to form and maintain interpersonal relationships with others is a fundamental human motivation that drives identification with social groups. Ideally, people tend to seek out interpersonal contacts and cultivate possible relationships that are personally satisfying rather than distressing. However, once formed, people will resist breaking social bonds even when they become difficult to maintain and when there are no material or pragmatic reasons to preserve them (Baumeister & Leary, 1995).

By implication, we suggest that individuals generally will seek to cultivate and preserve relationships with their work organization, even when they perceive that it is less desirable or possesses less attractive features relative to other organizations (Dutton et al., 1994). The desire to belong and to identify with one's work organization, however, can be a challenging task for individuals with ambiguous memberships. As we describe below, individuals in these situations often exert considerable effort to resolve their membership status and create feelings of belonging.

## THE EXPERIENCE OF AMBIGUOUS MEMBERSHIPS

Membership ambiguity is not a stable descriptor of one's organizational standing, but a perceptual and emotional state experienced in particular social contexts. Ambiguity exists when an individual's membership status is unclear to him- or herself as well as other people in the social context. Ambiguous organizational memberships can emerge in several ways. Ambiguity can stem from tenuous organizational connections, such as when individuals are distanced from an organization in time and space. Virtual workers and telecommuters, for example, work off-site and often lack the physical and social ties that promote feelings of membership. Without clear evidence to suggest strong membership status, such individuals as well as others in the social context are often unsure about the degree to which they possess insider standing.

Ambiguous organizational memberships also arise when situational cues create boundaries that push individuals to go beyond the periphery. Individuals often find themselves in situations in which their organizational membership status is ambiguous because physical boundaries do not prescribe clear insider and outsider distinctions. Further, organizations themselves may have ambiguous features (e.g., M. S. Feldman, 1991), incommensurable technologies, unclear solutions and contradictory beliefs (Meyerson, 1991) that contribute to a sense of ambiguous membership for certain individuals. The pervasiveness of "boundarylessness" in organizations has inspired new conceptualizations of work and careers (Arthur & Rousseau, 1996a). Traditional views portray organizations as bureaucracies in which individuals climb steep hierarchies, whereas modern perspectives depict organizations as networks of connected goals and structures in which individuals move laterally across provisional and permeable boundaries. Our argument is that these structural changes have psychological consequences for understanding how people struggle to create feelings of membership in the organization.

Temporary workers, for example, perform tasks within an organization yet often face differential treatment by other members and exclusion from organizational routines or activities (Henson, 1996). Such situations promote ambiguity as individuals confront conflicting messages that confirm and deny membership simultaneously. Similarly, organizational volunteers, who work off-site to provide services directly to other groups (e.g., social service agencies, educational institutions) on behalf of their work organization, often wrestle with issues of membership as the boundary between work and community is blurred. These volunteers often experience ambiguity about the degree to which they perceive themselves as organizational members when performing community service. For example, an organizational volunteer noted the following:

> When I initially started it was hard to know who I should be. I'm not really a regular volunteer because I didn't come to be at [the service agency] through traditional means. I'm a part timer that's here for [my work organization]. To me, that's who I represented but I wasn't sure that's how [the service agency] saw me. I didn't know who to be. I was hoping someone would help me, to just tell me up front how I fit in here. It would've made that first day a lot easier. (Bartel, 2001)

In situations where organizational memberships are ambiguous, the process of organizational identification becomes difficult. Our discussion takes the perspective of social identity theorists (Abrams, 1999; Hogg & Terry, 2000; J. C. Turner, 1985; J. C. Turner et al., 1987) that perceptions of organizational membership are context dependent. Identification is a perception of belonging to an organization that is triggered when situational cues highlight common interests or shared outcomes between an individual and the organization (Ashforth & Mael, 1989). However, situational cues (e.g., cooperative tasks, shared experiences, perceived similarities to others) often do not clarify whether and to what degree an individual is an organizational member. Individuals lack sufficient information to conduct cognitive evaluations of their organizational relationship and, thus, often rely on alternative means to resolve the ambiguity. Social interactions constitute another mechanism through which individuals may come to perceive themselves as organizational members.

We emphasize that membership ambiguity is more than a perceptual puzzle, it presents an emotional dilemma as well. The term ambiguity reflects the degree to which individuals *perceive* themselves as organizational members and how much they *feel* like organizational members. Baumeister and Leary (1995) noted that real, potential, or imagined changes in one's belongingness status can produce emotional responses, with positive feelings associated with inclusion and negative feelings linked to exclusion. In fact, social exclusion has been identified as a basic source of anxiety (Leary, 1990). Williams' (1997; Williams & Sommer, 1997) work on social ostracism illustrates the effects of social exclusion in the workplace. Social ostracism is a perception of being ignored, excluded, or rejected by others in one's presence that deprives people of feelings of belongingness to an organization and weakens their perceived control over interactions with others (Williams & Sommer, 1997, p. 694). Accordingly, the greater the ambiguity surrounding one's organizational memberships status, the more likely it is that a person will perceive him- or herself as an outsider and experience feelings of insecurity and instability.

The feeling of exclusion and devaluation associated with temporary worker status is portrayed vividly in Henson's (1996) research. A temporary worker whom he interviewed noted that "it is kind of bleak in that respect. I mean, you're always marginal. You're totally peripheral. You're not part of anything" (p. 104). Other temps shared similar sentiments, noting that "the life of the temp is eating lunch alone every single day" (p. 105) and that the work can be "a debilitating and a painful reminder of one's place in the world" (p. 112). Such comments illustrate that ambiguous memberships often lead oneself and others to perceive one as existing at the margins; not feeling like an outsider, but barely as an insider. Attempts to marginalize members of one's own social group and the perceptual and emotional consequences that ensue for those individuals are implicated in research on the "black sheep effect" (Marques & Paez, 1994). Such research applies social identity theory to show how negative perceptions about atypical ingroup members are often more extreme than negative perceptions about outgroup members. By implication, individuals with ambiguous memberships are likely to encounter more frequent and more extreme acts of exclusion from other organizational members than do people whose membership clearly places them outside the organization (e.g., suppliers, customers, competitors). Accordingly, we assert that individuals with ambiguous memberships are generally motivated to gain greater clarity about themselves and to clarify their status to others, with the goal of repairing negative self-perceptions and emotional states. We suggest that individuals aim to accomplish this task through social interactions.

## SOCIAL INTERACTIONS AND SITUATED ORGANIZATIONAL IDENTIFICATION

Relationships with others play an important role in how information about the self is organized. Theorists have long considered social interactions as the origin of the self, with other people's thoughts, feelings, and behaviors providing important information about who we are (Blumer, 1966; Cooley, 1902; Mead, 1934). Work in this tradition has examined how social identities are created, used, and changed through social interactions (e.g., Potter & Wetherell, 1998; Prus, 1996; S. Reicher, 1995; Schlenker, 1985; Swann, 1987). In terms of organizational memberships, conceptualizing the process of identification as an interpersonal achievement emphasizes that other people are coproducers of self-understanding and self-feeling (Dachler & Hosking, 1995; Gergen 1994; Somers, 1994). That is, interactions are arenas in which individuals collectively construct a person's membership status in the organization.

We draw on Goffman's (1959) idea of "working consensus" to elaborate the role of social interactions in resolving membership ambiguity. Goffman argues that participants in an interaction aim to simplify and order the social environment by establishing the nature of their relationship to each other. This process requires "identity work," a collaborative effort to give meaning to one's self and others in a given context. We suggest that people do identity work in clarifying their membership status in an organization. We borrow the idea of identity work from Snow and Anderson (1987), who studied homeless persons' efforts to construct a particular personal identity. However, we alter their definition by using identity work to refer to the joint work done by the self (in claiming) and the "other" (in granting) that creates, presents, and sustains a particular social identity. That is, we are interested in the identity work involved in creating perceptions of membership in and belonging to an organization.

In the remainder of this chapter, we focus on the structure of social encounters and processes through which identity work helps resolve ambiguous organizational memberships. We describe efforts of individuals to "claim" membership status in a given context as well as the efforts of others to "grant" membership status to individuals. We focus on overt behaviors as well as verbal expressions, given that both forms of expression are infused with social and political implications and meaning that affect individuals' perceptions of themselves and others (McKinlay, Potter, & Wetherell, 1993; Reicher, 1995). Throughout, we utilize examples of individuals in two types of circumstances where their organizational membership is likely to be ambiguous: temporary workers and organizational volunteers. In building our theoretical storyline, we borrow from the stories of temporary workers and volunteers, which are part of the data sets from ongoing projects of both authors.

## CLAIMING ORGANIZATIONAL MEMBERSHIP STATUS

The social creation of membership status in an organization is a type of performance (Goffman, 1963). For people who are unclear about whether and to what degree they belong as a member, the performances can take significant effort and be met with mixed degrees of success. The moves or acts that individuals engage in for the purpose of displaying their status as members are what we call membership-claiming behaviors. Membership claiming describes an individual's efforts to communicate that he or she is a legitimate organizational member of a particular work organization.

Membership claiming can be attempted through both verbal and physical displays. In direct contrast to passing or attempting to "get by" without being identified with a particular group or organization (Goffman, 1963), claiming involves active efforts to have others see oneself as a viable organizational member. Using the terms of Creed and Scully (2000), claiming involves both stating and owning a particular social identity. In this sense, claiming can be thought of as a strategic use of words and acts to assert that one is a legitimate organizational member. As we will suggest below, the achievement of organizational member status is not done on the basis of claiming alone. Rather, organizational identification depends also on whether or not other people affirm or validate this social claim of organizational membership through different forms of identity granting.

The simplest and most direct form of claiming an organizational identity comes in the form of *declaring*. Declaring occurs when an individual makes verbal assertions that he or she is a member of a certain organization. In Snow and Anderson's (1987) terms, declaring resembles role embracement, as it is a form of "identity talk" that expresses an acceptance of and/or attraction to a particular social role. In this case, the role is organizational member. Sometimes membership claiming is done voluntarily, as when individuals have a choice and choose to exercise it by stating their organizational membership. For example, organizational volunteers often talk about the degree to which they feel comfortable displaying and asserting their organizational affiliation within social service agencies. When working with agency clients, such individuals must decide whether they will present themselves as "just another volunteer" or whether they will distinguish themselves by announcing their organizational membership. As an organizational volunteer at a homeless shelter noted,

> You need to make a quick choice about who you're going to be. It's a tough call; you never know how people will react. Sometimes [the clients] think it's great that local companies are trying to help out, but other times they get very cynical. They don't know who you are and they question your motives. Sometimes it's just better to check your company hat at the door, that way you don't have to constantly prove yourself.

As a contrasting example, office and clerical temporary employees often talk about exercising discretion in the degree and timing of declaring their membership in a client organization, all the while knowing that any claims of organizational "member" would be short-lived. Even if client assignments for a temporary employee are of long duration, individuals in these types of jobs face the constant challenge of claiming and legitimating their organizational affiliation. Even for the high-end, professional temporary employee (e.g., researchers, lawyers, lab technicians) the challenge of claiming and feeling like an organizational member is never-ending. As an experienced contingent employee who is a mechanical design engineer explained:

> You go to a new company, they look on you as an outsider. They don't tell you much, and you are a stranger in the beginning, and it takes a while to get to know them. You have to prove yourself all over again. It takes a while to establish yourself. By the time you establish yourself, you're out of the company. Your work is done and you're gone. So that is the downside. (Kunda, Barley, & Evans, 1999, p. 18)

Verbally declaring one's membership in an organization is the simplest form of claiming, but it is certainly not the only one. *Questioning* is a form of active inquiry used to shape one's own view of the self as well as the impressions that others form of oneself. This can be accomplished in at least two ways. First, becoming an active inquirer can convey an image of competence, interest, and dedication. Such qualities are more typical of organizational insiders than outsiders and, thus, support claims that one possesses membership status. For example, organizational volunteers often report that their supervisors perceive them as "slackers" and treat them as marginal members (e.g., delegating important assignments to others) when they use opportunities to volunteer on company time. One way volunteers maintain or restore their good standing is through questioning. For example, an organizational volunteer noted that:

> It's critical that you persuade your boss that you're still a player, that you haven't gone soft. Make sure you find out what went on while you were gone, ask everyone. Following up shows them that out of sight doesn't mean out of mind, at least when it comes to the office.

Questioning can also uncover similarities between oneself and organizational insiders in terms of traits and qualities characteristic of organizational members. Individuals can then use this information to display how and to what degree they possess such features. This, in turn, influences an individual's feelings of membership and shapes other people's perceptions of his or her status. For example, temporary clerical workers discussed the ways that they asked questions and sought information upon entry into a new client assignment (Henson, 1996). They sought information about key organizational players, sacred organizational values, favored organizational language, and behavioral norms that would allow them to effectively "fit in" as new organizational members.

Membership claiming can also take the form of *revealing* when individuals use information gathered through questioning. Revealing acts involve showing others that one has the knowledge and attitudes befitting an organizational insider. For example, individuals can verbally acknowledge aspects of the organization's culture that become part of the backdrop for insiders' interactions, such as specialized language and jargon, organizational rituals and celebrations, and commonly shared values and ideology. Revealing is an important way that people present themselves as "possessors of culturally appropriates selves" (Kunda, 1992, p. 171). Through revealing, individuals whose membership is ambiguous strive to create and sustain membership status by displaying interest and creating the impression that they fit the prototypical image of an organizational member. In Henson's (1996) terms, revealing is a way temporary workers transform "their temporary status of their current employment and pass for normals" (p. 151). Passing for normals means creating a valid sense in one's own eyes and the eyes of others that one is more an organizational insider than an outsider.

Membership claiming is accomplished through more ways than talk. Individuals can *equip* themselves with the material and symbolic resources that help to legitimate their assertions that they do, indeed, belong. Claiming by equipping can take the form of behavioral and artifactual displays that help to communicate the validity of an organizational self (Kunda, 1992). For example, individuals can use dress to claim organizational membership. Dressing appropriately for organizational membership can be an effortful activity involving physical, emotional, and cognitive work (Rafaeli & Pratt, 1993; Rafaeli, Dutton, Harquail, & Mackie-Lewis, 1997). Focus group interviews with temporary clerical and administrative employees were brimming with stories of failed membership claiming through botched organizational dressing. Temporary employees are typically given limited, if any, information about what to wear in new client assignments other than the noninformative request to where business or casual business attire. The information vacuum about appropriate dress can lead to dressing mishaps that botch or limit current or future attempts at claiming organizational membership. A seasoned clerical temporary described a typical instance:

> That situation when I walked into that environment where everyone is casual, in jeans and that, and I'm like, I look like, you know, I looked like the boss, and immediately, I was dead, was dead. I knew it too. I was there a couple of days and they'll find some reason that's totally unrelated to your performance and they will dismiss you. But you know, half the time, you know it. You're doomed. You feel it.

This temporary worker sensed immediately that her chances for claiming valid status as organizational member were eliminated through improper dress. From the moment she walked in, she was poorly equipped to construct a viable claim that she was a legitimate organizational member. As a result, we would expect that creating perceptions of membership would be nearly impossible in this social encounter.

Individuals also equip themselves as a form of membership claiming through the display of artifacts that communicate their association or disassociation with the organization. As Kunda (1992) put it, "office space contains numerous clues to the inhabitants' stance toward the organization." Individuals can play an active role in providing clues about their stance. Administrative temporary workers talk about the difficult decisions they have to make in taking over someone's desk on a contingent basis. On the one hand, having control over the office space gives individuals a physical platform to use in the claiming of an organizational identity. On the other hand, because of temporary workers' status, they have to be careful not to disturb or violate physical materials that may belong to the permanent desk owner or place holder. Nonetheless, displaying physical artifacts is an important means for claiming membership status.

## GRANTING ORGANIZATIONAL MEMBERSHIP STATUS

If the social creation of membership status in an organization is a performance in which individuals act out through words and behavior the part they wish to claim, then the success of such performances is partly dependent on audience reactions. As Sampson (1993) put it, " the other endows us with meaning and clothes us in comprehensibility" (p. 106). Thus, other people in the social setting actively participate in the construction of organizational membership.

Goffman (1959) argued that interaction partners strive to create "working consensus" or agreement about the degree to which a person's claims will be honored in a given context. This agreement does not reflect consensus about what truly exists, but rather, an agreement about whose claims will be temporarily honored. Accordingly, we suggest that individuals with ambiguous organizational memberships can use claiming tactics to attain greater insider status, but that others must confirm such claims to resolve the ambiguity. We refer to interaction partners' affirmation of membership status as membership granting. Membership granting refers to efforts to acknowledge that another person is a legitimate organizational member. In social interactions, people can grant to others both the content (what it means) and value (what it is worth) of their organizational membership. This is often accomplished through verbal and behavioral acts that mirror various claiming tactics.

Individuals can grant others membership status through *declaring* and *questioning*. Declaring involves verbal assertions acknowledging that an individual maintains a strong position as an organizational insider. Organizational volunteers, for example, note that staff members at social service agencies often announce their company affiliation when introducing them to clients. Such announcements smooth the way for volunteers to successfully make the claim of organizational member. Sometimes staff members will also include value statements about volunteers' organizational membership, providing further information about what individuals represent or stand for in that context. A volunteer who worked for an agency that builds homes for low-income families noted that the agency director told him:

> We really count on [your company's] support to build these homes. It's not just a matter of getting bodies to help out. A company is only as good as the people who work for it. [Your company] is responsive to community needs and wants to help others out because its employees, like you, think it's important. That's why we count on [your company], because we know its people are concerned, are reliable, and will do a good job.

Declaring acts can help remove ambiguities about the degree to which an individual holds membership status in a given context. We propose that membership ambiguity is attenuated and working consensus is achieved when a person's declarations match closely the content and value of another individual's claims of organizational membership. That is, individuals involved in an interaction can partly resolve membership ambiguities when their claiming and granting acts are mutually reinforcing.

Granting can also occur through acts of questioning. Individuals can make inquiries that help to establish that another person is a legitimate organizational member. Questioning is a dialogical tool that brings forth and sustains a particular construction from another (Sampson, 1993). Questioning allows individuals to proclaim their organizational affiliation and define their degree of membership. For example, when agency personnel ask volunteers to explain the structure and goals of their organization's community service programs, it provides opportunities for them to proclaim their membership status by revealing insider knowledge of the organization's strategic initiatives regarding social responsibility. Questioning can also elicit information that an individual possesses characteristics typical of members with a strong insider standing, thus helping to further resolve his or her membership status.

Granting is not limited to the spoken word, but can also occur through *equipping* behaviors that fortify an individual's membership status. Individuals can equip others with tangible and intangible resources that organizational insiders possess. Tyler and Lind (1992) argued that supervisors are potent status grantors because they often control the distribution of valued resources that signal whether someone is a legitimate organizational member. Temporary workers, for example, often speak of how their immediate supervisors fail to equip them with material resources that help create feelings of membership. Notably, supervisors often provide less compensation, benefits, and promotion opportunities relative to permanent employees. In other cases, temporary workers express frustration with inadequate work spaces and equipment. Failure to equip an individual with such materials provides direct feedback about the degree to which an individual is (or is not) perceived as an organizational member. The absence of material resources that signal one is more "outside" than "inside" the organization can make difficult the social accomplishment of membership status.

Supervisors can also equip others with intangible resources, such as information that only organizational insiders are usually privy to. This includes task-related technical information as well as cultural information regarding shared ideologies, specialized language, customs and rituals, and appropriate member etiquette and demeanor (Van Maanen & Schein, 1979). Granting such information to individuals with ambiguous memberships may promote feelings of inclusion by better enabling them to accurately diagnose, understand, and take part in task and social processes within the organization. A temporary worker vividly expresses the value of information in the following quote:

> The boss I had was extraordinary at taking me under his wing. He did things for me as a temp that I wasn't used to. It was as if the minute I walked through the door I wasn't . . . you know, I was a permanent employee, even if I really wasn't. He took me to lunch the first day. I mean, he went over everything [the company] did in detail, he brought out all the materials, and he even talked about all the political relationships of everyone in the

department—his allies, management, this person and that person. This was the most delightful experience I've ever had.

This temporary worker went on to explain how such acts brought her "into the fold" and made her feel "part of the system," suggesting that information provided informally to others holds symbolic value that increases the degree to which individuals view themselves as organizational members. Individuals with ambiguous memberships, however, are often granted nonmembership status, being excluded from rites, rituals, and customs (e.g., awards ceremonies, annual meetings, and office parties) where social information is learned through both observation and conversation. Such acts also reduce opportunities for individuals to form relationships with organizational insiders, which can reinforce feelings of isolation often associated with ambiguous memberships.

In addition to informal means, individuals can equip others with task and social information though formal mechanisms such as training. For example, a temporary worker expressed this point:

> They brought me in and gave me very rudimentary training. I really didn't know what I was doing. I was told specifically that I had to be very careful with the information I gave out on the phone, yet they wouldn't tell me the information I was supposed to give out on the phone. I was there for two days, there were no back-ups, no other information, and the boss was gone. So the employee who trained me went to management and said this person isn't working out, so they fired me.

Failure to equip an individual with pertinent task or social information does more than convey a lack of respect for the person or position, it creates barriers to successfully creating a sense that one belongs. It also reduces the likelihood that others will grant him or her the status of organizational member.

Authority and political clout are other types of intangible resources that individuals can provide, increasing the chances that recipients will be granted membership status. Such resources are a primary source of power in organizations (Pfeffer, 1982), which we see as a critical factor in determining degrees of organizational membership. For example, Kunda et al. (1999) found that technical contract workers were often reminded of their outsider status because they lacked the ability to "speak for the company." Even though the work of contract employees actively promotes organizational goals and interests, others may attempt to keep such individuals at or beyond the periphery by preventing them from fully enacting the role of organizational representative. For example, a contract worker whom Kunda et al. (1999) interviewed noted:

> When it comes to representing the company, I can make recommendations and all that. But when it comes down to it, I can't speak for the company. I don't have the authority to do things in their name even though I have a job description that says, OK, this contract employee is the one who will recommend go—no-go on this kind of thing. (p. 18)

Other examples of equipping include providing individuals with political resources by involving individuals in activities that are highly visible and central to an organization's operations, or providing employees with vital political resources such as access to opportunity structures for expressing support or dissent about the organization's activities. For example, Lautsch's (2000) study of temporary workers at SarCo. described circumstances in which management restricted temporary workers from opportunities to express concerns. In doing so, management denied, rather than granted, them the necessary political "equipment" for constructing a viable sense of organizational membership. In the words of one manager:

> I won't tolerate contractors making disparaging remarks about SarCo. and management though. They need to come in and do their work and mind their own business. SarCo employees do have the right to comment. Contractors don't." (Lausch, 2000, p. 14)

We summarize in Table 8.1 the repertoire of claiming and granting acts that individuals use to resolve ambiguous organizational memberships in social interactions.

TABLE 8.1. Summary of membership claiming and granting acts.

|  | Verbal acts | Behavioral acts |
|---|---|---|
| Membership claiming | *Declaring*<br>• Asserting that one is a member<br><br>Questioning<br>• Active inquiry to shape other people's impressions<br>• Active inquiry to gather information about members<br><br>Revealing<br>• Showing that one has member knowledge | *Equipping*<br>• Material resources (securing office space)<br>• Symbolic resources (displaying artifacts, dress) |
| Membership granting | *Declaring*<br>• Asserting that another person is a member<br><br>Questioning<br>• Active inquiry to gather information that shows another person is a member | *Equipping*<br>• Material resources (pay, benefits, office space, equipment/technology)<br>• Symbolic resources (task and social information)<br>• Social resources (contact and interaction with other members)<br>• Political resources (power and authority) |

## GRANTING AND CLAIMING AS TWO SIDES OF THE MEMBERSHIP COIN

Crafting one's membership status in a given context is often an interdependent rather than an independent process. Through claiming and granting, social interactions can transform ambiguous memberships, providing the impetus for organizational identification. Such interactions are critical when the cognitive act of self-categorization (J. C. Turner et al., 1987) fails to illuminate the degree to which an individual holds insider status. In these situations, social interactions are locales in which self-understanding is mutually constructed. This involves one's own attempts to claim membership status as well as other people's efforts to grant membership status. We see the fusion of such acts as an improvised performance that can create feelings of membership in and belonging to an organization.

Cocreating situated identification is a complex process. To achieve a successful outcome, both granting and claiming must be intelligible. That is, the identity work results in a social fact that is accepted by all participants involved in the interaction. This can be difficult to achieve. Participants do not always partake in membership claiming and granting acts with equal vigor. Our discussion addresses individuals who are motivated to resolve their ambiguous memberships and will draw upon a repertoire of claiming tactics to accomplish this. We realize, however, that people are not equally motivated to do so. In the same vein, other people in the social context vary in terms of their willingness to reciprocate an individual's claims with comparable granting acts. The absence of granting precludes feedback from others that is necessary to complete the performance and bring some closure to the identification process. Creating a working consensus becomes more difficult, perhaps impossible, to achieve, and ambiguity about one's membership status is likely to persist.

In other situations, membership claiming and granting may operate at cross-purposes. That is, the degree to which an individual claims organizational membership may differ from the degree of membership status that another person wishes to grant. Although it may be common to see discrepant forms of claiming and granting at the start of an interaction, participants can synchronize their efforts successfully and achieve consensus on a person's membership status. In other contexts, participants may be unwilling to adjust their definition of a person's status. Or, participants may be unable to grant a certain degree of membership status due to contextual constraints, such as normative beliefs about particular organizational roles or occupations. We expect that ambiguity about one's organizational membership will endure in such settings.

This chapter provides an initial mapping of the specific strategies that social interaction partners use to resolve ambiguous organizational memberships. We focused on the "tools" that people use, but additional work is needed to understand how these tools are practiced in everyday organizational life. For example, we do not expect that various claiming and granting acts are equally effective in all situations. We recommend research to examine conditions under which certain tactics exert substantial influence on perceptions of a person's membership status. Identifying attributes of the individuals involved in an interaction and the social context features that affect which claiming and granting acts are likely to be used is another important issue to be explored. Finally, we echo Pratt's (1998) position that a deeper understanding of organizational identification must consider how emotions affect the process. The experience of organizational membership involves an inseparable mix of perceptions and sensations, thus we recommend research to focus on how individuals experience and cope with ambiguous memberships in their minds and in their hearts through claiming and granting encounters with others.

## CONTRIBUTIONS

The perspective that we have outlined makes organizational identification a form of social accomplishment. The key word in this claim is the word "social." We wrote this chapter in part to resocialize accounts of organizational identification that tend to underspecify the role of others in actively creating and sustaining one's organizational membership status. Our perspective builds on prior claims that perceptions of the self unfold in social interactions to suggest that individuals play distinct roles in the identification process as both claimers and granters of membership status. Thus, our perspective expands how we think about verbal and behavioral strategies that individuals use to create their own sense of organizational membership. It also elaborates the specific actions that other people undertake to intentionally, or otherwise, allow for the granting of membership status to individuals. Our prediction is that richer conceptualizations of organizational identification processes could emerge from greater consideration of the different ways that people actively contribute to the social creation of organizational identification. Ibarra's (1999) recent study of novice investment bankers and consultants reflects such an effort, describing how these individuals initially define their membership status or "provisional selves" by seeking out role models, experimenting with behaviors, and soliciting feedback. Guild's (1999) study of the creation of order through the linking of authority and identity claims for ski patrollers and lift operators in a California ski resort also brings rich texture to the idea that identity is socially constituted in situ through interactions with others.

We also emphasize that identity work is not limited to people who are affiliated with "spoiled" organizational identities, as suggested by studies of stigmatized occupations and work organizations in which individuals seek to rectify or redignify the status of their organization, job, or role (Ashforth & Kreiner, 1999; Snow & Anderson, 1987). Like Van Maanen (1998), we argue that identity work is a normal process of identity negotiation that occurs in all jobs. We also suggest that identity work is particularly central to understanding identity dilemmas of people who experience ambiguous organizational memberships. Thus, our perspective has broad application that further elaborates how individuals come to think, feel, and act like organizational members.

Finally, our perspective may also expand how socialization processes are conceptualized. Organizational researchers (D. C. Feldman, 1981; Louis, 1990; Morrison, 1993; Van Maanen & Schein, 1979) have described the types of information that organizations impart to newcomers, or that newcomers actively seek out, to become effective and participating members. Implicit in such perspectives is the idea that newcomers cross a clear organizational boundary and can readily identify themselves as members. As we point out, new forms of work challenge such assumptions. Organizational memberships are often unclear and unstable. Thus, organizational entry and socialization may also require substantial identity work. We provide an account of the social interaction tactics that novice and veteran members may exhibit.

Ongoing changes in how organizations structure and execute their activities will continue to raise questions about how individuals construe their relationship with their employers. We highlighted a specific dilemma facing individuals with nontraditional work arrangements and asked the question, "How do individuals with ambiguous memberships achieve a sense of membership in and belonging to their work organization?" Our answer suggests that we cannot understand the achievement of organizational identification without considering the social processes that undergird its production. We believe that the perspective on claiming and granting opens new ways of looking at identification for people in unambiguous membership situations as well. Future research will need to address how these granting and claiming activities are situated in particular organizational and subgroup contexts (Guild, 1999). With new forms of work and the multiplication of forms of attachment to work organizations, there is fertile ground for growing new ways to look at the important process of organizational identification.

## ACKNOWLEDGMENT

We thank Batia Wiesenfeld for her helpful comments on an earlier version of this chapter.

# 9

# Organizational Identification:
## Psychological Anchorage and Turnover

DOMINIC ABRAMS
GEORGINA RANDSLEY de MOURA
*University of Kent at Canterbury*

*E*mployee turnover presents significant economic and psychological challenges to organizations. Investment in selection, training, and promotion is wasted if valued workers leave. Thus it is useful to understand the
social and psychological variables that affect turnover intentions (see Mobley,
Griffeth, Hand, & Meglino, 1979). The present chapter considers the role of
various distal and proximal influences on turnover intentions, drawing on the
theory of reasoned action (TRA; Fishbein & Ajzen, 1975), theories of organizational commitment (e.g. Meyer & Allen, 1997), and social identity theory (SIT;
Tajfel & Turner, 1979). We also discuss the meaning and measurement of different measures of organizational identification (see also Ellemers, Chapter 7
of this volume and Tyler, Chapter 10 of this volume).

The TRA has been used widely to predict individuals' intentions from their
attitudes and normative beliefs, thus emphasizing the subjective expected utility of intended actions. SIT has been used predominantly to predict group-
serving behavior, emphasizing the relationship between behavior and identity.
Both theories have been used separately, but not in combination, to predict
turnover intentions in organizations (e.g. Fishbein & Stasson, 1990; Mael &
Ashforth, 1995). Recent research also suggests that there may be important
cross-cultural differences in psychological aspects of workers' turnover intentions (e.g. Besser, 1993). We review our own research, which suggests that organizational identification remains important across cultures but that the impact of norms may differ in the individualistic culture of the United Kingdom
and the collectivist culture of Japan.

We propose that strength of organizational identification is probably a, and perhaps the major, determinant of turnover intention. In the second part of the chapter we consider its position in a causal sequence. We examine how, across several different data sets, identification and job satisfaction may mediate one another, and we propose that identification is the more influential mediator for predicting turnover intention. We offer a model for understanding where identification fits in the sequence of variables affecting turnover and other organizational participation variables.

## THEORY OF REASONED ACTION

The TRA (Ajzen & Fishbein, 1980; Fishbein & Ajzen, 1975) distinguishes among different "calculative" influences on intentions, including the attractiveness of the behavior or its outcomes (attitude) and the direction and subjective importance of normative pressure to engage in the behavior. According to the TRA, behavioral intentions are the result of the weighted additive combination of attitudes toward the behavior and subjective norms. The TRA has been used previously to predict workers' turnover intentions (I. M. Lane, Mathews, & Presholdt ,1988; Mobley et al., 1979; Presholdt, Lane, & Mathews, 1987). I. M. Lane et al. (1988) found that attitudes and subjective norms were both associated with turnover intentions among nurses, and intentions mediated the path to turnover behavior. Consistent with the TRA, Steel and Ovalle (1984) reported a meta-analytic correlation of $r = .50$ between turnover intentions and turnover behavior.

Ajzen (1991) augmented the TRA by adding perceived behavioral control as a predictor of intentions. Perceived control is particularly relevant to situations where control over behavior might be uncertain. This does not seem to be the case for intentions associated with organizational commitment. Hinz and Nelson (1990) found that attitudes and subjective norms of U.S. academic faculty were significant predictors of turnover intentions but that perceived behavioral control was not. Fishbein and Stasson (1990) studied a complementary intention, that of seeking additional job-related training among nonacademic university employees. They found that attitudes and subjective norms, but not perceived control, were significant predictors of intentions. Interestingly, Meyer, Allen, and Smith's (1993) measure of continuance commitment, which includes items such as, "It would be very hard for me to leave my organization right now, even if I wanted to," also shows only a weak or nonsignificant relationship with turnover intention. We think perceived control may be of limited relevance to turnover intentions because people may have complete control over the behavior. Technically, it would be easy to resign if one wished to. In this respect, turnover differs from addictive or habitual behavior such as smoking, for which perceived behavioral control might be expected to vary across individuals (Ajzen, 1991). In the light of past findings concerning perceived control and turnover intentions, our research limited its focus to attitudes and subjective norms within the framework of TRA.

# ORGANIZATIONAL COMMITMENT

The term "organizational commitment" is commonly used to describe employee-organization linkages and has been variably and extensively defined, measured, and studied (Reichers, 1985). A frequently used measure has been L. W. Porter, Steers, Mowday, and Boulian's (1974) Organizational Commitment Questionnaire (OCQ). The OCQ measures three components of commitment: belief in and acceptance of organizational goals and values, willingness to exert effort towards organizational goal accomplishment, and desire to maintain organizational membership. Items assessing this last component include, "It would take very little change in my present circumstances to cause me to leave this organization," and "I would accept almost any type of job assignment in order to keep working for this organization." These seem to imply turnover intentions, so perhaps it is not surprising that research using the OCQ consistently reveals a negative correlation between organizational commitment and turnover (e.g., Ben-Bakr, Al-Shammari, Jefri, & Prasad, 1994; Hom, Katerberg, & Hullin, 1979; Mathieu & Zajac, 1990; L. W. Porter, Crampon, & Smith, 1976) and also with related behaviors such as absenteeism (Koch & Steers, 1978; Mathieu & Zajac, 1990).

Mathieu and Zajac's (1990) review revealed a meta-analytic relationship between organizational commitment and turnover intentions of $r = -.47$. Mathieu and Zajac emphasized the distinction between the "attitudinal" and "calculative" components of organizational commitment. The OCQ primarily taps attitudinal commitment, which can be thought of as affective and affiliative orientations to the organization as a whole. In contrast, calculative commitment reflects the side bets or sunk costs associated with membership in an organization. Calculative commitment can be increased by factors that are unrelated to the organization itself but that make it harder to leave and more attractive to stay. These factors include having established a family and being older (Hrebiniak & Alluto, 1972; Meyer & Allen, 1984). Mathieu and Zajac (1990) found that turnover was more strongly associated with attitudinal than with calculative commitment. However, as mentioned above, attitudinal commitment measures were often confounded with other constructs such as intention. Also, these measures often focus on general attitudinal commitment rather than attitudes specifically associated with turnover behavior.

Meyer and Allen's work (e.g., 1997) on organizational commitment involves measurement of three factorially distinct constructs: continuance, affective, and normative commitment. Continuance commitment is primarily a reflection of the sunk costs and investments that prevent a person from considering an alternative organization. Affective commitment is a reflection of emotional attachment to the organization. Normative commitment is concerned with the sense of moral obligation and debt to the organization that militates against leaving. It is clear that continuance and affective commitment correspond well with the constructs of calculative and attitudinal commitment that Mathieu and Zajac (1990) used. However, the normative commitment measure is not clearly of either type but seems to share some of the antecedents of affective commitment (Hackett, Bycio, & Hausdorf, 1994; Meyer & Allen, 1997).

Within the TRA, attitudes focus on evaluations of an act or evaluations of an outcome associated with an act. In our view, the operationalization of attitudes in the TRA is closer to the calculative than the attitudinal aspects of commitment referred to in the organizational commitment literature (Mathieu & Zajac, 1990). If this is the case, then we would not expect attitudes towards quitting to be a predominant predictor of intentions.

## ORGANIZATIONAL IDENTIFICATION

The traditional organizational commitment approach and the TRA do not explicitly consider the sense of identification or "oneness" with an organization in turnover intentions (Ashforth & Mael, 1989; Dutton et al., 1994; Meyer & Allen, 1997). According to SIT (Tajfel & Turner, 1979), identity can be described along a continuum ranging from personal identity at one end to social identity at the other. Personal identity refers to self-conceptions in terms of unique and individualistic characteristics, for example, "I am a friendly sort of person" or "I am good at playing the guitar." Social identity, in contrast, derives from category memberships, for example, "I am British" or "I am a member of this university." Category and group memberships are important because they also contribute to a person's identity (cf. Abrams & Hogg, 1990b). Mael and Ashforth (1995) pointed out that whereas organizational commitment tends to be conceptualized as a general orientation (to a set of organizational goals or values), organizational identification involves psychological attachment to a *specific* company.

Given the importance of group memberships for self-conceptions, we hypothesize that turnover intention will be negatively associated with organizational identification. Ashforth and Mael (1989) proposed that the consequences of identification should include support for the organization and social attraction to ingroup members. These should be manifested as increased commitment to remain within the organization. We concur, and, like Ashforth and Mael, we think it is important to distinguish identification from behavioral commitment.

Mael and Ashforth's (1995) measure of identification seems to emphasize the *public* aspects of identification. In their study of members of the Armed forces the scale included the following items: "When someone criticizes the Army it feels like a personal insult," "I am very interested in what others think about the Army," "When I talk about the Army I usually say 'we' rather than 'they'," "The Army's successes are my successes," and, "When someone praises the Army it feels like a personal compliment." Mael and Ashforth (1995) found that turnover was significantly predicted by organizational identification, even after accounting for various factors such as previous experience, teamwork, delinquency, achievement orientation, and educational level. Mael and Tetrick's

(1992) factor-analytic study verified the statistical independence of organizational identification and organizational commitment measures.

Meyer et al.'s (1993) affective commitment measure is quite close to traditional measures of social identification (though we have some reservations, discussed later). Consistent with SIT and with Mael and Ashforth's work, research on the three components of organizational commitment consistently reveals that affective commitment is more strongly related to turnover intentions (Allen & Meyer, 1996). Therefore, we feel confident in asserting that organizational identification is one of the most important variables associated with turnover intention.

## CROSS-CULTURAL DIFFERENCES IN FACTORS RELATED TO ORGANIZATIONAL TURNOVER INTENTIONS

Research suggests that the level of individualism and collectivism of a culture may moderate turnover intentions and its correlates (Triandis, 1995). Japanese organizations may maximize employee commitment through factors such as security of employment, welfare programs, and strong company ideology (e.g., Lincoln & Kalleberg, 1990; Shook, 1988). Behaviorally, Japanese workers seem more willing to maintain organizational membership and exert effort toward organizational goals than workers in Western countries, as evidenced by lower rates of turnover and absenteeism (Lincoln & Kalleberg, 1990), longer working hours relative to North American workers (Keizai Koho Center, 1987), and very low unexpected absenteeism (Sengoku, 1985).

In contrast, self-reports suggest a more mixed picture. Some surveys reveal Japanese workers express *less* commitment to their organizations (e.g. Cole, 1979; Luthans, McCaul, & Dodd, 1985; Near, 1989). Although it is possible that such findings could reflect measurement problems and a modesty response bias in Eastern cultures (Farh, Dobbins, & Cheng, 1991), these biases seem to be weak and/or domain specific (Lincoln and Kalleberg, 1985; Yu & Murphy, 1993).

Of greater interest is Besser's (1993) suggestion that there are cultural differences in the role of structural and normative *processes* affecting organizational turnover and commitment. Besser suggests one reason for the weaker association between organizational commitment and turnover rates among Japanese workers is the relatively greater importance of other ties (including duties to family, community, and specific others) in Japanese relative to North American culture (Takezawa & Whitehill, 1981).

Besser's analysis is consistent with Markus and Kitayama's (1991) account of cross-cultural differences in the way people construe the self, others, and the interdependence between the two. In Western cultures, people seek *independence* from others. Relationships with others are relatively unimportant for self-definition. In Eastern cultures, the emphasis is on attending to others, fitting in, and harmonious *interdependence*. The self is defined through relationships with others (Cousin, 1989; Hofstede, 1980; Lebra, 1976; Triandis, Bontempo, Villareal, Asai, & Lucca, 1988). As a result, anticipated reactions from others can be expected to play a more important role in determining intentions to leave a work organization in a collectivist culture (cf. Rohlen, 1974).

## Two Studies of Cross-Cultural Variation in Antecedents of Turnover Intention

Previous research in the United States demonstrated reliable relationships among turnover intentions, attitudes, and subjective norms. Other research demonstrated reliable effects of organizational identification on turnover intentions. However, previous research had not examined whether variables specified by the TRA and organizational identification were able to account for unique portions of the variance in turnover intentions. Thus, a conceptual and empirical gap remained to be explored. Specifically, because studies using the TRA had not included a measure of organizational identification, it was conceivable that effects associated with attitudes and norms were actually due to shared but unmeasured variance with identification. Similarly, studies investigating organizational identification had not included a measure of subjective norms, leaving open the possibility that the association between identification and turnover intentions was partially due to normative pressure for loyalty to the organization. Indirect support for this idea comes from research using Meyer and Allen's (1997) measures of affective and normative commitment, both of which tend to be related to turnover intention. However, we note that their normative commitment measure focuses on personal morality and sense of obligation, whereas the TRA operationalization of subjective norms is about normative pressure from specific others in relation to a specific act. Thus we think the subjective norm measure might be more distinct from the identification measure than normative and affective commitment measures are. In addition, because the subjective norm measure is more specific and therefore corresponds more closely to the intention, it offers a more useful index of normative processes than Meyer and Allen's normative commitment scale does.

In light of these issues we conducted two parallel studies (Abrams et al., 1998). The first goal of our research was to examine the utility of a model that employs both the TRA and organizational identification variables to predict turnover intention and thus to analyze the relative contribution of each predictor variable. Our second goal was to investigate cross-cultural differences in the predictors of turnover intentions. The two studies compared workers in parallel organizations in Japan and Britain. In Study 1 we distributed questionnaires to employees of matched Japanese service sector organizations in the United Kingdom and Japan. We obtained a 67% response rate. In Study 2 we distributed questionnaires to academic faculty in Japanese and UK universities, with a response rate of 43%. The two studies employed essentially the same measures and procedures. We produced parallel British and Japanese versions of the questionnaire, verified by back-translation. We used multi-item measures to produce composite scores to reflect the TRA constructs and organizational identification.

**Measurement issues.** We expected favorable attitudes to turnover to predict intentions, as found in previous studies (see also Becker et al., 1995). Our attitude measure concerns the favorability towards the outcomes of leaving the organization, rather than attitudes towards the organization per se. Subjects were asked how much their pay and their opportunities for advancement would change (for better or worse) if they left the company in the next few years. In this respect it may be closer to calculative than attitudinal commitment as defined by Mathieu and Zajac (1990).

Subjective norm was measured using questions asking how much the partner, family members, colleagues, and work supervisor would approve of the respondent leaving the organization in the next few years.

Recall that Mathieu and Zajac (1990) discovered that calculative commitment was the less important of the two forms. Meyer and Allen (1997) found that normative commitment is a better predictor of turnover intention than continuance (calculative) commitment. Therefore, we expected subjective norms to be more strongly associated than attitudes with turnover intentions.

We had considered various measures of identification, but several seemed to confound the sense of attachment and linkage between self and group with other issues. For example, Allen and Meyer's (1990) affective commitment measure originally included an item about behavior ("I enjoy discussing my organization with people outside it"), and the revised 6-item scale (Meyer et al., 1993) still included items that relate to planning ("I would be very happy to spend the rest of my career in this organization") and attribution ("I really feel as if this organization's problems are my own"), although the other items are more directly based on traditional measures of social identity ("strong sense of belonging"). As discussed previously, Mael and Ashforth's (1995) scale is predominantly concerned with public expressions of identification rather than its subjective meaning. Thus, we opted to use our own measure of organizational identification, developed within a SIT framework (Abrams, 1985, 1990, 1994; Abrams & Emler, 1992; Hinkle, Taylor, Fox-Cardamone, and Crook; 1989). Versions of this measure have been used by us or our colleagues in several previous studies of organizational contexts (e.g. Abrams, 1992; R. J. Brown, 1978, Brown, Condor, Wade, Mathews, & Williams, 1986; Hinkle & Brown, 1990).

The items in our scale focus exclusively on feelings about membership in the organization and the importance of the organization to the individual, reflecting Tajfel's (1978c) definition of social identity: "the individual's knowledge that he/she belongs to certain social groups together with some emotional and value significance to him/her of the group membership." A further criterion for item selection was that all items should be closely translatable between English and Japanese. In contrast to our measures of attitudes and subjective norms, our identification measure was not specifically focused on turnover intention. However, to the extent that a person's membership in an organization is a positive part of his or her identity, that person should be less willing to lose that part of their identity (Tajfel & Turner, 1979) and hence less willing to quit.

Our organizational identification measure consisted of seven items. Two questions, "I feel strong ties with this company" and "This company is important to me" were selected from Hinkle et al.'s (1989) in-group identification scale. Five questions, "I feel proud to be a member of my company," "I often regret that I belong to this company" (reversed), "I feel a strong sense of belonging to this company," "Belonging to this company is an important part of my self-image," and "I am glad to be a member of this company," were taken from previous research by Abrams (1985, 1990, 1992).

Turnover intention was measured using four items concerning plans to leave or remain within the organization: "In the next few years I intend to leave this company," "In the next few years I expect to leave this company," "I think about leaving this company," and "I'd like to work in this company until I reach retirement age."

Various researchers have suggested that biographical factors may be important either as antecedents of organizational identification (Mael, 1991) or as side-bet determinants of commitment and turnover intentions (Alluto, Hrebiniak, & Alonso, 1973; Loscocco & Kalleberg, 1988; Meyer & Allen, 1984). We thus controlled for the effects of marital status, number of children, and age by including them as covariates in our analyses.

We found our measures to be highly reliable. In Study 1 and 2, respectively, Cronbach's alphas for the various scales were as follows: turnover intention (.88, .89), attitude toward leaving the organization (.73, .77), subjective norm (.74, .79), and organizational identification (.87, .93).

**National differences.** In the service organization study, Japanese respondents had higher turnover intentions, lower identification, and attitudes and subjective norms that were more favorable towards leaving. In comparison with the neutral scale midpoint, British participants were significantly positive about the organization on all measures, whereas Japanese participants were only positive in terms of identification and attitudes.

In the university study, Japanese respondents had lower turnover intentions, stronger identification, and attitudes and subjective norms that were less favorable towards leaving. Compared with the neutral scale midpoint, British participants held significantly negative attitudes, whereas Japanese respondents held significantly positive levels of identification, subjective norms, and turnover intentions.

There was no evidence of any particular cultural bias in responses or differences in levels of organizational commitment. In this respect our data suggest that differences in commitment between Japanese and Western workers (Besser, 1993; Cole, Kalleberg, & Lincoln, 1993) may depend on particular organizational settings. It appears that in some organizations, Japanese workers express more, and in others less, commitment than their Western counterparts.

**Prediction of turnover intention.**   Of greater interest was the relationship between the different predictors and turnover intention. Previous evidence suggested that the weak relationship between self-reported commitment and turnover among Japanese workers may have resulted from the relatively increased importance of interpersonal norms within Japanese culture. If the intentions of Japanese workers are more heavily influenced by expectations from others, it follows that subjective norms would have greater importance in determining turnover intentions in Japan than in Britain.

In both studies we found a relatively weak correlation between attitude and intention ($r = 0.07$ in study 1 and $r = .28$ in Study 2) and a strong correlation between identification and intention ($r = .55$ in Study 1 and $r = .68$ in Study 2). However, the relationship between subjective norm and intention varied depending on the country in which the sample was based. In the United Kingdom, the relationships were quite weak ($r = .20$ across studies), whereas in Japan they were stronger and significant ($r = .58$ across studies).

In order to examine the distinct impact of each variable on turnover intention we conducted hierarchical regressions. After the covariates, we first entered attitude, subjective norm, identification, and country. Next we entered the interaction of each measured variable with country. As shown in Table 9.1, both studies produced a similar pattern of results, with a substantial main effect of identification and an interaction between country and subjective norm.

**Theory of reasoned action.**   In both studies, attitudes consistently accounted for less variance in turnover intentions than did subjective norms. Previous stud-

TABLE 9.1. Study 1 and 2. Hierarchical standardized regression weights for predictors of turnover intentions.

| Step | Variables entered | Service organizations | | | Universities | | |
|------|-------------------|:---:|:---:|:---:|:---:|:---:|:---:|
| | | β | $t$ | $\Delta R^2$ | β | $t$ | $\Delta R^2$ |
| 1 | | | | $.40^{\circ\circ\circ}$ | | | $.55^{\circ\circ\circ}$ |
| | Attitude | −.11 | 0.98 | | .15 | 2.16° | |
| | Subjective norms | .29 | 3.18°° | | .28 | 3.96°°° | |
| | Identification | −.60 | 5.31°°° | | −.53 | 7.41°°° | |
| | Country | −.32 | 2.37° | | −.07 | 1.07 | |
| 2 | | | | .05° | | | .03+ |
| | Country x Attitude | .16 | 1.90 | | −.01 | 0.15 | |
| | Country x Norms | −.21 | 2.44° | | −.15 | 2.18° | |
| | Country x Identification | −.10 | 0.80 | | −.11 | 1.59 | |

Note. $+ p < .11$; $^{\circ}p < .05$; $^{\circ\circ}p < .01$; $^{\circ\circ\circ}p < .001$.

ies that revealed significant associations between attitudes and turnover intentions have employed considerably larger samples than ours (e.g., Hinz & Nelson, 1990; I. M. Lane et al., 1988), which raises the possibility that our present research may have lacked sufficient statistical power. However, the pattern of correlations between attitudes and intentions was inconsistent across our studies, with no hint of a systematic relationship. We were slightly surprised that there was not a stronger relationship with turnover intention, given that we had measured attitude as a specific construct related directly to the particular intention (i.e., we measured attitude toward leaving and not attitude toward the organization). Our operationalization should have maximized the chances for the attitude-intention relationship to be revealed.

Given the rather "calculative" nature of our attitude measure, our results are fairly consistent with Mathieu and Zajac's (1990) conclusion that the relationship between calculative commitment and turnover intentions is weak. Nevertheless, a more comprehensive measure of attitudes, administered to a larger sample, might reveal a more consistent or subtle relationship with turnover intentions. It is also conceivable that cross-cultural differences in the attitude-intention relationship could be revealed.

Our prediction that subjective norms would play a more important role in shaping turnover intentions in Japan than in Britain was confirmed in both Study 1 and Study 2. Mean levels of subjective norms did not differ systematically between Japan and Britain, but they were substantially associated with turnover intentions in both Japanese samples and only weakly associated with turnover intentions in the British samples. These findings are consistent with the view that the committed behaviors of Japanese workers can be partially explained by the pressures of the work group, family, and community, rather than by strong feelings of commitment to organizations (Besser, 1993; Near, 1989) and that strong social ties in Japan make people more sensitive to others' expectations for their actions (Markus & Kitayama, 1991).

**Organizational identification.** Consistent with expectations derived from SIT, organizational identification was strongly related to turnover intentions. In both organizational and both national contexts, organizational identification was the most important predictor of turnover intentions. These two studies extended our previous work combining components of SIT with the TRA (Abrams, 1990; Abrams, Hinkle, & Tomlins, 1999; Hinkle, Fox-Cardamone, Haseleu, Brown, & Irwin, 1996). This finding is consistent with SIT, which would predict that when group membership is important for their self-concepts, people will try to maintain that membership.

The correlations between subjective norms and identification with the organization were generally moderate ($r = -.21$ in study 1, $r = -.26$ in Study 2) and significant only in the Japanese university sample ($r = -.33$). This suggests that acceptance of external social norms regarding turnover intentions does not strongly imply parallel levels of identification with the organization. For some individuals, subjective norms may even press in one direction (e.g., to stay) and identification in another (e.g., to leave). Thus, our data seem consistent with the view that identification and subjective norms are two different psychological constructs that should remain conceptually and empirically distinct as determinants of turnover intentions (cf. Meyer & Allen, 1997). Our views on this issue are consistent with Cole et al.'s (1993) analysis that committed behaviors, and thus turnover intentions, can stem from social pressures but that the effects of these pressures depend on a high degree of individual acceptance and compliance, which are ultimately internalized as commitment.

It is conceivable that while being equally important the value associated with group membership arises through different processes in Japan and Britain (Markus & Kitayama, 1994), and that this might affect the quality of the relationship between identification and intention. For example, in a study of intentions to leave Hong Kong after the transition from British to Chinese sovereignty, we found that individual differences in collectivism/individualism moderated the identification-intention relationship (Abrams, Hinkle, & Tomlins, 1997). The positive association between identification and intention to remain in Hong Kong was higher among collectivists than individualists. Future research could compare the effects of such ideological and cultural differences on the identification–turnover intention relationship within individualistic and collectivist cultures (cf. Triandis et al., 1988).

## JOB SATISFACTION AND IDENTIFICATION AS PREDICTORS OF TURNOVER INTENTION

The literature on job satisfaction is voluminous and does not require repetition in this chapter. Suffice to say that job satisfaction has frequently been used as a key predictor of turnover intention (e.g., Eby, Freeman, Rush, & Lance, 1999; Rosse & Hulin, 1985). Although there are many different measures and foci of job satisfaction (Becker & Billings, 1993), most may reflect issues such as a person's sense that they are fairly treated and that they are not being denied better alternatives (e.g., Eby et al., 1999; Farrell & Rusbult, 1981). One obvious response to dissatisfaction is to leave one's job, and it is therefore reasonable to expect that job (dis)satisfaction should be associated with stronger turnover intentions due to either personal satisfaction levels (Porter & Steers, 1973; Spencer & Steers, 1981) or group level indices of satisfaction (Jinnet & Alexander, 1999). However, it is unclear precisely how or why this relationship exists. Job satisfaction may arise from many different sources, and it is not always evident that these would change if one left. For example, role ambiguity, autonomy, a good manager, good social relationships, and support in the workplace may all contribute to job satisfaction. However, leaving a job does not guarantee that any of these will improve, or indeed that the net improvement will be tangible or large. One may risk exchanging one set of dissatisfying aspects with a different set (Rusbult, Farrell, Rogers, & Mainous, 1988).

As we observed in the Abrams et al. (1998) study, organizational identification appears to be a strong predictor of turnover intention. This suggests that we should consider the relationship between job satisfaction and identification. There is evidence that both variables are associated with turnover intentions. For example, Covin, Sightler, Kolenko, & Tudor (1996) found the three measures to be correlated in their study of nearly 3,000 employees in a merger situation. Eby et al.'s (1999) meta-analysis revealed that both affective commitment and job satisfaction predicted turnover, though affective commitment was the stronger predictor. However, it is possible that one of these two variables plays a more proximal, and the other a more distal, role. Meyer and Allen's (1997) model of organizational commitment (e.g., p. 106) does not locate job satisfaction explicitly. We think that the literature and Meyer and Allen's model suggest two models that are plausible.

Meyer and Allen's (1997) model defines work experiences, role states, and psychological contracts as distal variables that affect judgments about norms, costs, and affective feelings. These in turn influence forms of commitment, which then determine retention, productive behavior, and well-being. If we consider identification to be somewhat close to Allen and Meyer's construct of affective commitment it follows that identification should be a relatively proximal influence on turnover intention.

In our Model 1, satisfaction is considered to be an aspect of employee well-being that could be influenced by commitment. Thus, satisfaction is an even more proximal cause of turnover than identification. The strong version of Model 1 posits that identification is merely an antecedent of satisfaction with one's job (Reichers, 1986, Becker & Billings, 1993). Together with issues such as pay, conditions of service, and social relationships in the situation, identification could affect satisfaction, which could then determine turnover intentions. Thus, the strong version of Model 1 holds that the effect of identification on turnover intention is mediated by job satisfaction.

Our Model 2 assumes that job satisfaction is most closely associated with the more distal variables in the Allen and Meyer model (i.e., with work experiences, role states, and psychological contracts) and thus should precede commitment. The strong version of Model 2 posits that job satisfaction is one of several possible antecedents of identification, along with variables such as wide job scope (Hackett et al., 1994), just policies (Folger & Kanovsky, 1989; Schaubroek, May, & Brown, 1994), good working relationships, prototypical leaders and participative decision processes (Morris, Hulbert, & Abrams, 2000), and perhaps clear intergroup boundaries (Hogg, 1993). In Model 2, the effects of job satisfaction on turnover intention are mediated by identification.

A weaker version of Model 1 would allow both job satisfaction and identification to influence turnover intention but the effect of identification to be mediated partially by job satisfaction. A weaker version of Model 2 would allow both job satisfaction and identification to influence turnover intention but the effect of job satisfaction to be mediated partially by identification.

In order to test these competing models we examined data from 5 different data sets that measured organizational identification, job satisfaction, and turnover intention (Abrams, Randsley de Moura, Vaughan, Gunnarsdottir, & Ando, 2001). These studies all involved organizational surveys, but sampled quite different populations of workers. Study 1 revisited the Abrams et al. (1998) data from workers in the service industry, Study 2 revisited the Abrams et al. (1998) data from university academics. Study 3 involved employees in a large urban hospital, Study 4 involved workers in a large national mail service, and Study 5 involved workers in a legal firm. Although the demographic and gender profile of each sample varied somewhat, our primary concern was to examine variation in the relationships among the three key variables. For the purposes of this analysis we were not concerned with absolute levels of identification, satisfaction, and turnover intention. However, we should note that data from Studies 3, 4, and 5 were generally in line with the data from Abrams et al. (1998).

Our analytic strategy was to conduct two mediation analyses, one to test each model. Table 9.2, shows the regression coefficients for the mediation analyses. The first column of data reveals that, in all the samples, turnover is significantly related to both identification and job satisfaction. This establishes that there are effects of both variables that can potentially be mediated. The final column reveals that identification and satisfaction are significantly correlated with each other. This establishes that each is a potential mediator of the other. The second column of data provides the coefficients for identification and satisfaction controlling for the other predictor (i.e., the direct effect of each predictor). If these statistics are significant it demonstrates that, as mediators, they affect turnover even when the independent variable is accounted for. The third column provides the change as a result of the potential mediator (the indirect

TABLE 9.2. Regression weights for assessing the relationships among identification, job satisfaction and turnover intention.

| Study | Predictor | Total effect on turnover intention ($b$) | Direct effect on intention ($b$) | Amount of mediation ($b$) | Relationship between Identification-Satisfaction ($b$) |
|---|---|---|---|---|---|
| Hospital | Satisfaction | −.59°°° | −.37°°° | −.22°°° | .37°°° |
| (N = 870) | Identification | −.67°°° | −.60°°° | .07°°° | |
| Postal | Satisfaction | −.52°°° | −.21° | −.31°°° | .53°°° |
| (N = 171) | Identification | −.69°°° | −.60°°° | −.09° | |
| Legal Survey | Satisfaction | −.75°°° | −.40°° | −.35°°° | .49°°° |
| (N = 129) | Identification | −.81°°° | −.71°°° | −.10° | |
| University | Satisfaction | −.64°°° | −.03 | −.61°°° | .77°°° |
| (N = 117) | Identification | −.81°°° | −.79°°° | −.02 | |
| Commercial | Satisfaction | −.72°°° | −.22° | −.50°° | .72°°° |
| (N = 99) | Identification | −.80°°° | −.69°° | −.11° | |

*Note:* ° $p < .05$, °° $p < .01$, °°° $p < .001$.

effect of each predictor). This is a measure of the amount of mediation. Baron and Kenny's (1996) adaptation of the Sobel (1982) test provides a Z test to determine whether the amount of mediation is significant.

If the strong version of a model is supported there should be complete mediation, meaning that the coefficient in column 1 is significant, the coefficient in column 2 is nonsignificant, and the mediation in column 3 is significant. If the weak version of a model is supported the coefficient in column 2 may remain significant. Table 9.2 shows clearly that the mediating effect of identification is larger than the mediating effect of satisfaction, although both sustain direct effects even when the indirect effect is accounted for.

In order to assess the effect sizes for the different mediators we performed a meta-analysis on these data. The meta-analytic effect size (weighted by sample size) for the mediation of identification by job satisfaction gives mean $R = .14$, $Z = 4.87$, $p = 5.88\text{E-}7$. The meta-analytic effect size for the mediation of job satisfaction by identification gives mean $R = .28$, $Z = 8.48$, $p = 1.69\text{E-}16$. A focused comparison of the effect sizes for the two mediators yields a significant $Z = 4.53$, $p = 3.006\text{E-}6$, indicating that identification mediates job satisfaction significantly more than job satisfaction mediates identification.

In view of these findings we feel fairly confident about accepting the weak version of Model 2 as depicted in Figure 9.1. When identification is a mediator it reduces the impact of job satisfaction quite substantially, whereas when satisfaction is the mediator it does not affect the impact of identification so markedly.

## RESEARCH QUESTIONS AND A MODEL

An important aspect of our research strategy, and one of the key recommendations in Mathieu and Zajac's (1990) review, was to sample from different types

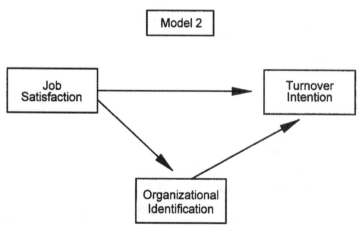

**FIGURE 9.1.** Model 2: Job Satisfaction affects Turnover Intention directly and mediated by Identification.

of organizations. Sampling from multiple organizations helps to avoid problems of homogeneity of experience (and hence restriction of variance and covariance among measures). For example, adding a powerful factor, such as culture, increases the confidence with which we can generalize not only across organizations but within and between nations as well.

Our research leaves some questions unanswered. For example, the relationships we have explored are correlational rather than causal. Previous research has established causal links from other indicators of organizational commitment to turnover intentions and from intentions to turnover behavior (Mathieu & Zajac, 1990). In the light of three decades of research on the TRA, we think it reasonable to believe that attitudes, subjective norms, and identification have a greater causal effect on turnover intentions than vice versa. Future research could address these issues directly using a longitudinal design and by including a measure of turnover behavior.

A further issue is where attitudes and subjective norms might fit in the causal sequence. Using Meyer and Allen's framework it would seem that attitudes could be a highly proximal variable that emerges from various calculative processes and identification. Similarly, subjective norms could be a function of the individual's reporting of their attitudes to significant others, and thus both could be highly relevant at the crucial time when a person decides to quit. Alternatively, more global attitudes and subjective norms (or perhaps global calculations) about quitting (any) job might result from job characteristics, culture, and other more distal variables that feed into commitment. From our own data, all we are able to say is that organizational identification accounts for more variance than attitudes or subjective norms. However we have also shown that identification can influence intentions indirectly through attitudes (Abrams, 2000).

Our findings also reaffirm the relevance of social identity for organizational turnover (Mael & Ashforth, 1995). The existence of a substantial relationship between identification and intention across all our studies is consistent with the idea that social identity involves the subjective value of group membership (Tajfel & Turner, 1979). There is every reason to believe that in the absence of a completely engulfing situation (e.g., war, strike, protest), group membership can vary greatly in importance among group members, regardless of the particular group or the particular culture.

We concur with Ashforth and Mael (1989) that there may be multiple antecedents of group identification, and we have demonstrated that job satisfaction is one candidate variable. Pertinent to this, our measure of organizational identification differs from Mael and Ashforth's, because of our focus on private rather than public recognition of social identity. Our measure also turns out to be slightly more reliable (alphas were .87 and .93 as compared with Mael and Ashforth's (1995) alpha of .74). Future research might benefit from using the two measures in conjunction. It would then be possible to explore whether there are distinct antecedents and consequences of these two measures of organizational identification.

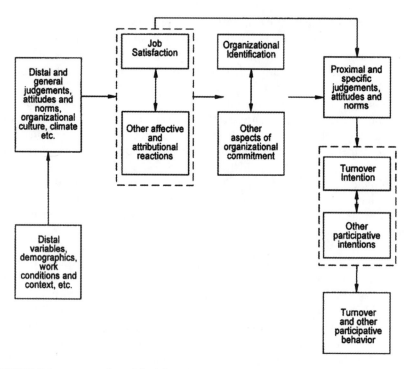

**FIGURE 9.2.** A general model of the relationship between organizational context and participative intentions and behavior.

In the light of previous research and our own findings we would like to conclude by offering a general and somewhat provisional model of turnover (and other participative) intentions, as shown in Figure 9.2. We expect that organizational conditions and other contextual variables might affect the more general or global attitudinal and normative orientations toward an organization (measures that we did not take in the reported studies). These, in turn, may affect aspects of job satisfaction and other conclusions about the organization. We are confident that the impact of job satisfaction on intentions is largely mediated by organizational identification, and our model therefore includes job satisfaction as an antecedent of identification and other aspects of commitment. We also allow for satisfaction to have some small direct impact on organizational partipation. We also believe that evidence will confirm our view that the impact of identification is mediated partly by specific attitudes and norms that correspond more closely and are more proximal to actual turnover decisions. Further research will be needed to determine how well this model fares in comparison with alternatives.

# CONCLUSIONS

In conclusion, we have shown how different aspects of self-to-group relationships have implications for turnover intentions in different cultures. Subjective norms reflect pressure from *tangible* social relationships with family, coworkers, and supervisors. This appears to be a more influential determinant of turnover intentions in a collectivist culture, where people place more weight on interdependent relationships in matters of importance to the self (Markus & Kitayama, 1991). Regardless of culture, membership in an organization influenced turnover intentions through the process of social identification. Social identification is based on a subjective *conceptual* relationship between the self and the group (cf. J. C. Turner et al., 1987), together with a strong affective link. We think organizational identification provides a powerful and crucial mediator between general organizational conditions and satisfaction or evaluations of those conditions on the one hand, and organizationally committed intentions and behavior on the other.

# 10

# Cooperation in Organizations:
## A Social Identity Perspective

TOM TYLER
*New York University*

A core question within the study of groups, organizations, and societies is why people are motivated to cooperate with organizations to which they belong. This question is central to people's relationships with a wide variety of organizations, including the political and legal system; work organizations; families; and informal associations, such as clubs, teams, churches, and gangs. Whenever people are members of organized groups, they make decisions about the extent and nature of the efforts they will make to behaviorally engage in those organizations by acting in cooperative ways that benefit those organizations. My purpose here is to highlight the role that processes of social identity play in shaping the degree to which people are motivated to cooperate in organizations.

Social identity theories suggest that an important function that organizations play for the individuals within them is to help those individuals define themselves and assess their self-worth (Deaux, 1996; Tajfel & Turner, 1979). Social categorization theory and research have demonstrated that group memberships play an important role in defining the self, with people using the salient dimensions of the groups to which they belong to define the salient dimensions of themselves (Hogg & Abrams, 1988). So, for example, the members of sports teams define themselves in terms of athletic ability, the defining attribute of their group, while the members of elite colleges define themselves in terms of their intelligence and insightfulness. Self-categorization theory describes the process through which such self-definitions are created and maintained (J. C. Turner et al., 1987).

In addition, people are motivated to develop and maintain a positive view

**149**

of their self-worth. They do so, to the degree possible, by joining and identifying with high-status groups and by avoiding membership in and/or identification with low-status groups. Further, people are motivated to enhance their status by increasing their judgments of the status of the groups to which they belong and/or by derogating the status of other groups. Social identity theory argues that such comparative judgments are central to the creation of a favorable identity, a concept referred to as "positive distinctiveness."

This chapter reviews studies demonstrating that social identity processes also explain people's behavioral engagement within organizations. In particular, studies suggest that social identity processes shape the degree to which people are motivated to act in ways that benefit the organizations to which they belong, i.e., to cooperate with organizations. People cooperate with organizations to the extent that those organizations are important in their efforts to create and maintain a favorable social identity.

This examination of cooperative behavior draws upon the core argument of social identity theory: that people use groups and organizations as a source of information when constructing and maintaining their identities. They do this by combining the social identity information that they draw from the organizations to which they belong with unique information about themselves (i.e., their personal identity). Together, these types of identity combine to form the self, and to establish its valence.

## TYPES OF COOPERATIVE BEHAVIOR IN ORGANIZATIONS

There are two key types of cooperative behavior on the part of organization members that are beneficial to organizations. Those are: (a) the willingness to act in ways that are beneficial to the organization (proactive behavior); and (b) the willingness to refrain from acting in ways that hurt the organization (limiting behavior).

One important function served by organizations is to organize and coordinate people's positive, proactive behaviors in ways that will most effectively facilitate organizational tasks. To do so, organizations develop roles and leaders. Roles coordinate the actions of organization members in many ways. They specify the tasks that various people will perform, the responsibilities they will have, and the manner in which their efforts will be evaluated. Leaders implement organizational rules by defining their meaning and by providing members with specific directives about what they should do. Such specifications define in-role behaviors: the actions that are expected of the particular members who have specific positions within the organization. People within organizations are encouraged to cooperate with the organization by engaging in such in-role behaviors. For example, workers are encouraged to do their jobs, teachers to attend and be prepared for their classes, and parents to supervise their children. When they do so, they are acting in ways that benefit their organization by fulfilling their organizational roles.

The psychological literature on prosocial behavior is an example of a literature of this type. It is concerned with understanding the factors that facilitate the occurrence of behaviors that help the group (i.e., behaviors that are prosocial in the sense that they aid society or social groups). The issue for society is how to develop ways that lead people to engage in those behaviors. They can range widely in nature, being as clear and specified as doing one's job or as vague as acting to help others in emergencies in which the question of who has the responsibility to help is unclear (Mussen & Eisenberg-Berg, 1977).

A second function of organizations is to recognize behaviors that, while potentially beneficial to the short-term interests of particular individuals within an organization, are damaging to the organization. An example of such a behavior is using organizational resources for personal gain, as when people steal supplies from their work organizations. Such behaviors are typically defined as inappropriate by organizational rules and/or by organizational authorities. People are encouraged to limit their behavior so as not to engage in behaviors that violate organizational rules. When they do follow rules, they are refraining from engaging in actions that, if engaged in, would benefit them but hurt their organization.

The problem of trying to limit behavior that hurts the organization is a core issue within all organizations and is addressed by the literature on social dilemmas (see Foddy, Smithson, Schneider, & Hogg, 1999). That literature recognizes that there are many situations in which the people within organizations have reasons to engage in actions that, if widely engaged in, would interfere with the success of the organization. For example, everyone would like to be free to leave work when they have personal errands or tasks to perform. However, if too many employees engage in such actions, the ability of the organization to complete work tasks is undermined. To prevent such difficulties, organizations typically have rules limiting people's activities.

Two types of behavior have been identified: engaging in actions that benefit the group and not engaging in activities that hurt the group. Two forms of each can also be distinguished: mandated and discretionary. Mandated behaviors are those linked to environment contingencies, i.e., rewards and punishments, while discretionary behaviors are those that are voluntary in the sense that they flow from people's attitudes and values.

## MOTIVATIONS FOR BEHAVIOR

We can distinguish between two types of motivation for behavior. The social psychological literatures noted do not take a position on the reasons that people have for engaging in cooperative behaviors. For example, the literature on prosocial behavior distinguishes itself from the literature on altruistic behavior.

Understanding prosocial behavior involves exploring how to encourage actions that help the group, however those actions are motivated, while the literature on altruism examines actions that help others for moral reasons, rather than out of concerns about personal gain or loss. Similarly, the social dilemma literature focuses on obtaining desired behavioral limits, i.e., catching fewer fish, using less electricity, etc., rather than on the reasons that people have for engaging in those actions. A wide variety of possible reasons for such actions are identified and studied.

Drawing upon the field theory model originally developed by Lewin, social psychologists usually separate the motivations for behavior into two components: first, the influence of environmental contingencies upon behavior, and, second, the influence of personal attitudes and values—i.e., the influence of a person's own motivational force (Lewin, 1997). These two forms of motivation combine to determine what a person will do within a given situation.

Environmental contingencies shape behavior by influencing people's instrumental reasons for acting. That is, those contingencies reflect the possibilities for gain and loss within a given situation. One motivation that people have for behaving is to seek gain and avoid loss, so this motivation is shaped by the possibilities for gain or loss within a given situation.

There are two potentially important aspects of instrumental strategies of motivation. The first is the possibility of providing people with gains. Such strategies create incentives, enhancing the possibilities of resource gains. Incentive strategies are central to efforts to encourage desired behaviors. People are paid to do their jobs, promoted if they succeed, and rewarded with bonuses and stock options ("pay for performance").

The second possible instrumental strategy is to create the risk of sanctions for engaging in particular types of behavior. For example, people know that if they are caught for stealing office supplies, they will be punished through fines, demotion, and other sanctions. These risks of punishment create disincentives and encourage people to limit their actions so as to conform to group rules. Disincentive strategies are central to efforts to discourage undesired behaviors.

The second set of motivational forces are internal to the person. They are those things that a person brings into the situation, as opposed to elements linked to the contingencies within any given situation. Two key internal forces are attitudes and values. Attitudes are those things that people want to do. For example, people might feel committed to their group, and to its well-being, and therefore want to work on behalf of the group. Values are the things that people feel obligated or responsible for doing. These include feelings of obligation to group authorities, as well as judgments about personal morality. Values represent the things that people feel that they ought to do.

Both attitudes and values are sources of motivation that are separate from concerns about immediate gains and losses. Hence, they are a long-term, cross-situational, motivational force that shapes people's behavior within given situations. This does not mean, of course, that they are necessarily distinct from long-term instrumental concerns. However, they are distinct from short-term situational judgments about gain and loss.

Behavior that is motivated by attitudes and values is voluntary or self-regulating in the sense that people's behavior flows from their own internal motivations, rather than from efforts to secure rewards or avoid punishments. That is, people are willing to help their organizations and to obey organizational rules because they feel a commitment or loyalty to the organization. Hence, discretionary forms of behavior are especially likely to develop from attitudes and values, and mandatory forms from environmental contingencies.

There are clear organizational advantages to behavior that is internally motivated. The organization does not need to utilize its resources to provide incentives or to engage in the surveillance needed to implement sanctioning systems. Instead, it can rely upon people to be motivated to engage in cooperative behaviors for internal reasons. Such internal motivations are especially valuable during difficult times, when organizations may be unable to provide incentives or enact sanctioning strategies. Every organization, whether a small group, an organization, or a society has periods of stagnation and decline. The survival of the organization requires that, during such times, people more fully engage themselves in the group, working longer and harder and investing more of themselves in the group, just when the personal risks of such an investment to the individual may be the greatest.

Consider, as an example, a study by Brann and Foddy (1988). Using a simulated commons dilemma, they examined how people reacted when they felt that a commonly held resource was being rapidly depleted in a community. Those people low in loyalty to their group reacted by taking more of the remaining scarce resource for themselves ("hoarding"). Such behavior is personally rational, since the individual then has some of the resource for their own use when the pool is depleted, but it accelerates collective disintegration. People high in loyalty, on the other hand, took less of the resource in response to scarcity. Those individuals took a personal risk in an effort to slow the deterioration of the group. Their response to crisis was to take more personal risks on behalf of the group, not fewer. Such individuals were motivated by internal values and attitudes to act in ways inconsistent with their own short-term interests.

This example also illustrates the way in which short-term and long-term interests diverge. By taking a short-term risk, people may be increasing the prospects for their long-term future. Conversely, by quickly grabbing some diminishing resources in pursuit of immediate self-interest, people may actually be hurting their own long-term prospects. It is just such a dilemma that is at the heart of the study of social dilemmas, which explores the ways in which people can protect themselves against their own short-term, self-interested tendencies.

The distinction between types of motivation illustrates two paths to cooperation. The first path involves the generation of cooperation through the use of incentives and sanctions. The second path encourages cooperation by developing and maintaining supportive attitudes and values.

## WHAT DO PEOPLE WANT FROM ORGANIZATIONS?

The link between cooperative behavior and issues of identity comes through an effort to address the question of the underlying motivation that shapes the extent to which people feel a willingness to cooperate with the organizations to which they belong. Two bodies of social psychological theory address this issue: social exchange theory (Thibaut & Kelley, 1959) and social identity theory (Hogg & Abrams, 1988; Tajfel & Turner, 1979). To understand why people cooperate, we need to examine the role of the factors identified by each of these two models in shaping cooperation.

One reason that people might participate in and cooperate with groups is to gain the resources associated with group membership. Traditional explanations of people's choices among possible behaviors in organizations, their decisions about whether or not to stay or leave an organization, their decisions about the enactment of organizational roles, and their decisions about rule following have been shaped by social exchange theory (Thibaut & Kelley, 1959).

Social exchange theory suggests that people's orientation toward organizations reflects their views about the favorability of the exchange of effort and resources between them and that organization. If people feel that they are receiving favorable resources from the organization, they stay within it, performing their organizational role and following organizational rules.

An example of the application of social exchange theory to behavior within groups and organizations is provided by the work of Rusbult on the investment model. The investment model explores loyalty to long-term relationships with other people, groups, and organizations (Rusbult & Van Lange, 1996). The key issue that is predicted by the investment model to shape personal decisions about whether to exit a group or to remain loyal to it is how dependent an individual feels they are on the organization for obtaining personally valued resources.

Studies based on the investment model suggest that greater dependence on an organization leads to heightened loyalty, with people being less willing to leave organizations that provide them with high levels of desired resources, that provide more resources than available alternatives, and/or in which they have invested time, energy, or resources. These studies support the argument that one way to understand people's behavior in organizations is via an instrumental perspective focusing on long-term assessments of resources likely to be obtained from the group.

## SOCIAL IDENTITY THEORY

Social identity theory provides an alternative conceptualization of the basis of the relationship between organizational members and organizations. It suggests that the key function served by an organization is not providing resources to the people within the organization. Instead, the key function is to provide those people with a social identity that allows them to define themselves in terms of attributes central to the organization and to develop and maintain a favorable sense of self-worth and self-esteem by drawing upon the status of the organization.

This use of the core ideas of social identity theory extends them from their original intergroup framework to an intragroup setting. That is, instead of considering how people's association with one group shapes their attitudes and behaviors toward that group in relationship to other groups, this analysis explores how people's membership within a group is shaped by issues of identity and status (see also Moreland, Levine, & McMinn, Chapter 6 of this volume).

The key distinction between intergroup settings and intragroup settings is the way that status is understood. In intergroup settings the central concern is the status of the organization to which one belongs, either intrinsically or in comparison to the status of other organizations. To enhance the status of the organizations to which they belong, people both seek to join and stay within high-status organizations and distort their views about status, enhancing the status of their own organizations and derogating the status of other organizations. In this discussion judgments about the status of an organization to which one belongs are referred to as *pride* in that organization (Tyler & Blader, 2000).

Early social identity studies focused on minimal groups, formed in arbitrary ways based upon the color of randomly assigned dots or preference for various forms of art. These classification schemes, as well as the temporary nature of the groups studied, were designed to minimize the possibility that groups would have actual resource-based interests that might drive the dynamics of intergroup relations. In minimal groups the key issue was group membership without shared resource interests. However, to achieve this objective, the groups studied were "minimal."

In contrast to minimal groups, actual real-world organizations have structures and hierarchies. This means that people are not only members of an organization, they also have status within that organization. Hence, when considering real-world organizations it is important to consider a second aspect of status—status within the organization. In this discussion, we will refer to people's judgments about their within-organization status as the *respect* that they feel they receive from others in the organization (Tyler & Blader, 2000).

## IDENTIFICATION

I have outlined several dimensions along which people's behavioral engagement in an organization can vary. I would now like to examine what accounts for this variation. One important issue is the degree to which people are psychologically engaged in the organization (see also Abrams & Randsley de Moura, Chapter 9 of this volume, and Ellemers, Chapter 7, & Pratt, Chapter 2 this volume). From a social identification perspective the core aspect of psychological engagement is the degree to which people identify with the organization.

Identification refers to the merger of the self and the organization, with people defining themselves in terms of their group membership. A person might, for example, say that being a professor at Harvard or a player on a soccer team is very important to their sense of themselves as a person, or that it is only peripheral.

Psychological engagement is a key antecedent to behavioral engagement. This is especially true for discretionary behaviors, which are more strongly linked to attitudes and values. We expect that those organizational members who are psychologically invested in the group will be more willing to act cooperatively toward the organization—investing their time and energy in working to see the group succeed (Tyler & Blader, 2000).

A number of studies within the social identity tradition support the argument that the degree to which people merge with or separate themselves from groups has important social consequences. For example, people who are more identified with groups are more likely to interpret their experiences as being due to their group memberships (Tyler, 2001). As a consequence, they are more likely to respond to injustices on a group or collective level (Grant & Brown, 1995; Kelly & Kelly, 1994; Lalonde & Silverman, 1994; B. Simon et al., 1998). In other words, a number of studies show that the form of people's behavior is shaped by the degree to which they identify with groups.

Here our concern is with the influence of identification on the degree to which people act on behalf of groups. Abrams et al. (1998) provided evidence that identification shapes behavior by demonstrating that those who identify with an organization are less likely to leave it.

Other studies demonstrate that those who identify with groups are more willing to defer to the decisions of group authorities based upon issues of justice, rather than in response to self-interested judgments (Huo et al., 1996; Tyler & Degoey, 1995; H. J. Smith & Tyler, 1996).

The relationship between identification and cooperation was directly addressed by Tyler & Blader (2000) in a study of employees in work organizations. They found that employees who identify more strongly with their work organization were more likely to engage in cooperative behavior of all four of the types outlined. On average, they found that 16% of the variance in cooperative behavior was explained by identification with the organization. In contrast, resource concerns on average explained 10% of the variance in cooperative behavior.

Interestingly, as we would expect, resource concerns were found to explain approximately 10% of the variance in mandated and 10% of the variance in discretionary cooperative behavior. In other words, resource concerns did not explain discretionary behavior more effectively than they explained mandated behavior. In contrast, identification 12% of the variance in mandated behavior, but 19% of the variance in discretionary behavior. This suggests that those people who identify with an organization were especially likely to do those things that were not required or rewarded, as well as being more willing to voluntarily defer to organizational rules.

These findings support a social identity perspective, which predicts that people who identify more strongly with their organizations will engage themselves more within those organizations by cooperating. They suggest that issues of both resource exchange and identity formation and change are important in shaping cooperation in organizations. However, identity formation and change seems more central to shaping such behaviors, especially when voluntary behaviors are the focus of concern.

## DIRECT MEASURES OF STATUS: PRIDE AND RESPECT

How does social identity theory differ from social exchange theory as an explanation for cooperative behavior? From a social exchange perspective, we expect people to cooperate with the organization to the extent that they see the possibility of gain and see the risk of loss. On the gain side, people should be responsive to incentives that reward them for fulfilling their organizational roles. On the loss side, people should focus on the possibility of being caught and punished for rule breaking. People's behavior should be responsive to their judgments about the potential resource gains and losses for them within their organizational environment. These same concerns have a long-term component, as illustrated in the investment model. People are not only responding to immediate gains and losses, but to the potential of long-term gains and losses as well. Within either the short-term or the long-term framework, however, the key issue underlying behavior engagement is the person's view about their potential for short- or long-term gain within their organizational environment.

The social identity perspective suggests that people focus on the role of the organization in defining their social self and in giving themselves a sense of self-worth through an organizational membership that has positive identity implications. From this perspective we would expect that judgments of pride and respect should be linked to the occurrence of cooperative behavior.

I have already noted the role of identification with organizations in stimulating cooperative behavior in groups. Based on the theoretical perspective outlined here, I would expect that identification with an organization would be responsive to judgments of pride and respect, rather than to assessments of the total rewards being acquired from an organization. Tyler and Blader (2000) test this argument in work settings. They find that identification was primarily linked to respect (beta = 0.41, $p < .001$) and to pride (beta = 0.35, $p < .001$), rather than to total reward assessments (beta = 0.12, $p < .01$). As expected, employees identify with organizations for reasons of maintaining a connection that enhances and maintains their favorable sense of self-worth and self-esteem, more than out of a desire to obtain desired resources.

## PRIDE, RESPECT, AND COOPERATIVE ENGAGEMENT IN ORGANIZATIONS

It is also possible to compare the two models outlined by examining the degree to which each type of judgment (pride, respect, rewards) shapes people's cooperative behavior in organizations. Tyler, Degoey, and Smith (1996) examined the influence of pride and respect on two types of cooperative behavior: compliance with group rules and extrarole behavior. They did so within four types of hierarchical settings: family, work, the university, and the political arena. Their study suggested that pride influenced compliance in all four settings (average amount of variance explained = 11%). Respect also influenced compliance in all four settings (average amount of variance explained = 8%). Further, pride influenced extrarole behavior in the three settings in which that variable was studied (family, work, the university), with an average of 17% of the variance explained. In the same three settings respect also influenced extrarole behavior (average amount of variance explained = 10%). These findings support the argument that pride and respect led to cooperative behavior. However, they did not directly compare the magnitude of this influence to the influence of resource based judgments.

Tyler (1999) compared the influence of status judgments to that of outcome favorability in two studies of employees, one conducted in Chicago ($n$ = 409) and the other using a multinational sample ($n$ = 649). In the case of willingness to engage in behavior that helps the group, he found that the average independent influence of pride and respect beyond the variance explainable by resource judgments was 0.23%. On the other hand, the average independent influence of resource judgments beyond what can be explained by status judgments was 0.1%. In the case of rule-following behavior, the average unique influence of status judgments was 9%, while that of resource judgments was 1%. In both cases status judgments dominated influence on cooperative behavior.

Tyler and Blader (2000) also directly compared the influence of status-based and resource-based judgments in their previously described sample of employees. They found that status judgments uniquely explained 11% of the variance in mandated behavior and 12% of the variance in discretionary behavior. In contrast, outcomes uniquely explained 0% of mandated behavior and 0% of discretionary behavior.

All of these studies support the predictions of social identity theory by demonstrating that people who feel greater pride in their organizations and greater respect from their organizations are more likely to engage in cooperative behavior within those groups and organizations. Such status judgments are found to have more influence on the degree to which people engage themselves behaviorally in organizations than do the assessments of reward levels that are central to resource exchange models.

# TYPE OF IMPACT

It is also possible that it is not simply the relative impact of the indicators of these two models that is of interest to us. It may be that the nature of the impact of status and resource judgments is different. One possibility is that social identity processes are especially important because they create an identity-based psychological dynamic that changes people's internal sense of themselves, i.e., changes their attitudes and values. These changes in identity may change who organizational actors think they are and, as a consequence, what they want or feel that they ought to do. That is, identity processes may be especially important in shaping voluntary, self-regulatory actions. As a consequence, they may most strongly shape discretionary behavior. This argument is similar to the argument already made and supported, that identification plays an especially important role in shaping discretionary behavior.

The argument that identity processes influence people's sense of themselves and of their self-worth receives support from the findings of Tyler, Degoey, and Smith (1996). Their results indicate that in family, university, and political settings, pride and respect influence self-esteem. The average amount of variance explained by pride is 5%, and by respect, 20%. Similarly, people's commitment to their organizations in work and university settings is linked to these status judgments. The average amount of variance explained by pride is 39%; the average by respect, 5%.

Tyler and Blader (2000) also found that status judgments were key to shaping self-esteem. In a regression equation, self-esteem was found to be shaped primarily by respect (beta = .40, $p < .001$), with a lesser influence of resources (beta = 0.11, $p < .05$), but no influence of pride (beta = −.03, n.s.). Their findings also suggest that status judgments shape commitment. They uniquely explained 37% of the variance in commitment to one's work organization, while resource-based judgments uniquely explained 1%. Further, status judgments uniquely explained 6% of the variance in people's views about their obligation to obey organizational rules. In contrast, outcomes uniquely explained 0% of the variance in obligation.

These findings support two key conclusions. First, cooperative behaviors are strongly linked to people's status judgments about the organizations to which they belong. These findings support the argument that cooperation is linked to the effort to engage with organizations that facilitate developing and maintaining favorable status judgments. Two judgments are important: the judgment that one belongs to a high-status organization (pride) and the judgment that one has high status within that organization (respect).

Second, status judgments are most directly linked to feelings about the self. This suggests that status judgments may differ in the nature of their influence on the individual, changing the person's sense of themselves. This argument is further supported by the finding that status judgments are linked to attitudes such as commitment. Status judgments influence people's feelings of support for the group, i.e., their feelings about whether or not they care if the group succeeds. Commitment, in turn, is linked to people's willingness to behave in ways that help the group. Status judgments also influence people's feelings of obligation toward the group—their feelings about whether or not they are obligated to defer to the group and its rules and authorities. Again, it is status judgments that are the key influence on these social values.

## THE RELATIONSHIP BETWEEN PRIDE AND RESPECT

High pride and high respect are typically found to occur together. People who are treated by others with respect feel more pride in their organizations. Conversely, people who feel more pride in their organizations also feel more respected. In the organizations that have been examined in the studies reported here, therefore, these two aspects of status are interrelated.

While typically found to be interrelated, pride and respect are also distinct. They are distinct from a conceptual perspective in that they reflect two aspects of the social self (Tyler & Smith, 1999). Pride reflects the categorical social self; respect the reputational social self.

The pride-based categorical social self reflects a focus on the attributes of the category, i.e., the organization to which the person belongs. In defining pride in the organization, people focus on their feelings about the prototypical norms and values that define the organization. Their emphasis is on the things that the members of the organization share, their common mission, values, lifestyles, etc. People's attention is directed to their feelings about the organization.

This focus on the organization encourages the motivation to be loyal to the group in one's values and behaviors, holding the values that define the group, and following group norms and rules in one's behavior. Studies suggest that the categorical social self shapes the acceptance of organizational rules and that people high in pride bring their behavior into compliance with organizational rules, producing a uniformity of behavior around consistency with group rules.

The respect-based reputational social self reflects a focus on the individual. A group member's attention is directed toward themselves and their unique features—the things that lead them to have a position with the group. In contrast to pride, which reflects a focus on the attributes of the group, respect reflects a focus on the attributions of the person. It reflects how the person thinks the group is judging them.

When they feel respected by the organization, people are motivated to act in ways that both express and develop their unique attributes and abilities in ways that will benefit the organization. The reputational social self, in other words, should motivate diverse and unique behaviors, all motivated by the desire to benefit the group. Further, unlike the rule orientation that is linked to the categorical social self, these unique behaviors should flow from people's internal values. That is, they will be self-motivated, with an emphasis on voluntary actions.

# PRIDE-BASED AND RESPECT-BASED ORGANIZATIONAL CULTURES

The recognition that pride and respect are conceptually and empirically distinct has important prescriptive consequences for organizations. Organizations may choose to develop organizational cultures that are linked to pride or to respect, and this choice has important consequences for the organization.

A pride-based culture focuses on developing a strong connection between the person and the group to which they belong. In that way, it is similar to the identification approach already outlined. It encourages people to follow organizational norms by uniform dress, thinking, and behavior. Encouraging such uniform rule-governed behavior is ideal for organizations that value uniform behavior. One example is the military, which seeks to develop uniform dress and behavior by instilling pride in the organization and its values. The benefit of such a pride-based model is that people's behavior is predictable and people can be counted on to perform their organizational tasks.

The characteristics of combat illustrate the value of a pride-based culture. Soldiers are expected to engage in difficult, dangerous, and onerous tasks. They must live in unpleasant conditions, risk their lives, and kill other people. How can people be motivated to engage in these tasks? One way is by loyalty to the organization that mandates them and through clear and routinized tasks. The military emphasizes pride in the service and loyalty to one's unit and engages in lengthy and repetitious engagement in the tasks of fighting to build a clear sense of what organizational tasks are and to create a motivation to follow organizational norms. These produce a pride-based organizational culture in which soldiers endure hardship and engage in the unpleasant and dangerous task of combat.

When might a pride-based culture be important? It is crucial in situations in which people are unlikely to be motivated by the intrinsic quality of their group tasks. Again, the military is a good example. Most soldiers are unlikely to be motivated by an intrinsic love of combat. Hence, their motivation must come from loyalty to their group. Such situations are widely found among workers with assembly-line jobs. There is little to the repetitive job of putting on fenders or wrapping packages that will inspire people to work. In addition, pride-based cultures are important when the quality of organizational performance is linked to doing organizational tasks well. The assembly line workers noted above need to take the job of putting on fenders seriously and do it well. That is, there needs to be a clear statement of what their job is and how to do it, and workers need to be motivated to follow those rules.

There are two downsides to pride-based cultures. The first is their lack of creativity and innovation. Consider the Japanese corporation, the prototypical pride-based culture. Such organizations are well known for worker loyalty and for their ability to maintain high quality control standards, since group members are motivated to adhere to task norms. On the other hand, such organizations are not especially innovative. The focus on group norms that leads to uniformity of behavior does not lead to a questioning stance toward those norms.

Hence, pride-based cultures may find it difficult to innovate and change.

The second downside of pride-based cultures is the problem of authorization (Kelman & Hamilton, 1989). People's loyalty to the organization and to organizational norms can replace their attention to their own moral values. As a consequence, people may engage in illegal and immoral actions on behalf of their organization. Kelman and Hamilton noted the dramatic case of soldiers killing women and children. However, other examples they mention, such as the willingness of corporate actors to engage in illegal and unethical behavior to advance their organization's goals, are probably more widespread. These behaviors occur when the norms of an organizational culture violate the law or moral principles. The difficulty is that loyalty to an organization leads people to focus on that organization's norms, rather than external norms (such as laws) or even personal moral principles. The focus of the categorical social self is on the organization, not the individual.

Respect-based cultures build upon the motivation of group members to make personalized and idiosyncratic contributions to the organization. Such contributions are encouraged by a culture that puts its focus on the people within the organization. Such a focus does not encourage uniformity of behavior or attention to organizational tasks and norms. Instead, it encourages group members to think about what they can contribute to solving group problems and achieving group objectives. It leads people to think about how they can bring their talents to bear in ways that help the group.

Respect-based cultures are likely to be most useful in situations in which novelty and innovation are important. For example, start-up companies need to be able to create both products and organizational forms. They need people who can work without clear definitions of their job tasks. Such people focus on organizational goals such as developing new products, defining new markets. The goals are clear, but there are often not clear and specified procedures for achieving those goals.

Consider the example of a university researcher embarking on a new project. There are no clear procedures for moving forward, since the person is doing something new and innovative that has not been done before. Instead, people rely upon their experience and intuitions, being guided by their "gut" feelings toward new studies and new ways of thinking about their findings. When someone visits a university department, they seldom see uniformity of behavior across faculty. Some people work early in the morning, others work late at night. Some people are engaged in a series of empirical studies or specific research projects. Others are thinking about theoretical ideas or writing textbooks or review papers. Everyone is engaged is trying to make a contribution to knowledge in their field, but everyone has defined the manner in which they can most effectively do so in a unique way.

What are the problems associated with respect-based strategies? It is difficult to establish and maintain common group goals. For the efforts of individuals to help the group, those efforts must be directed at common organizational goals. A start-up company wants everyone to be original and creative up to a point, but to also focus that creativity on common group goals. If everyone is simply following their own ideas, no common products will be created and produced. Similarly, while universities encourage individual innovation by faculty, there are mechanisms for trying to channel that innovation into productive areas—as defined by the organization. There must, for example, be agreement about what areas deserve funding or merit future faculty hiring. The tendency of individuals to move in their own directions must be counteracted by ways to maintain common direction.

Organizations, of course, develop procedures for finding a common direction within respect-based cultures. However, anyone who has attended a faculty meeting at a university and then visited a military base recognizes that respect-based cultures are not especially well designed to handle situations in which uniform and unquestioning behavior is desirable. They are best designed to handle situations in which innovation and change are desirable and valued. In a respect-based organization, highly motivated people will be making idiosyncratic and innovative contributions to a broad set of organizational goals. Those people will often dress differently, work different hours, have unique styles of working, and have trouble following rules. But, they will also bring high levels of intelligence and energy to achieving organizational objectives.

This presentation of respect-based cultures is not intended to suggest that they require group tasks that are intrinsically rewarding or interesting. While university professors or high technology innovators are often motivated by their own intrinsic interest in their work, respect-based cultures do not depend upon such motivation. Rather, they draw upon people's desire to be respected for their contributions. A janitor or maid is similarly motivated by the desire to be respected and valued in their work, and individuals in such situations can also be motivated by their sense that their own contribution to the organization is valued. Stories abound of building superintendents, maintenance workers, and clerical workers or administrators who are highly valued by their organizations and clients or customers and who respond to that respect by being helpful and "going out of their way" to meet people's needs and solve people's problems. Respect for a person and their contribution to an organization can occur at any level and with any type of job. When people feel respected in their roles, they respond by trying to help their customers, clients, and organizations.

## WHERE DOES STATUS COME FROM?

One of the most interesting findings of the research outlined is that status judgments are typically largely distinct from resource judgments. For example, Blader and Tyler (2000) measured the level of resources that people are receiving from the group in a variety of ways. When the relationship between those indices and status judgments was examined, the average correlation was $r = 0.29$. This suggests that people were not judging either the status of their organization or their status within that organization simply through a consideration of the level of resources they were obtaining, although the level of resources being received was certainly linked to status judgments.

If the level of resources being obtained from an organization is not the key to people's judgments about it, what is? The studies outlined have examined this issue in a variety of ways, including a consideration of the influence of different aspects of personal experience on status judgments and a consideration of the influence of overall judgments about the organization on status judgments. Irrespective of these variations, the findings are similar. The key antecedents of status judgments are assessments of the fairness of organizational procedures (i.e., procedural fairness).

For example, Tyler and Blader (2000) found that judgments about procedural justice (beta = 0.35, $p < .001$), distributive justice (beta = 0.14, $p < .05$), and outcome favorability (beta = 0.16, $p < .01$) all shaped pride (total amount of variance explained = 33%). Similarly, judgments about procedural justice (beta = 0.29, $p < .001$) and outcome favorability (beta = 0.23, $p < .001$) shaped respect (but distributive justice had no influence, beta = $-.03$, n.s.; total amount of variance explained = 19%).

Two aspects of procedural fairness are important influences on status judgments: judgments about the quality of decision-making and judgments about the quality of the treatment that organizational members received from organizational authorities. Tyler and Blader (2000) found that procedural justice itself was influenced by the quality of decision making (beta = 0.44, $p < .001$), the quality of the treatment received (beta = 0.34, $p < .001$), and outcome fairness (beta = 0.24, $p < .001$), but not by the favorability of outcomes (beta = $-0.02$, n.s.) These factors explained 81% of the variance in procedural justice judgments.

Pride was also directly linked to the quality of the treatment received (beta = 0.36, $p < .001$); to outcome fairness (beta = 0.15, $p < .001$), and to the favorability of decisions (beta = 0.11, $p < .05$), but not to the quality of decision making (beta = .04, n.s.; total amount of variance explained = 34%). Similarly, respect was shaped by the quality of the treatment received (beta = 0.54, $p < .001$), and by the favorability of decisions (beta = 0.12, $p < .05$), but not by the quality of decision making (beta = $-.04$, n.s.) or by outcome fairness (beta = $-0.11$, n.s.) (the total amount of variance explained was 26%).

These findings suggest that the roots of attitudes, values, and cooperative behaviors lie in status assessments. Such status assessments, in turn, are linked to people's views about justice in groups and organizations. In particular, people base their status assessments on procedural justice—the fairness of the processes used to make decisions within the organization. Organizations that make decisions fairly and treat those within them fairly are more likely to be viewed as organizations to which people are proud to belong. Further, those experiences of justice lead people to feel respected and valued by their organizations. Both judgments lead people to want to cooperate with their organization.

# SUMMARY

My goal has been to provide evidence for the argument that people's cooperative behavior can best be understood, at least in part, as an effort to create and maintain a favorable view of the self. People's view of their "self" is rooted, to some important degree, in being a member of high-status organizations. People seek to join such organizations and, when in them, seek to maintain their high status by working to build and enhance the organization. Such efforts involve both mandated activities and voluntary actions. By working on behalf of their group, people are maintaining their own feelings of pride and, thereby, maintaining a favorable self-image. Further, by working on behalf of their organization, people become respected members of their group. This further enhances their feelings of self-worth.

While the findings outlined provide strong support for the value of applying ideas from social identity theory to the study of organizations, it is also clear that resource exchange plays an important role in intragroup dynamics. In other words, people are not only interested in issues of identity. They also want resources, and one reason for being in groups is to gain them. Ultimately, a model of cooperation in organizations must pay attention to both identity, and resource-based motivations for joining and remaining within groups. However, since past approaches to this question have been dominated by resource models, it is important to recognize the value of expanding our conceptual framework to include issues of identity.

# 11

# Identity and Trust in Organizations:
## One Anatomy of a Productive but Problematic Relationship

RODERICK M. KRAMER
*Stanford University*

*Trust rarely occupies the foreground of conscious aware-
ness. We are no more likely to ask ourselves how trusting
we are at a given moment than to inquire if gravity is still
keeping the planets in orbit. However, when trust is
disturbed it claims our attention as urgently as would any
irregularity in the gravitational field.*
— D. Brothers (1995, p. 3).

rust has been defined as a psychological state that encompasses an
individual's "expectations, assumptions, or beliefs about the likelihood
that another's future actions will be beneficial, favorable, or at least not
detrimental to one's interests" (S. L. Robinson, 1996, p. 576). Social scientists
have long recognized the importance of such trust within organizations (Barber,
1983; Zucker, 1986). They have argued, for example, that trust plays a crucial
role in the productive and efficient exchange of valuable resources among interdependent actors pursuing diverse goals within an organization (Arrow, 1974;
Williamson, 1993).

Recognizing its importance, organizational theorists have recently begun
to explore with renewed interest the nature of trust and trust-related phenomena in organizations (e.g., Creed & Miles, 1996; G. Fine & Holyfield, 1996; R.
M. Kramer, 1999; C. Lane & Bachmann, 1998; Rousseau, Sitkin, Burt, &
Camerer, 1998). The ascension of trust as a prominent focus of contemporary
organizational research can be attributed, at least in part, to recent and pro-

167

vocative evidence regarding the substantial and varied benefits associated with high levels of trust (e.g., Coleman, 1990; Fukuyama, 1995; Putnam, 1993).

Despite widespread appreciation of its importance, however, the particular *kind* of trust that matters within organizations, and the *bases* of such trust, have been much less obvious (Creed & Miles, 1996; R. M. Kramer, 1999; Rousseau et al., 1998; Zucker, 1986). In particular, it has been recognized that the decision to trust others in organizational contexts is different from, and in many respects more problematic than, judgments about trust that arise in many other social contexts. Because of the size and structural complexity of most organizations, for example, organizational members do not have the opportunity to engage in the sort of incremental and repeated exchanges that have been shown to facilitate the development of trust in more intimate settings, such as dyadic relations (Lindskold, 1978; Rotter, 1980). Relatedly, it is evident that many of the social mechanisms and interpersonal processes that foster trust development in small, relatively homogeneous groups (e.g., G. Fine & Holyfield, 1996) are likely to lose their efficacy in the larger, more differentiated, and more diffuse environments of large organizations (Fox, 1974). Moreover, the often political and highly competitive nature of organizational life increases greatly the costs of misplaced trust to those who trust too readily or indiscriminately: In sharp contrast to the relatively benign penalties associated with misplaced trust encountered in experimental games, getting the "sucker's payoff" in real-world organizational encounters is not only aversive; it can be fatal to one's career.

Given these problematic features, the critical question arises, "On what basis can or do individuals predicate trust in other organizational members?" Under what circumstances, for example, are they likely to presume that other organizational members are trustworthy or that their own acts of trust will not be exploited? Contemporary organizational theory has articulated a number of useful perspectives on these important questions. Considerable attention has been afforded, for instance, to explicating the role of various institutional mechanisms in the production of trust within organizations (Zucker, 1986). These mechanisms include structural arrangements and governance regimes that contribute to the creation of trust. Other research has focused on the role that social structures, such as network ties, play in the development and diffusion of trust among organizational members (Burt & Knez, 1995; Granovetter, 1985).

Although drawing on these contributions, the present chapter takes a rather different point of departure for conceptualizing the origins of trust among organizational members. In particular, I propose that individuals' identification with an organization and its members enhances both their propensity to trust others in the organization and their willingness to engage in acts of trust when interacting with members. According to this conception of trust, individuals' awareness of a shared organizational identity fosters a form of *presumptive trust* in other organizational members.

This conception of *identity-based trust*, I should note, is based on a considerable body of previous theory and empirical research linking social identity, generalized interpersonal trust, and cooperative behavior (Brewer, 1981; Brewer & Kramer, 1986; Brewer & Schneider, 1990; Elsbach & Kramer, 1996; R. M. Kramer, 1991, 1994, 1996a, 1996b; R. M. Kramer & Brewer, 1984; 1986; R. M. Kramer, Brewer, & Hanna, 1996; R. M. Kramer & Goldman, 1995; R. M. Kramer, Pommerenke, & Newton, 1993; Messick, Wilke, Brewer, Kramer, Zemke, & Lui, 1983). Because space constraints preclude an exhaustive review of this prior work, I will offer instead a somewhat synoptic account of the major ideas and findings that have emerged from it. Specifically, I will provide an overview of some of the psychological and social underpinnings of identity-based trust in organizations. I will then suggest some of the reasons why that linkage is sometimes rather tenuous and fragile. Viewed together, these two sides of the identity-trust relation reveal why identity and trust enjoy a potentially productive but sometimes problematic relationship.

To set the stage for this argument, it may be helpful to begin by defining what is meant by identity-based trust in organizations and describing what we know about its determinants.

## PSYCHOLOGICAL AND SOCIAL UNDERPINNINGS OF IDENTITY-BASED TRUST IN ORGANIZATIONS

As social identity theorists have long appreciated, all individuals possess multiple social identities, corresponding to the various social categories and groups to which they belong (Brewer, 1996; Hogg & Abrams, 1988). These identities serve many useful functions, including helping individuals define themselves and their relationships to others.

The idea that individuals' mutual awareness of a shared social identity might provide a basis for presumptive trust in each other was first articulated by Brewer (1981). In elaborating on this notion, Brewer reasoned,

> Common membership in a salient social categorization can serve as a rule for defining the boundaries of a low-risk interpersonal trust that bypasses the need for personal knowledge and the costs of negotiating reciprocity with individual others. *As a consequence of shifting from the personal level to the social group level of identity, the individual can adopt a sort of "depersonalized" trust based on category membership alone.* (p. 356, emphases added)

Research on the cognitive consequences of social categorization and ingroup formation provides support for this argument. For example, research has demonstrated that people tend to perceive other members of their "ingroup" in relatively positive terms (as being, for example, more cooperative, honest, and trustworthy) compared to outsiders. Relatedly, it has been shown that ingroup members often expect more positive behavior in their exchanges with other ingroup members compared to outgroup members (e.g., Brewer, 1996; R. M. Kramer & Goldman, 1995; R. M. Kramer, Prahdan-Shah, & Woerner, 1995; Rothbart & Hallmark, 1988; Thompson, Valley, & Kramer, 1995).

Other evidence suggests the cognitive benefits of shared social categorization and common identity extend as well to the causal attributions and dispositional inferences group members draw regarding the motives and intentions of other group members. Research has shown, for example, that individuals are more likely to attribute negative behaviors by ingroup members to external, unstable causal factors, while the same behavior by an outgroup member is more likely to be attributed to stable, internal influences (Hewstone, 1992; Pettigrew, 1979). Thus, even when ingroup members appear to act in a less than fully trustworthy fashion, there may be a tendency to grant them the benefit of the doubt (Brewer, 1996).

Complementing evidence that ingroup categorization processes influence how individuals perceive and judge other individuals within the group is evidence that similar processes influence how individuals view themselves as well. J. C. Turner et al. (1987) characterized these as *self-categorization* effects. When individuals' identification moves from the personal level to the collective level, he noted, there is a "shift towards the perception of self as an interchangeable exemplar of some social category and away from the perception of self as a unique person" (p. 253). Consequently, they are likely to draw less sharp a disjunction between their own outcomes and those that accrue to other group members.

Consistent with this argument, laboratory studies have demonstrated that, when superordinate or collective-level social identities are made salient to individuals, they are more likely to act in a trustworthy and cooperative fashion when interacting with other members of that collective (Brewer & Kramer, 1986; R. M. Kramer & Brewer, 1984; R. M. Kramer et al., 1993; see also Tyler, Chapter 10 of this volume). Field research has replicated these experimental findings (Tyler & Degoey, 1996).

Early attempts to make sense of these assorted empirical findings (Brewer & Kramer, 1986; R. M. Kramer, 1991; R. M. Kramer & Brewer, 1984, 1986; R. M. Kramer et al., 1996) drew attention to evidence that expectations alone did not provide a sufficient explanation for the observed relationship between an individual's salient social identity and the emergence of cooperation and trust-related behavior. In other words, the effects observed in these studies could not be explained simply from the standpoint of the sort of "calculative" considerations emphasized in expectation-based conceptions of trust. Accordingly, it was necessary to invoke other mechanisms when trying to explain this pattern.

One explanation which seemed to fit the data was that individuals' willingness to engage in trusting acts when interacting with other ingroup members reflected the fact that they construed such acts as decisions with symbolic and expressive meaning. Specifically, it could be posited that, from the standpoint of individuals who identify positively with a group or organization, engaging in acts of trust when interacting with other group members can serve a number of important psychological and social motives as well.

According to this perspective, behavioral displays of trust provide a way for individuals to affirm the importance they associate with their membership in the organization. Engaging in acts of trust thus provide organizational members with an opportunity to communicate to others the symbolic value they attach to their organizational identity. From this perspective, the psychological significance of trust acts resides not only in the sort of strategic or calculative considerations emphasized in economic conceptions of trust (e.g., the material payoffs that flow from reciprocated trust), but also the *social* motives and *affiliative* needs of group members that are met through such actions. Thus, trust behaviors in group settings had to be understood not just as "economic" decisions about risk and benefit, but as social decisions (R. M. Kramer et al., 1996).

One important implication of this formulation of the psychological and social underpinnings of identity-based trust is that individuals' willingness to confer trust on other group members presumptively (i.e., with minimal evidence of their trustworthiness), along with the willingness to engage in acts of trust, can be understood as socially expressive actions that have social meaning and that lead to desired social consequences (cf. Fine & Holyfield, 1996). Another way of stating this idea is that identity-based forms of trust are associated with perceived hedonic consequences. Thus, doing one's duty or fulfilling one's moral obligations in trust dilemma situations can lead to feelings of satisfaction and pleasure. As H. A. Simon (1991) observed in this regard, "Identification with the 'we,' which may be a family, a company, a nation, or the local baseball team, allows individuals to experience satisfactions (to gain utility) from successes *of the unit thus selected*" (p. 36, emphases added). Conversely, the failure to do one's duty or violations of one's obligations can produce shame, guilt, and remorse.

## Summary

The perspective on trust-related judgment and choice behavior developed in this section provides a reasonably coherent account of a diverse set of empirical findings across a variety of trust-related domains of organizational action, ranging from free-rider problems to bargaining contexts to simple exchange situations. The framework implicates, moreover, a number of distinct cognitive, motivational, and affective processes that facilitate the emergence of presumptive trust among other organizational members. The analysis would be incomplete, however, without some attempt to probe the limitations and boundary conditions for such trust. Would we necessarily expect, for example, all individuals who ostensibly share the same organizational identity to experience comparable levels of presumptive trust in others? Do all group members come by— and benefit from— such trust to the same degree? Stated differently, do all individuals find presumptive trust predicated on psychological salience of a shared identity equally easy to come by?

## TROUBLE IN PARADISE: SOCIAL UNCERTAINTY AND THE FRAGILITY OF IDENTITY-BASED TRUST

A first cut at an analysis of sources of intragroup variation in the propensity toward presumptive trust produces, as a reasonable working hypothesis, the conjecture that individuals' degree of presumptive trust in others will correspond to their level of positive identification with the organization and its members.

Several prima facie arguments can be marshaled in support of this proposition. First, individuals' level of psychological identification with a group or organization reflects, presumably, the extent to which they maintain a positive "ingroup stereotype" about the group or organization (Elsbach & Kramer, 1996). There is, additionally, some evidence that such stereotypes can facilitate generalized trust in others (see, e.g., Yamagishi & Yamagishi, 1994). Second, it can be argued that identification with an organization is likely to be related to individuals' beliefs regarding how readily they "fit" into the organization and its culture.

From this perspective, individuals within an organization can more readily confer trust on others when they feel a sense of psychological security or "safety" in their interactions with other group members (Edmondson, 1998). In particular, trust acquires a "taken-for-granted" quality for those individuals in the organization whose identities are central and secure. Paraphrasing the observation from Brothers (1995) at the beginning of this paper, when identities are secure, trust recedes to the background of conscious awareness, much like our lack of awareness, moment-to-moment, of gravity's constraining pull on our movements. Trust becomes, in Gestalt terms, ground.

In contrast, when individuals lack a sense of security regarding their status or "fit" within a group, then trust may not be so readily forthcoming. For such individuals, confidence in their footing in the social landscape is less secure and, concomitantly, a sense of psychological safety remains more elusive. Trust has a more tenuous quality. Rather than presumptive trust, a rather "uneasy" form of trust is likely to obtain in their relations with others. Concerns about trust loom large or become, in Gestalt terms, figural.

This argument can be developed more systematically by introducing the notion of *social uncertainty*. In a perceptive analysis of the role of social uncertainty in intergroup contexts, Hogg and Mullin (1999) elaborated on human requirements for social certainty in the following terms:

> People have a fundamental need to feel certain about their world and their place in it—subjective certainty renders existence meaningful and thus gives one confidence about how to behave, and what to expect from the physical and social environment within which one finds oneself. (p. 253)

Social uncertainty, they go on to suggest, is aversive because "it is ultimately associated with reduced control over one's life and thus it motivates behavior that reduces subjective uncertainty" (Hogg & Mullins, p. 253; see also Hogg, 2000b, 2000d).

Drawing on these observations, we can characterize *social certainty* within organizations in terms of organizational members' subjective confidence and clarity (lack of ambiguity) regarding their place in the social order of the organization. *Social uncertainty*, in turn, can be construed in terms of their lack of confidence and/or greater ambiguity regarding their place in that order.

The concept of *perceived standing* in a group or organization provides useful traction for explicating more fully the effects of social uncertainty on the development of trust within organizational relationships (or perhaps more accurately, its role in impeding trust development). Standing refers to the "information communicated to a person about his or her status within the group . . . communicated both by interpersonal aspects of treatment—politeness and/or respect—and by the attention paid to a person as a full group member" (Tyler, 1993, p. 148). Numerous studies by Lind and Tyler on the group-value model have shown that people often attach considerable importance to their standing within social systems, whether they be social groups or formal organizations (e.g., Lind & Tyler, 1988).

According to Lind and Tyler's model, and consistent with social identity theory more generally, individuals are presumed to care about their status in the groups to which they belong. Consequently, they are motivated to actively seek evidence diagnostic of their standing in the group. In other words, they are assumed to be motivated to reduce uncertainty about standing. In support of such ideas, it should be noted, there already exists considerable evidence suggestive of the importance individuals attach to their status within social systems (Frank, 1985) and the extent to which they are motivated to reduce uncertainty about that status (Ashford & Cummings, 1985). This connection is supported, moreover, by evidence regarding the deleterious effects of loss of certainty on psychological and social functioning (e.g., Baumeister & Tice, 1990; Janoff-Bulman, 1992).

## When in Doubt: Coping with Social Uncertainty

Under what conditions are organizational members likely to experience social uncertainty in their intraorganizational relations and dealings? To develop an answer to this question, it is useful to briefly describe a rather clever and conceptually elegant study by Zimbardo, Andersen, and Kabat (1981). Their study provides some suggestive clues regarding the inherent aversiveness of social uncertainty and its potentially catastrophic effects on trust-related cognitions and behavior.

Zimbardo et al.'s (1981) study was inspired by a rather provocative, although at the time poorly understood, clinical observation. Clinicians working within institutional settings had often noted a correlation between gradual hearing loss and the onset of paranoid ideation. For example, it was noted that elderly hospitalized patients diagnosed as paranoid often had significantly greater deafness compared to patients with other affective disorders. Moreover, paranoid perceptions appeared to be more prevalent among those hard-of-hearing individuals whose deafness had a gradual, and therefore undiagnosed, onset and course.

Drawing on such observations, Zimbardo et al. (1981) theorized that when hearing loss is unexpected and gradual, patients are likely to remain relatively oblivious of their hearing loss and its impact on their social relationships. This leads, they argued, to the emergence of paranoid-like thinking as the hard-of-hearing individual tries to explain the "perceptual anomaly" of not being able to hear what people around them are apparently saying (p. 1529). Judging others around them to be whispering, the individual begins to ask, "About what?"

These initial responses by the hard-of-hearing person can be construed, it should be emphasized, as reasonable attempts to make sense of a discomforting, but apparently quite genuine, experience. Consistent with the notion of social perceivers as "intuitive scientists" (Kelley, 1973) trying to understand and explain others' behavior, the hard-of-hearing person ponders, "Why are people suddenly whispering?" Such ruminations inevitably turn selfward: "Are they talking about me—and, if so, why?"

Attempts to find an answer to this question are frustrated, however, by those around the hard-of-hearing person, who vehemently deny they are whispering. As Zimbardo et al. (1981) noted, the persistent denial by others that they are whispering is likely to be construed by the hard-of-hearing person as an intentional lie since it is so clearly at odds with the evidence seemingly provided by their own senses. Thus, while intended to be reassuring, these protestations of innocence by others that nothing is amiss only spur the hard-of-hearing person to press more vigorously to find out what's really going on.

The increasingly persistent behavior of the hard-of-hearing person to make sense of their predicament creates, in turn, a rather disconcerting predicament for those around the hard-of-hearing person. As Zimbardo et al. (1981) reasoned, "Without access to the perceptual data base of the person experiencing the hearing disorder, [innocent bystanders and observers] judge these responses to be bizarre instances of thought pathology" (p. 1529). As a consequence, they actually *do* begin to whisper about the hard-of-hearing person, and *do* increasingly shun them, because the suspicions and accusations about their alleged whispering become more and more upsetting.

These reciprocal misattributions, and the behaviors they engender, lead persons experiencing hearing loss and those around them to become locked in a spiraling pattern of mutual wariness and escalating hostility, punctuated by periodic social withdrawal. As a consequence, "the individual experiences both isolation and loss of the corrective social feedback essential for modifying false beliefs" (p. 1529). The system thus assumes a life of its own, becoming, as Zimbardo et al. (1981) aptly put it, a "self-validating, autistic system" in which "delusions of persecution go unchecked" (p. 1529).

Construed broadly as a parable regarding the perils of loss of certainty regarding one's standing in a social group, Zimbardo et al.'s (1981) study suggests how readily the disruption of presumptive trust can occur as soon as situational or contextual factors weaken or tear one's otherwise largely tacit and taken-for-granted connection to others. This raises the question of whether there are structural or functional "equivalents" of this "hard-of-hearing" dynamic found within organizations.

One answer to this question can be derived, I argue next, from an analysis of those sorts of social identities and identity relations that are likely to prompt doubts about one's standing within the organization.

## PERCEIVED DISTINCTIVENESS, SOCIAL UNCERTAINTY, AND UNEASY TRUST: ONE LIABILITY OF MERELY BEING DIFFERENT FROM OTHERS

Because individuals in organizations possess multiple social identities, they can categorize themselves—and be categorized by others—in a variety of different ways. These include categorizations based upon their obvious physical attributes (such as age, race, or gender) as well as categorizations based upon various social attributes, such as their religious affiliation, socioeconomic status, and educational background. Additionally, individuals may be categorized on the basis of organization-specific groupings (e.g., departmental affiliation, branch location, tenure, etc.).

Recognizing their importance, researchers have afforded a great deal of attention in recent years to exploring how these categorization processes influence social perception and behavior within social groups and organizations (e.g., Kanter, 1977b; R. M. Kramer, 1991; Tsui et al., 1992; Wharton, 1992). Several conclusions emerge from this research. First, salient social categories can influence how individuals define themselves in a given social situation. This research has shown, along these lines, that individuals often categorize themselves in terms of those attributes that happen to be distinctive or unique in a given setting (Cota & Dion, 1986; Kanter, 1977a, 1977b; Swan & Wyer, 1997; S. E. Taylor, 1981). For example, if an individual is the only female in a group, her gender status may be afforded disproportionate emphasis when explaining her behavior, affecting not only how she is seen by other organizational members, but how she sees herself as well. From a cognitive standpoint, the distinctiveness of this category makes gender-based attributions and causal stories involving gender more available during social information processing. As a result, they tend to "loom larger" during social interaction, affecting the social inference process for both actor and observer.

Extrapolating from such evidence, it can be argued that individuals who belong to distinctive social categories within an organization are more likely to be self-conscious when interacting with other organizational members, and especially when interacting with those from the (statistically) dominant group. Because they feel that they are different or "stand out" in the organization, such individuals tend to overestimate the extent to which their behavior is being noticed and that they are under a sort of judgmental or evaluative scrutiny by other group members.

The argument that self-categorization on the basis of distinctive or exceptional identity can contribute to the perception of being under evaluative scrutiny is consistent with a considerable body of evidence regarding the cognitive and social consequences of merely "being different" from other members of a social group or organization (Brewer, 1991; Kanter, 1977a, 1977b; Kramer, 1994; Taylor, 1981; Tsui et al., 1992). Such evidence suggests that such distinctiveness can be aversive (Frable et al., 1990; C. G. Lord & Saenz, 1985). As Brewer (1991) noted, "being highly individuated leaves one vulnerable to isolation and stigmatization (even excelling on positively valued dimensions creates social distance and potential rejection)" (p. 478). Distinctive individuals thus occupy a potentially undesirable social "no man's land" in the organizational landscape.

In social information processing terms, one consequence of individuals' awareness of "being different" from other organizational members is that it prompts attempts to make sense of the experience, including "spontaneous" attributional search (Weiner, 1985) for the causes of their self-consciousness. Such self-consciousness will be especially pronounced and aversive when individuals are uncertain about precisely how much "being different" from others really matters (e.g., its impact on whether they will be accepted by others and the kind of treatment they will receive from them).

In many respects, so-called "token" members of organizations exemplify this quandary. Token status in organizations is based upon "ascribed characteristics (master statuses such as sex, race, religion, ethnic group, age, etc.) or other characteristics that carry with them a set of assumptions about culture, status, and behavior that are highly salient for majority category members" (Kanter, 1977a, p. 966). In her now classic discussion of the effects of token status on social perception and interpersonal relations within organizations, Kanter (1977a, 1977b) noted that individuals who are members of token categories are likely to attract disproportionate attention from other organizational members, particularly those who enjoy dominant status in terms of their greater numerical proportion.

In support of Kanters' ethnographic observations, S. E. Taylor (1981) demonstrated experimentally that observers often do allocate disproportionate amounts of attention to individuals who have token status in groups, especially when making attributions about group processes and outcomes. C. G. Lord and Saenz (1985) subsequently provided an important extension of this early work by showing how token status affects the cognitive processes of tokens themselves. On the basis of their evidence, they concluded that, "Tokens feel the social pressure of imagined audience scrutiny, and may do so even when the 'audience' of majority group members treat them no differently from nontokens" (p. 919). For example, she argued that females in many American corporations often feel as if they are in the "limelight" compared to their more numerous male counterparts.

This evidence supports the argument that individuals who have token status in a social system are more likely to experience higher levels of social uncertainty and, in response, will be more self-conscious and perceive themselves to be under evaluative scrutiny to a greater extent than nontoken members. As a consequence, they will tend to overestimate the extent to which they are the targets of others' attention. This tendency to overperceive the extent to which people are paying attention to the self has been shown to foster a state of paranoid-like social suspicion and distrust of others (see R. M. Kramer, 1998, for a review). Thus, in sharp contrast to the sort of easy, presumptive trust facilitated by ingroup identification, those whose status in the group is problematic are more likely to experience only a kind of fragile, tentative, or "uneasy" sort of trust.

## A SOCIAL IDENTITY MODEL OF UNEASY TRUST

On the basis of such findings, it is possible to sketch the outlines of a framework for conceptualizing how identity-linked forms of social uncertainty can adversely affect trust-related judgment and behavior within organizations. According to this framework, social uncertainty is presumed to foster a state of dysphoric self-consciousness. Dysphoric self-consciousness refers to an aversive form of heightened public self-consciousness characterized by the feeling that one is under intense social and evaluative scrutiny. In contrast with positive (identity-enhancing) forms of public attention, dysphoric self-consciousness can be construed as a negative (identity-threatening) form of attention (Elsbach & Kramer, 1996; Sutton & Galunic, 1996).

One consequence of such self-consciousness, as noted above, is that it activates attributional search aimed at helping individuals make sense of their experiences. In other words, when individuals become self-conscious, they look for reasons why they are self-conscious: If one is self-conscious, then someone must be watching. And if someone is watching, then something might be amiss. One consequence of their self-consciousness, then, is that people are motivated to figure out what (or who) is causing it and what to do about it.

According to the model, these attempts at sense making promote a hypervigilant and ruminative mode of social information processing. The relationship between hypervigilance and rumination, moreover, can be viewed as one of reciprocal causation. Specifically, hypervigilant appraisal of social information tends to generate more "raw data" about which the already suspicious social perceiver ruminates. At the same time, rumination helps generate additional hypotheses suggesting that suspicion is warranted, prompting more vigilant scrutiny of the situation, and especially of others' behavior.

Hypervigilance and rumination are posited to contribute to several distinct modes of social misperception that can impede the development of presumptive trust. These include a tendency toward the overly personalistic construal of social interactions and a tendency to make unrealistically "sinister" attributions regarding others' actions and inactions. Although space constraints preclude a detailed discussion of the evidence, it should be noted that numerous studies have documented associations between self-consciousness, hypervigilance, rumination, and the tendency towards overly personalistic construal of social interactions (Buss & Scheier, 1976; Greenwald, 1980; Kramer, 1994; Pyszczynski & Greenberg, 1987). For example, Fenigstein (1984) postulated the existence of a general *overperception of self-as-target bias*, arguing that self-consciousness increases the extent to which individuals' construe others' behavior in self-referential terms (i.e., as intentionally focused on, or directed towards, them). In support of this proposition, Fenigstein and Vanable (1992) showed that individuals high in public self-consciousness were more likely than individuals low in public self-consciousness to feel they were being observed in an experimental setting involving a two-way mirror.

These perceptual biases or proclivities, in turn, stimulate behavioral responses consistent with a psychological state of uneasy trust in others. For example, because they are uncertain about their standing in the organization, such individuals are more likely to be uncomfortable in their informal interactions with other organizational members; they are more likely to experience social inhibition and more likely to avoid personal self-disclosures when interacting with other group members. Their behavior can be construed, in one sense, as "defensively motivated" and "avoidant," in so far as it is intended to avoid exposing the self to perceived vulnerability and social risks. One of the unintended, and ironic, consequences of such risk-averse interpersonal behavior is that it tends to elicit the very responses from others that lead to further uncertainty and concerns about trust. Thus, there is a self-sustaining and escalatory dynamic associated with uneasy forms of trust, comparable to the sort of escalatory "spirals" described by others (Deutsch, 1986). Much like the experience of Zimbardo et al.'s (1981) hard-of-hearing patients, these individuals engage in actions that produce the very consequences they most dread and most wish to avert.

## GENERAL DISCUSSION

The primary purpose of this chapter was to develop some ideas regarding possible linkages between individuals' identification with an organization and their resultant level of generalized trust in its members. The chapter initially focused on articulating the psychological and social underpinnings of identity-based trust, arguing that psychological awareness of a shared social or organizational identity can provide the basis for a form of diffuse, depersonalized trust, consistent with Brewer's (1981) original suggestion. I then argued that such presumptive trust might be more difficult for certain individuals whose identities render their relationship to the organization and its members problematic.

On the positive side of the equation linking organizational identity and trust, this analysis has a number of implications with respect to how such collective trust might be created and sustained in organizations. One approach to heightening awareness of shared or "collectivizing" identities is through structural arrangements that draw attention to, or increase the salience of, cooperative norms and expectations. As March (1994) observed, organizational arrangements function much like "stage managers" by providing "prompts that evoke particular identities in particular situations" (p. 72). G. J. Miller (1992) offered an excellent example of this kind of socially constructed and self-reinforcing dynamic. In discussing the underpinnings of cooperation at Hewlett-Packard, he noted that, "The reality of cooperation is suggested by the open lab stock policy, which not only allows engineers access to all equipment, but encourages them to take it home for personal use" (p. 197).

Note that this is a very straightforward structural arrangement which, from a strictly economic perspective, simply reduces monitoring and transaction-costs. However, from the standpoint of the sort of identity-based logic advanced in this chapter, its consequences are more subtle, more pervasive, and more enduring. G. J. Miller (1992) went on to observe along these lines,

> "the open door symbolizes and demonstrates management's trust in the cooperativeness of the employees. . . . The elimination of time clocks and locks on equipment room doors is *a way of building a shared expectation among all the players that cooperation will most likely be reciprocated* [creating] *a shared "common knowledge" in the ability of the players to reach cooperative outcomes.* (p. 197, emphases added)

Moreover, because such acts are so manifestly predicated on confidence in others, they tend to breed confidence in turn.

As a consequence, over time, this collective identity of "us" as "trustworthy" becomes institutionalized in terms of shared norms and practices regarding such things as turn-taking, relaxed monitoring, and presumed reliability. In addition to the external institutionalization of a regime of cooperative *practices*, however, individuals' identities also lead to internalized (cognitive) changes in terms of members' tacit expectations and beliefs regarding their duties, rights, obligations, entitlements, and mutual understandings. In this respect, awareness of a shared collective identity becomes a potent form of "expectational asset" (cf., Knez & Camerer, 1994) on which members can draw and depend when trying to decide what to do in trust dilemma situations.

# ACKNOWLEDGMENTS

This research was supported by a James and Doris McNamara Faculty Fellowship. I am grateful to Jonathan Bendor, Marilynn Brewer, John Darley, Russell Hardin, Bernard Weiner, and Philip Zimbardo for their contributions to the development of these ideas. Comments and reprint requests should be addressed to the author care of The Graduate School of Business, Stanford University, Stanford, CA 94305 or via e-mail at Kramer_Roderick@GSB.Stanford.edu.

# 12

# How Status and Power Differences Erode Personal and Social Identities at Work:
## A System Justification Critique of Organizational Applications of Social Identity Theory

JOHN T. JOST
*Stanford University*
KIMBERLY D. ELSBACH
*University of California, Davis*

Although they are seldom diagnosed accurately by insiders, most organizations suffer from problems of intergroup relations. It is a relatively common problem, for instance, that people from marketing and engineering departments may dislike or distrust one another, or they may misperceive what motivates, challenges, and interests members of the other department. Stereotypes abound concerning lawyers, accountants, professional women, CEOs, investment bankers, union members, and so on. In many different organizational contexts, people should be working together, but they are not; instead, "us versus them" mentalities persist, thwarting harmony and productivity at work (e.g., Pfeffer & Sutton, 2000). If group differences are not handled by management with tact and sensitivity, as well as with an informed awareness of the complexity of group dynamics and intergroup relations, then distrust and competition among groups may grow and fester, spreading intractable conflict and organizational discord (e.g., Blake & Mouton, 1984; R. M. Kramer, 1991).

In this chapter, we focus specifically on the roles of status and power differences between groups and how these complicate and exacerbate intergroup relations at work. Systems and procedures using grades, classes, rankings, negative feedback, performance evaluations, and external critiques all have the potential to devalue members of one group relative to others. Negative consequences may be expected to strike members of devalued groups most severely, causing them to withdraw from academic and professional pursuits and, in some cases, to internalize a sense of their own inferiority (e.g., Dutton & Dukerich, 1991; Elsbach, 1999; Jost & Burgess, 2000; Pfeffer & Sutton, 2000; Rosenthal & Jacobson, 1968; Steele, 1997; Steele & Aronson, 1995). Thus, hierarchical relationships in society and at work threaten the self-concepts and social identities of members of devalued groups (e.g., Elsbach & Kramer, 1996; Jost & Banaji, 1994; Sidanius & Pratto, 1999).

We argue that focusing on status and power differences between groups is the key to a viable theory of intergroup relations. Extant analyses of intergroup relations in organizations tend to emphasize symmetrical forms of competition and "ingroup bias," so that "we" are always preferred to "them." In today's organizations, however, status and power differences are often used and cultivated as a means of evaluation, motivation, promotion, identification, and commitment (Elsbach & Kramer, 1996; Dutton & Dukerich, 1991; Pfeffer & Sutton, 2000). Organizational hierarchies also tend to be legitimated by "expert evaluators" and other respected authorities who provide seemingly "objective" evidence that some groups are inferior to others. Under such circumstances, it would seem to be difficult and unlikely for members of devalued groups to maintain positive images of themselves and of their fellow group members (e.g., Hinkle & Brown, 1990; Jost & Banaji, 1994; B. Major, 1994; Tajfel & Turner, 1979).

An emphasis on symmetrical forms of intergroup bias can be traced to the foci and assumptions of a particularly influential theory in social and organizational psychology: social identity theory (Ashforth & Mael, 1989; R. M. Kramer, 1991; Tajfel & Turner, 1979). We argue here that a viable theory of intergroup relations must reconcile and integrate findings in support of social identity theory with evidence that status hierarchies and organizational systems tend to be internalized and justified. Theory and evidence from a "system justification" perspective (Jost & Banaji, 1994), for instance, address the ways in which status and power inequalities have deleterious social and psychological consequences for members of devalued groups (Jost & Burgess, 2000; Jost & Thompson, 2000).

In what follows, we first summarize the main applications of social identity theory to organizational contexts, stressing three theoretical assumptions: (a) the assumption that ingroup bias is a general or default motive or strategy, (b) the assumption that low-status-group members compensate for identity threats by increasing levels of ingroup bias, and (c) the assumption that people prefer to interact with members of their own group than members of other groups. All three of these assumptions are challenged by system justification theory (Jost & Banaji, 1994; Jost & Burgess, 2000), which is an alternative theory of intergroup relations with relevance for organizational behavior. We then relate theory and evidence concerning system justification processes, demonstrating that, for members of devalued groups, these processes work against tendencies to maintain or enhance individual self-esteem ("ego justification") and to develop positive social identities and to favor the ingroup ("group justification"). Finally, we address structural or systemic aspects of organizations (such as performance evaluation systems) that are likely to exacerbate status and power differences between groups, thereby eroding the personal and social identities of members of groups that are devalued at work.

## SOCIAL IDENTITY THEORY AT WORK

Since the 1970s, there has been one social psychological theory of intergroup relations that has been most influential and most useful for understanding the plethora of problems that can arise between members of different groups. This theory, known as "social identity theory," was originally articulated by Tajfel and Turner (1979), and it has been extended in various ways by a good many of the authors brought together in this book, and some others as well. The basic assumptions of the theory are relatively straightforward, although derivations and additions to the theory make matters far more complicated (e.g., see Hogg & Abrams, 1988; Spears, Oakes, Ellemers, & Haslam, 1997; J. C. Turner et al., 1987). In a nutshell, social identity theory holds that (a) we derive a great deal of personal value and meaning from our group memberships, so that our self-concepts depend in significant ways upon the ways in which our groups are regarded by ourselves and by others, and (b) the only way to assess value and regard in the social world is through processes of comparison, so that the value and worth of one group is always relative to the value and worth of another reference group.

Drawing extensively on Festinger's (1954) social comparison theory, social identity theorists have argued that, because people need to evaluate themselves favorably and because group memberships are an important constituent of the self-concept, group members tend to evaluate their ingroups more favorably than they evaluate other groups (e.g., Tajfel & Turner, 1979). This phenomenon is referred to as "ingroup bias" or "ingroup favoritism" (e.g., Brewer, 1979; Hogg & Abrams, 1988; Tajfel & Turner, 1979), and it may take the form of trait ascription, resource allocation, and the evaluation of group products (e.g., Hinkle & Schopler, 1986; Mullen, Brown, & Smith, 1992; Tajfel & Turner, 1979). The display of ingroup bias has been regarded largely as a strategy for maintaining or enhancing one's individual and collective self-esteem (e.g., Lemyre & Smith, 1985; Oakes & Turner, 1980). According to some very prominent interpreters, social identity theory holds that there is a general drive to enhance individual and collective self-esteem by making favorable comparisons between the ingroup and relevant outgroups (e.g., Abrams & Hogg, 1988; Rubin & Hewstone, 1998).

Although the motivational assumption that ingroup bias is a universal or ubiquitous tendency has been doubted and challenged by a number of researchers of intergroup relations (e.g., Abrams & Hogg, 1988; Hewstone & Ward,

1985; Hinkle & Brown, 1990; Jost & Banaji, 1994; Sidanius & Pratto, 1999), this skepticism has not yet found its way into the organizational literature. To date, organizational researchers examining intergroup relations have embraced in a relatively uncritical manner the assumptions of (a) *ingroup bias,* (b) *self-esteem enhancement in response to threat,* and (c) *homophily on the part of group members.* We address each of these assumptions in light of theory and evidence concerning system justification (Jost & Banaji, 1994), and we question their applicability to situations involving status and power differences between groups.

## The Assumption of Ingroup Bias

We readily grant that social identity theory is extremely useful for understanding many common manifestations of intergroup conflict (e.g., Blake & Mouton, 1984; R. M. Kramer, 1991; Pfeffer & Sutton, 2000), particularly symmetrical conflict among parties that are approximately equal in status or power. In such situations, group members frequently exhibit ingroup bias (e.g., Hinkle & Schopler, 1986; R. M. Kramer, 1991; Mullen et al., 1992), especially when norms for fairness are low in salience (e.g., Diekmann, Samuels, Ross, & Bazerman, 1997; Jetten, Spears, & Manstead, 1996; Jost & Ross, 1999). Social identity theory also does a very good job of predicting the behavior of established high-status and powerful group members, who exhibit strong levels of ingroup bias in experimental and field studies of intergroup relations (e.g., Mullen et al., 1992; Sachdev & Bourhis, 1984, 1987, 1991) as well as in organizational studies of job classification, employee treatment, and salary determination (Baron & Pfeffer, 1994; Bielby & Baron, 1986).

The assumption that group members favor their own does not apply nearly as well to members of low-status and powerless groups. Here, an ever-increasing body of evidence suggests that members of devalued groups often exhibit *out*group favoritism in the ascription of traits and stereotypes, the evaluation of group products, and the allocation of resources (e.g., Boldry & Kashy, 1999; R. J. Brown, 1978; Hewstone & Ward, 1985; Hinkle & Brown, 1990; Jost, in press; Jost & Banaji, 1994; Jost & Burgess, 2000; Reichl, 1997; Sidanius & Pratto, 1999). Outgroup favoritism is especially likely on status-relevant dimensions (e.g., Mullen et al., 1992; Skevington, 1981; Spears & Manstead, 1989) and when status and power differences are perceived as highly legitimate (e.g., Ellemers, Wilke, & van Knippenberg, 1993; Jost, in press; Jost & Burgess, 2000; J. C. Turner & Brown, 1978).

Findings of outgroup favoritism have been a persistent thorn in the side of social identity theorists. Hewstone and Jaspars (1984) responded to early evidence of outgroup favoritism by acknowledging that according to social identity theory, "ingroup devaluation would be an unlikely response pattern" (p. 393). Hinkle and Brown (1990) similarly pointed out that "the mere fact of out-group favouritism is inconsistent with the notion of groups engaging in intergroup comparison processes to create and maintain positive social identities" (p. 52). Although Tajfel and Turner (1979) acknowledged the existence of outgroup favoritism, several commentators have argued that the explanatory mechanisms of social identity theory are not well suited to account for the phenomenon (e.g., Hewstone & Ward, 1985; Jost & Banaji, 1994; Sidanius & Pratto, 1999).

To provide a more complete account of the causes and consequences of outgroup favoritism among members of low-status groups, Jost and Banaji (1994) developed *system justification theory*. The guiding assumption of the theory is that people engage in a social and psychological justification of the status quo, even at the expense of individual and collective self-esteem. System justification theory thus suggests that members of both high- and low-status groups engage in thoughts, feelings, and behaviors that reinforce and legitimate existing social systems, and that outgroup favoritism is one such example of the legitimation of inequality between groups. Evidence of outgroup favoritism garnered in support of system justification theory (e.g., Jost, in press; Jost & Burgess, 2000; Jost & Thompson, 2000) contradicts the assumption that ingroup bias is a general or default motive or tendency, and, a fortiori, it contradicts the motivational assumption that members of devalued groups compensate for identity threats by exhibiting elevated levels of ingroup bias.

## The Compensation Assumption

Many interpreters of social identity theory have argued that members of devalued groups should exhibit greater ingroup favoritism than members of highly valued groups, as a way of compensating for identity threat (e.g., Brewer, 1979; Sachdev & Bourhis, 1984). This notion has also made its way into Ashforth and Mael's (1989) application of social identity theory to organizational contexts. They proposed that:

> while a low-status group (such as a noncritical staff function or cadre of middle managers) may go to great lengths to differentiate itself from a high-status comparison group (such as a critical line function or senior management), the latter may be relatively unconcerned about such comparisons and form no strong impression about the low-status group. (p. 33)

Although Ashforth and Mael (1989) may be right that members of low-status groups will under some circumstances seek positive distinctiveness as way of resolving identity crises, in general it is high-status groups who are most eager to differentiate themselves from their subordinates (e.g., Jost & Banaji, 1994; Sidanius & Pratto, 1999). On the whole, research contradicts the notion that members of devalued groups would attempt to compensate for identity threats by displaying increased ingroup favoritism. Rather, as we have noted above, evidence suggests that members of high-status groups are more likely to exhibit ingroup favoritism and that members of low status groups frequently exhibit outgroup favoritism, admitting their own inferiority at least on status-related dimensions (see, inter alia, Boldry & Kashy, 1999; R. J. Brown, 1978; Hewstone & Ward, 1985; Hinkle & Brown, 1990; Jost, in press; Jost & Burgess, 2000; Reichl, 1997; Spears & Manstead, 1989).

Once again, this raises problems for social identity theory's account of hierarchical social relations. Hinkle and Brown (1990), for instance, noted that "the common occurrence of out-group favouritism among low-status groups is actually contrary to the hypothesis, derivable from SIT, that low-status groups have the greatest motivation to enhance their social identities and thus should be particularly likely to manifest pronounced in-group favouritism" (p. 52). Sidanius and Pratto (1999) similarly argued that if "the need for positive social identity motivates discrimination, then we should expect people in low-status groups to be even more motivated to discriminate than will people in high-status groups" (p. 20). The reality in society and in business organizations is that members of high-status groups are far more likely to engage in discrimination and ingroup bias against lower status group members than vice versa (e.g., J. Baron & Pfeffer, 1994; Bielby & Baron, 1986; Jost & Banaji, 1994; Sachdev & Bourhis, 1984, 1987, 1991; Sidanius & Pratto, 1999).

It is relatively easy to assume on the basis of social identity research, as Ashforth and Mael (1989, p. 33) have done, that members of devalued groups display outgroup favoritism only on dimensions that are unimportant to them. Evidence strongly supports the notion that members of low-status groups are far more likely to display outgroup favoritism on status-relevant or achievement-related dimensions than on status-irrelevant dimensions (e.g., Jost, in press; Mullen et al., 1992; Skevington, 1981; Spears & Manstead, 1989), but this does not mean that they reject the value of status-relevant characteristics (see B. Major & Schmader, 2001). This point is perhaps more consequential in work organizations than in other settings, because achievement-related characteristics are those that are most likely to be highly valued in business environments. On a day to day basis, it would be extremely difficult for workers to sustain the belief that characteristics such as intelligence, competence, responsibility, and industriousness are not very important within the organizational system.

Although we have criticized social identity theorists for suggesting that members of devalued groups would be more likely than members of other groups to exhibit ingroup bias, the theory's motivational focus does help to explain how people sometimes do maintain favorable images of themselves and their groups in the face of identity threat. Specifically, it has been hypothesized that when presented with negative evaluations of one's own group, people will attempt to preserve ingroup-favoring comparisons by switching to alternative dimensions on which they are more successful than other groups or by engaging in "downward social comparison" with reference groups that are even worse off, thereby reasserting their own superiority (Tajfel & Turner, 1979). Evidence does support the notion that low-status group members engage in ingroup bias on status-irrelevant or socioemotional dimensions such as honesty, friendliness, and warmth (e.g., Mullen et al., 1992; Skevington, 1981; Spears & Manstead, 1989). However, Jost (in press) has pointed out that this choice of alternative comparison dimensions may not be due to compensation strategies per se, given that neutral observers also attribute greater interpersonal warmth and emotionality to members of low status groups (e.g., Glick & Fiske, 2001). There is also no consistent evidence that low-status-group members compensate for identity threats by showing stronger ingroup bias on alternative dimensions than high-status-group members show on status-relevant dimensions (e.g., Jost, in press).

Despite the fact that several theoretical and empirical questions remain open, organizational researchers have obtained some support for the predictions of social identity theory with regard to identity management. For instance, Elsbach and Kramer (1996) found that in the wake of disappointing national rankings, business school professors strategically redefined their institutions to maintain the belief that their schools were at the top of some category or another (e.g., public university, regional powerhouse, or metropolitan business school). In an analysis of "dirty work," Ashforth and Kreiner (1999) argued that because their work is not respected by others, people whose jobs are widely viewed as disgusting or gruesome (garbage collectors, butchers, janitors, exterminators, funeral directors, etc.) tend to have extremely strong organizational cultures and to maintain very favorable self-evaluations and group evaluations. Citing prior research, Ashforth and Kreiner (1999) also used tenets of social identity theory such as social creativity and reframing to argue, for instance, that "exotic dancers and prostitutes claim they are providing a therapeutic and educational service, rather than selling their bodies" (p. 421). Thus, the takeaway message of social identity theory, especially in terms of its organizational applications, has been that people stubbornly maintain favorable identities and ingroup bias even in the face of evidence indicating that their group is low in status, power, or prestige (e.g., Ashforth & Kreiner, 1999; Ashforth & Mael, 1989; Dutton et al., 1994; Elsbach, 1999; Elsbach & Kramer, 1996).

In some ways, then, social identity theory provides a relatively optimistic message concerning the effects of status and power on personal and social identities at work. There is indeed evidence that identity threat can lead group members to exhibit pride and ingroup bias, especially when these groups are situationally rather than chronically devalued, as in the case of Elsbach and Kramer's (1996) study of academics and other studies of management executives whose companies are failing or declaring bankruptcy (e.g., Bettman & Weitz, 1983; Staw, McKechnie, & Puffer, 1983; Sutton & Callaghan, 1987). Under such circumstances, people do seem to defend themselves against imagined or real attacks, and they find ways of maintaining positive images of themselves, their groups, and their organizations.

But there is an important difference between how members of ordinarily high-status groups react to identity threats and how members of chronically devalued groups react to such circumstances, just as there is a major difference between how people with high self-esteem react to ego threats and how people with low self-esteem respond to those same threats (e.g., Swann, 1996). Social identity theory, like self-enhancement theories, tends to blur this distinction, treating "identity threat" as a blanket term covering the consequences of everything from negative performance feedback to systematic group-based discrimination. A huge program of research carried out by Swann and his colleagues indicates that individuals affirm and verify existing identities and expectations, even if those identities are devalued and the consequences for the self are extremely unfavorable (e.g., Swann, 1996; Swann, Griffin, Predmore, & Gaines, 1987).

With regard to intergroup relations, system justification theory makes an analogous argument at a higher level of analysis: members of systems and organizations tend to affirm and justify existing hierarchies, even if the consequences for the self and the group are extremely unfavorable (Jost, 1997, in press; Jost & Banaji, 1994; Jost & Burgess, 2000; Jost & Thompson, 2000). From this perspective, members of chronically low-status or powerless groups may not seek to maintain or enhance self-esteem under conditions of adversity, as social identity theory suggests. According to system justification theory, it would be quite difficult for people to reject and ignore such seemingly objective evidence of one's place in a status hierarchy such as that coming from job title, salary, performance evaluation, stock prices, and media rankings. As Dutton et al. (1994) put it:

> Organizational membership can also confer negative attributes on a member. If members interpret the external organizational image as unfavorable, they may experience negative personal outcomes, such as depression and stress. In turn, these personal outcomes could lead to undesirable organizational outcomes, such as increased competition among members or reduced effort on long-term tasks. (p. 240)

By stressing motivational drives for individual and collective self-enhancement, social identity theorists risk fully appreciating the deleterious effects of status and power differences on individuals and groups. It is easy to conclude, on the basis of claims concerning cognitive restructuring or reframing, selective social comparison, social creativity, and ingroup bias, that hierarchical relations at work and inequalities among industries and companies do not necessarily cause social or psychological harm to members of devalued groups and organizations. We disagree with this conclusion, arguing instead that status and power differences between groups contribute to a host of socially and psychologically detrimental outcomes, precisely because it is so difficult to challenge the legitimacy and stability of social and organizational systems (e.g., Baron & Pfeffer, 1994; Jost & Burgess, 2000; Jost & Thompson, 2000; Lerner, 1980; B. Major, 1994; J. Martin, 1986; Pfeffer & Sutton, 2000; Steele, 1997; Steele & Aronson, 1995).

### The Assumption of Homophily

In the field of organizational behavior, social identity theory and its intellectual heir, self-categorization theory (e.g., J. C. Turner et al., 1987), have often been treated as theories of homophily or similarity. For instance, organizational researchers have used concepts of social identification and ingroup bias to argue that people prefer to interact with and work with people who are demographically similar to them and who share common category memberships with them (e.g., Baron & Pfeffer, 1994; Hogg & Terry, 2000). Summarizing this body of work, Tsui, Egan, and O'Reilly (1992) concluded that, "Research consistently has shown that individuals choose to interact more often with members of their own social group than with members of other groups" (p. 550). Our reading of the literature is that, just as with the assumption of ingroup bias, the assumption of homophily applies more to the preferences of high-status or powerful group members than to the preferences of low-status or low-power-group members. Thus, Whites and males are more likely than minorities and females to respond negatively to increased diversity and contact with demographic outgroup members at work (e.g., Tsui et al., 1992; Wharton & Baron, 1987).

A recent study carried out by Jost, Pelham, and Carvallo (2000) directly contradicted the assumption of homophily insofar as it applies to ethnic minority groups. Results indicated that Latinos, Asian Americans, and European Americans all expressed significant preferences to interact with European Americans over the other two groups. Thus, the high-status group of European Americans did exhibit preferences for homophily, but the lower status minority groups preferred to interact with outgroup members. We do not argue on the basis of findings such as these that theories stressing similarity or ingroup preferences are wrong, only that they are one-sided in that they tend to neglect increasing evidence of cognitive, affective, and behavioral preferences for members of higher status outgroups (e.g., Boldry & Kashy, 1999; Hinkle & Brown, 1990; Jost & Banaji, 1994; Reichl, 1997; Sidanius & Pratto, 1999). System justification theory, we argue, does a better job of accounting for some of the social psychological effects of status and power differentials, such as the internalization of inferiority, depressed entitlement, outgroup favoritism, and preferences to interact with outgroup members (e.g., Jost, 1997, in press; Jost & Banaji, 1994; Jost et al., 2000). It is also in a better position than social identity theory to appreciate the deleterious consequences of hierarchical work arrangements on the self-concepts and social identities of members of devalued groups (e.g, Jost, 1997, in press; Jost & Burgess, 2000; Jost & Thompson, 2000).

## A Summary of the Critique

We argue that there are three assumptions that have been consistently derived from social identity theory and that have been challenged directly or indirectly by system justification theory (e.g., Jost, in press; Jost & Banaji, 1994; Jost & Burgess, 2000; Jost & Thompson, 2000; Jost et al., 2000). The first assumption is that ingroup bias is a general or default tendency or motive (e.g., Hogg & Abrams, 1988; Mullen et al., 1992; Tajfel & Turner, 1979). The second assumption is that members of low-status groups show greater ingroup favoritism than do members of high-status groups as a way of compensating for threatened identities (e.g., Ashforth & Mael, 1989; Brewer, 1979; Sachdev & Bourhis, 1984). The third assumption is that preferences to interact with fellow members of one's own demographic group apply generically (e.g., Baron & Pfeffer, 1994; Tsui et al., 1992).

According to system justification theory, all of these assumptions apply fairly well to groups that are relatively high in social standing, but they do not apply so well to groups that are low in status or power. Rather, members of groups that are low in social standing frequently internalize a sense of their own inferiority, express outgroup favoritism, and in some cases prefer to interact with outgroup members who are higher in status or power (see Jost, in press; Jost & Banaji, 1994; Jost & Burgess, 2000; Jost & Thompson, 2000; Jost et al., 2000). Thus, system justification theory challenges the generality of three widely held assumptions that are derived from social identity theory: the assumption of ingroup bias, the compensation assumption, and the homophily assumption. Having summarized the system justification critique of social identity theory, we now seek to articulate the constructive aspects of the theory. Specifically, we have argued that social identity theories are incomplete in explaining intergroup relations at work. In the following sections, we provide evidence that system justification theory helps to fill some of the conceptual holes left by social identity theories.

# SUPPORT FOR A SYSTEM JUSTIFICATION THEORY OF INTERGROUP RELATIONS AT WORK

Social psychological research addressing outgroup favoritism, attitudinal ambivalence, internalization of inferiority, and ideological support for inequality provides the primary support for a system justification theory of intergroup relations (e.g., Jost, 1997, in press; Jost & Burgess, 2000; Jost & Thompson, 2000). In addition, organizational research having to do with processes of disidentification and schizoidentification among members of devalued groups supports the notion that people accept and internalize formal evaluations and professional rankings (Elsbach, 1999). Finally, work addressing the effects of formal evaluation systems and organizational stratification provides further evidence that status and power differences between groups tend to erode personal and social identities (Pfeffer & Sutton, 2000). We review all three bases of support for a system justification theory of intergroup relations in the workplace.

## Research on System Justification Theory

System justification theorists argue that motivated tendencies to enhance individual and collective self-esteem may or may not be in conflict with parallel motives to believe in a "just world" (Lerner, 1980) and to legitimize structural forms of social inequality (Major, 1994; J. Martin, 1986). Because people find it extremely difficult to challenge or reject the credibility and authority of systems and organizations, they tend to internalize others' negative evaluations of their own group, at least to some degree. Thus, women have been found to show signs of "depressed entitlement," believing that they deserve to be paid less money for their work than men believe they deserve to be paid (e.g., Jost, 1997; Major, 1994).

Work from several independent but related research programs on system justification theory supports the conclusion that *for members of high-status groups, motives for self-enhancement, ingroup bias, and system justification are consistent and complementary, whereas for members of low-status groups, these motives are often in conflict or contradiction with one another.* For example, Jost and Thompson (2000) found that among African-American respondents, the tendency to believe that economic differences are fair, legitimate, and justifiable was associated with decreased self-esteem, increased neuroticism, and increased outgroup favoritism. Among European Americans, by contrast, these same system-justifying variables were associated with increases in self-esteem and ingroup favoritism and decreases in neuroticism (or guilt) among European Americans. Thus, attitudinal support for the system helped members of an advantaged group to feel good about themselves, but it harmed members of a disadvantaged group.

Jost and Burgess (2000) reasoned that the conflict between motives for ingroup bias and system justification would lead members of low-status groups to express greater attitudinal ambivalence about their group than would members of high-status groups. This hypothesis was supported in an experimental study involving students at different universities. Furthermore, Jost and Burgess found that increased levels of system justification were associated with increased levels of ambivalence among members of low-status groups but decreased ambivalence among members of high-status groups. Thus, women who scored high on a scale of just world beliefs were more likely than women who scored low on the scale to express ambivalence about a female plaintiff who was suing her university for gender discrimination and therefore posing a challenge to the overarching social system

Elsbach (1999) has also argued that previous theories of organizational identification need to be supplemented and extended in order to account for the full range of psychological outcomes, including various syndromes of disidentification and schizoidentification. Although this research was not carried out under the rubric of system justification theory, it does stress the social and psychological costs associated with being a member of a devalued group more than is customarily acknowledged by social identity theorists. Thus, we summarize the work of Elsbach and her colleagues to further illustrate the ways in which status and power differences between groups can erode personal and social identities at work.

## Research on Disidentification and Schizoidentification at Work

Recent research on identity management in organizational contexts suggests that current frameworks for understanding social and organizational identification do not capture several important aspects of intergroup relations at work (Pratt, 1998). Elsbach (1999) argued, for instance, that existing models do not adequately explain how individuals cope with organizational situations in which they are chronically devalued. Examples include members of labor unions who are openly criticized by management but need their jobs or employees of companies that are unpopular because of what they do or what they produce. Under such circumstances, group members may agree with the negative evaluations, and they may distance themselves psychologically from their organization, either partially or wholly (Elsbach & Bhattacharya, 2000; Elsbach, 2000).

In line with the assumptions of system justification theory (e.g., Jost, in press; Jost & Banaji, 1994), disidentification seems to be most likely when credible authorities and legitimate systems promote public status hierarchies. For example, Elsbach and Bhattacharya (2000) found that unfavorable media coverage caused people to distance themselves from the National Rifle Association (NRA). This was especially true among Americans who identified themselves as "Southerners" and who identified with Southern political ideals such as civil liberties and less governmental interference with private life. Many of these individuals felt that their groups (e.g., Southerners, Georgians) were tarnished by perceived associations with the NRA.

Elsbach (2000) similarly studied the effects of opinion polls that were published in the *Los Angeles Times* and that revealed overwhelming dissatisfaction with elected state officials (who received only a 22% to 44% approval rate during the 1980s and early 1990s). Because of the media coverage, California Legislative staffers could not deny that the Legislature as a whole and politicians as a group were devalued by the public. As a result, these employees simultaneously identified and disidentified with different aspects of their organization. For example, several staffers claimed to identify with the "policy-making" dimension of the Legislature but to actively disidentify with "partisan, political maneuvering" dimensions. As one staffer noted:

> You know, there's a certain segment of the policy-making process that's pretty sleazy, pretty questionable. And I do my best to stay away from that. I don't like to work on those bills. Most of the bills that I've worked on are not 'juice bills,' as that term is used. That is, they don't involve big insurance companies; they don't involve trial lawyers; they don't involve horse racing or gambling or liquor licenses. . . . And I was proud to point out that I was working for the least juiced committee of that index. At the time, that was one of my defenses to criticisms about excessive campaign contributions: 'Hey, no, wait a minute, let me tell you who I work for . . . the guys I work for can't even raise money!'" (Elsbach, 2000, p. 23)

Such disidentification and schizoidentification appears to be effortful and stressful to maintain. Most of the legislative staffers claimed that they routinely and consciously affirmed their disidentification by taking visible stands (e.g., refusing to be part of a story about movers and shakers at the capitol), using physical markers that differentiated them (e.g., customizing one's business cards to indicate that one worked for a particular legislator vs. the Democrats in general), and applying specific self-categorizations (e.g., always referring to oneself as a "wonk" rather than a "hack").

Similarly, many of the Southerners who distanced themselves from the

NRA mentioned how difficult it was to maintain the vigilance needed for disidentification. For instance, they had to make sure not to support any other groups or organizations that were affiliated with the NRA, which proved to be a difficult and time-consuming task. It seems likely that maintaining long-term disidentification, even if it is with only a part of the organization, would be emotionally taxing as well. Research on adolescence and alienation suggests that defining oneself in terms of what one "is not," as when adolescents go through a phase of defining themselves as "not their parents," can lead to isolation and depression over time (P. R. Newman & Newman, 1976).

In sum, while disidentification and schizoidentification appear to be adaptive responses on the part of individuals who find themselves in complex situations in which their groups are at least partially devalued, there are reasons to think that such responses are also mentally and emotionally taxing. In line with system justification theory, the need to disidentify with one's group or organization seems to be most acute when ratings or evaluations are seen as legitimate and widely shared. This is because it is difficult for members of devalued groups to maintain favorable images of themselves and the system at the same time (e.g., Jost & Burgess, 2000; Jost & Thompson, 2000). We argue that a similar situation arises in organizations that are highly stratified and that make heavy use of formal evaluation systems.

## Research on Organizational Stratification and Performance Evaluation Systems

In most cases, organizations are highly stratified systems. Although a lot of media attention has been given to the "flattening of the organization," and some industries such as the computer industry in Silicon Valley are run by small and relatively egalitarian teams, in most industries the wage dispersion between the CEO and the average worker has been growing steadily (see Baron & Pfeffer, 1994), increasing from a ratio of 40 to 1 in 1980 to a ratio of more than 400 to 1 by 1998 (Cassidy, 1999). Ostensibly for the sake of efficiency, chains of command are still very much in place, and evaluation systems such as "pay for performance" constantly stress differences in achievement or ability among individuals and groups, which can have extremely negative social and psychological consequences for organizational members (e.g., Pfeffer & Sutton, 2000). According to system justification theory, people develop justifications and rationalizations for social inequality and structural arrangements, coming to believe that systems and policies are largely fair and legitimate (Jost, in press). What this means is that stratification and performance evaluation systems at work will have deleterious consequences for members of devalued groups, just as they have been shown to have unfortunate consequences at school (e.g., Rosenthal & Jacobson, 1968; Steele, 1997; Steele & Aronson, 1995).

There is reason to believe, then, that many performance evaluation systems undercut the perceived worth of groups or teams. For example, many managers cite incentive pay systems, which tie large amounts of compensation (e.g., year-end bonuses, pay raises, stock options, or other perks) to predetermined performance goals such as meeting a company-wide or divisional productivity improvement goal, as a primary culprit in the devaluation of work groups. Incentive pay systems became popular in the 1980s as a means of encouraging creativity, innovation, and "healthy" competition among workers as they attempted to improve the profitability of their organizations. Yet, in most of these systems only a few teams can achieve the top performance goals, and others must settle for "average" or "below average" status. When companies reward only those employees who meet top performance goals, they may serve to devalue other workers by implicitly (or explicitly) communicating that they are inferior. As a result, recent accounts of incentive pay systems have become highly critical after little more than a decade of use. Surveys report that incentive pay promotes greed, short-sightedness, and decidedly unhealthy competition among employees (Brenner, 1995). According to an article about the failure of incentive pay systems at a small manufacturing organization:

> In the real world, pay for performance can also release passions that turn workers into rival gangs, so greedy for extra dollars they will make another gang's numbers look bad to make their own look good . . . some employees even argued over who would have to pay for the toilet paper in the common restrooms. One aspiring bean counter suggested that toilet paper costs should reflect the sexual makeup of the division, on the shaky theory that one gender uses more tissue than the other. (Nulty, 1995, p. 235)

Thus, even if members of devalued groups do not internalize a sense of their own inferiority, intergroup hostility and escalating conflict can result.

Such problems underscore the double-edged sword of performance rankings as motivators: while a few may claim the rank of "top-tier" employee, many more must suffer by comparison. This may help to explain why incentive pay systems have failed at many organizations. Research suggests that when only extreme performance is rewarded, many moderately high-level performers become dissatisfied and leave the organization (Zenger, 1992). By disappointing high-performing employees who may expect a large bonus, incentive pay systems dole out what is perceived as "punishment" to many employees (Kohn, 1993).

Pfeffer and Sutton's (2000) analysis of the "knowing-doing gap" in corporate culture documents many harmful consequences of status and power differences at work. Organizations that create internal competition among divisions, departments, and regional offices tend to foster negative feelings and poor performance in many of those groups. According to Pfeffer and Sutton (2000), many companies claim to value teamwork and collaboration but, in fact, create working environments that quickly categorize people and groups into "winners" and "losers." Pfeffer and Sutton (2000) observe that:

> Once a person, group, or division has lost in a performance contest and is labeled a "loser," research suggests that subsequent performance will be *worse*

because leaders and others will unwittingly act to fulfill the poor performance expectation. And, the loss of self-worth and motivation felt by those who are treated as losers leads to further decreases in their performance. (p. 193)

By focusing on "winning" rather than doing well, by rewarding individual performance as opposed to collaboration and team-building, and by motivating individuals to identify with their unit rather than the organization as a whole, business organizations spread conflict and resentment. In one example involving a failed merger between two restaurant chains ("Fresh Choice" and "Zoopa"), Pfeffer and Sutton (2000) observed that status differences exacerbated by a competitive culture and reward system were responsible for an overall lack of respect and cooperation. Thus, rather than learning from employees of the acquired company, managers at Fresh Choice began to derogate the people and practices of Zoopa, ultimately causing the resignation of most of Zoopa's longtime and best-performing staff.

Many of these findings, we suggest, are consistent with a system justification view of intergroup relations at work, according to which status and power differences serve to erode healthy forms of personal and social identification. When people are consistently evaluated in negative terms by leaders, bosses, and other representatives of social systems and organizations, or when they are faced with seemingly "objective" evidence of their inferiority, individuals and groups are faced with threats to their social and psychological well-being. Furthermore, if evaluation systems are highly formalized (i.e., by containing well-defined ranks or categories) and rationalized within the organization, then it may be relatively easy for people to begin thinking of themselves in terms of "inferior" category memberships. To the extent that people accept the legitimacy of systems and policies (Jost, in press; Lerner, 1980; Major, 1994; Martin, 1986), and to the extent that people behave in ways that confirm rather than challenge others' expectations of them (e.g., Rosenthal & Jacobson, 1968), performance evaluation systems can lead to a downward spiral that is self-perpetuating (Pfeffer & Sutton, 2000).

## CONCLUSION

Social identity theory has been an extremely influential theory within organizational behavior (e.g., Ashforth & Mael, 1989; Baron & Pfeffer, 1994; Dutton & Dukerich, 1991; Elsbach, 1999; Hogg & Terry, 2000; R. M. Kramer, 1991; Pratt, 1998), and for good reason. The theory is especially useful for explaining self-serving and group-serving responses to identity threat (e.g., Ashforth & Kreiner, 1999; Dutton et al., 1994; Elsbach & Kramer, 1996). Despite its many successes, we build on prior critiques of social identity theory (e.g., Abrams & Hogg, 1988; Hewstone & Jaspars, 1984; Hinkle & Brown, 1990; Jost & Banaji, 1994; Sidanius & Pratto, 1999) to challenge three of its most common assumptions: (a) the assumption of ingroup bias, (b) the assumption that members of devalued groups compensate for identity threats, and (c) the assumption of homophily.

By incorporating a system justification theory of intergroup relations (e.g., Jost, 1997, in press; Jost & Banaji, 1994), we argue that a fuller appreciation emerges of the deleterious consequences of status and power differences at work. From a system justification perspective, there is an inherent conflict among members of devalued groups between tendencies to support the legitimacy of existing hierarchies and motives to preserve individual and collective self-esteem (e.g., Jost & Burgess, 2000; Jost & Thompson, 2000). The existence of conflict and ambivalence is further supported by organizational studies addressing syndromes of disidentification and schizoidentification among members of devalued groups and organizations (e.g., Elsbach, 1999, 2000; Elsbach & Bhattacharya, 2000). Recent analyses of the effects of organizational stratification, incentive pay, and performance evaluation systems (e.g., Kohn, 1993; Nulty, 1995; Pfeffer & Sutton, 2000; Zenger, 1992) also support the contention of system justification theory that status and power differences negatively affect the well-being of members of devalued groups. As a whole, the work we integrate points to the sober conclusion that unless and until organizations are capable of developing economically viable systems and practices that stress equality and cooperation, there will be significant social and psychological costs to pay.

# 13

# Social Identification, Group Prototypicality, and Emergent Leadership

MICHAEL A. HOGG
*University of Queensland*

*L*eadership is a key feature of social groups, ranging from small groups such as families through work teams and organizations to nations. It is actually very difficult to think about groups without thinking about who leads or manages them and about how well they are led or managed. Not surprisingly, the study of leadership has long been a core concern of social scientists. The literature is enormous, stretching back to Plato and beyond. My own goal in this chapter is a modest one: to describe how social identity theory can explain some aspects of leadership (see Hogg, 1996b, 2001, in press c), and to sketch out some implications of this analysis for organizational contexts (e.g., Hogg & Terry, 2000; also see Haslam & Platow, Chapter 14 of this volume).

## SOCIAL IDENTITY AND THE FIELD OF LEADERSHIP RESEARCH

Leadership was an important focus of social psychological research for many years, particularly during the boom years of small group dynamics (e.g., D. Cartwright & Zander, 1968; Shaw, 1981), and it was a component of some of social psychology's classic research programs; see for example, Bales (1950); Hollander (1958); Lippitt & White (1943); Sherif (1966); Stogdill (1974). This tradition of leadership research culminated in Fiedler's (1965, 1971) contingency theory: the leadership effectiveness of a particular behavioral style is contingent on the favorability of the situation to that behavioral style.

During the 1970s and 1980s there was a new emphasis in social psychology on attribution processes and then social cognition (e.g., Devine, Hamilton, & Ostrom, 1994; Fiske & Taylor, 1991). These developments were associated with a very well documented decline in interest in groups (e.g., Steiner, 1974, 1986), that carried across to the study of leadership. The last edition of the *Handbook of Social Psychology* had a chapter dedicated to leadership (Hollander, 1985), whereas the current edition (Gilbert, Fiske, & Lindzey, 1998) does not. The study of small group processes and of leadership shifted to neighboring disciplines, most notably organizational psychology (Levine & Moreland, 1990, 1995; McGrath, 1997; Sanna & Parks, 1997; Tindale & Anderson, 1998).

## Social Cognition and Leader Categorization Theory

One exception to this trend has been Lord and colleagues' leader categorization theory (e.g., R. G. Lord, Foti, & DeVader, 1984; Nye & Forsyth, 1991; Palich & Hom, 1992; Rush & Russell, 1988; also see Nye & Simonetta, 1996). Based on implicit leadership theory (Hollander & Julian, 1969) and on contemporary social cognition principles, leader categorization theory states that people have preconceptions about how leaders should behave in general and in specific leadership situations. These preconceptions are cognitive schemas of types of leader (i.e., categories of leader that are represented as person-schemas) that operate in the same way as other schemas. When someone is categorized on the basis of their behavior as a leader, the relevant leadership schema is engaged to generate further assumptions about behavior. Leadership schemas vary in situational inclusiveness. Subordinate schemas apply only to specific situations, whereas superordinate schemas apply to a wide range of situations and embody very general leadership characteristics. Effective leaders are people who have the attributes of the category of leader that fits situational requirements.

This perspective treats leader categories as cognitive groupings of instances that share attributes but do not have any psychological existence as a real human group. Pol Pot, Adolf Hitler, Josef Stalin, Idi Amin, and Ghengis Khan probably share leadership attributes that place them in the same leader category, but are they really a human group in the sense of having a shared identity and a set of group membership–defining emergent normative properties? In addition, there is no analysis of the intragroup dynamics that produce leaders and followers. Leader categorization theory views leadership as a product of individual information processing, not as a structural property of real groups, nor as an intrinsic or emergent property of psychological ingroup membership.

## Organizational Psychology and New Leadership Research

Most of the activity in leadership research occurs in organizational psychology or in organizational settings (e.g., Bass, 1990a; Yukl, 1998; Yukl & van Fleet, 1992). This tradition rests on the view that leadership is a dynamic outcome of transactions between leaders and followers (Bass, 1990b; Hollander, 1985; Lord

& Maher, 1991; Nye & Simonetta, 1996): because leaders play a significant role in helping followers achieve their goals, followers bestow power and status on leaders to restore equity. Relatedly, followers may try to redress the power imbalance in groups by gaining personal information about the leader, an attribution process that imbues the leader with charisma and additional power (Fiske, 1993; Fiske & Dépret, 1996). Leaders may also accumulate "idiosyncrasy credit" with the group by conforming to group norms, subsequently allowing leaders to be innovative and effective (Hollander, 1958; Hollander & Julian, 1970).

Recent leadership perspectives focus on transformational leadership. Charismatic leaders are able to motivate followers to work for collective goals that transcend self-interest and transform organizations (Bass, 1990b; Bass & Avolio, 1993; see Mowday & Sutton, 1993, for critical comment). This focus on "charisma" is particularly evident in "new leadership" research (e.g., Bass, 1985, 1990b, 1998; Bryman, 1992; Burns, 1978; Conger & Kanungo, 1987, 1988), which proposes that effective leaders should be proactive, change-oriented, innovative, motivating and inspiring, and have a vision or mission with which they infuse the group. They should also be interested in others and be able to create commitment to the group and extract extra effort from and empower members of the group.

## Commentary on the State of Leadership Research

Recent research on leadership has mainly been conducted outside contemporary mainstream social psychology, and so has not fully benefitted from conceptual advances made within social psychology over the last 20 years, particularly the development and emerging synthesis of social cognition, group processes, and intergroup relations research. Although most perspectives on leadership now acknowledge that leadership is a relational property within groups (i.e., leaders exist because of followers, and followers exist because of leaders), the idea that leadership may emerge through the operation of ordinary social-cognitive processes associated with psychologically belonging to a group has not really been elaborated.

Instead, the most recent analytic emphasis is mainly upon (a) individual cognitive processes that categorize individuals as leaders, that is, the social orientation between individuals is not considered, and thus group processes are not incorporated, or (b) whether individuals have the charismatic properties necessary to meet the transformational objectives of leadership, that is, leadership is a matter of situationally attractive individual characteristics rather than group processes. Both these perspectives have attracted criticism for neglecting the effects of larger social systems within which the individual is embedded (e.g., R. J. Hall & Lord, 1995; R. J. Lord, Brown, & Harvey, 2001; Pawar & Eastman, 1997; also see Chemers, 2001; Haslam & Platow, Chapter 14 of this volume). Lord, Brown, and Harvey (2001) explained that leadership cannot be properly understood in terms of a leader's actions or in terms of abstract perceptual categories of types of leader and that a paradigm shift in how we understand leadership is required. Haslam and Platow (this volume) echo this concern and warn against any explanation of leadership that rests too heavily, or at all, on invariant properties of individuals and their personalities.

### Social Identity and Group Processes

These concerns about leadership research are consistent with wider metatheoretical stances concerning the explanation of group processes in general. The warning that a focus on personality, a-social cognition, and decontextualized groups does not provide an adequate explanation of group processes and the collective self is one that forms the metatheoretical context for social identity theory (see, Taylor & Brown, 1979; also see Hogg, 2001b; Hogg & Williams, 2000).

The approach to leadership taken in this chapter integrates two notions: (a) leadership is a relational property; that is, leaders and followers are interdependent roles embedded within a social system bounded by common group or category membership; and (b) leadership is a process of influence that enlists and mobilizes others in the attainment of collective goals; that is, it imbues people with the group's attitudes and goals and inspires them to work towards achieving them (e.g., Chemers, 2001; R. G. Lord, Brown, & Harvey, 2001). The integration is tackled from a social identity theory perspective that considers a group to exist psychologically when people share a collective self-definition. This approach has said a great deal about influence within psychologically salient groups, but as yet has said less about role differentiation and leadership within groups.

I do not give a detailed overview of the social identity approach here, there are already many such published overviews (e.g., Hogg, 2001; Hogg & Abrams, 1988; Hogg, Terry, & White, 1995; Tajfel & Turner, 1986; J. C. Turner, 1999), and Chapter 1, by Terry and myself, in this volume, provides such an overview. In recent years the social identity approach has been a key player in a marked revival of interest among social psychologists in the study of group processes and intergroup relations (see Abrams & Hogg, 1998; Hogg & Abrams, 1999; Moreland, Hogg, & Hains, 1994). Very recently, building on self-categorization theory (e.g., J. C. Turner, 1985), this approach has been applied to the explanation of leadership (e.g., Hogg, 1996a, 2001, in press c).

## SOCIAL IDENTITY PROCESSES AND LEADERSHIP

A key insight of the social identity approach is that the basis of self-conceptualization, perception, attitudes, feelings, and behavior is contextually fluid. Self-conception can vary from being entirely based on idiosyncratic personal attributes and the unique properties of a specific interpersonal relationship to being entirely based on a shared representation of "us" defined in terms of an ingroup prototype. The more that social cognition contextually resembles the latter, the more that the situation represents a group situation, and perceptions, attitudes, feelings, and behavior acquire the familiar characteristics of inter- and intragroup behaviors: conformity, normative behavior, solidarity, stereotyping, ethnocentrism, intergroup discrimination, ingroup favoritism, and so forth. Another way to put this is that the more that an aggregate of people is a salient basis for self-definition as a group member, the more strongly is self-definition, perception, cognition, affect, and behavior based upon prototypicality. When group membership is the salient basis of self-conception people, including self, are represented and treated in terms of the relevant in- or outgroup defining prototype. Self-categorization depersonalizes self in terms of the ingroup prototype (producing self-stereotyping, conformity, normative behavior, social attraction, social identification, and so forth), and it depersonalizes perception of others so that they are seen as more or less exact matches to the relevant prototype. Prototypicality is the yardstick of life in salient groups.

The implication of this idea for leadership is quite straightforward. As group membership becomes increasingly salient, leadership perceptions, evaluations and effectiveness are increasingly based on how group-prototypical the leader is perceived to be. Let us look in more detail at the underlying process (also see Hogg, in press a, in press c).

Where group membership is contextually or enduringly salient, people self-categorize in terms of the ingroup prototype and become depersonalized; that is, they conform to the ingroup prototype and exhibit normative behavior. In a highly salient group the prototype is likely to be relatively consensual, and thus the group as a whole appears to be influenced by a single prototype which prescribes a single norm or goal. Social identity research on conformity and social influence shows that self-categorization produces conformity to an ingroup prototype that may capture the central tendency of the group or may be polarized away from a relevant outgroup (for reviews, see Abrams & Hogg, 1990a; J. C. Turner, 1991; J. C. Turner & Oakes, 1989).

## Relative Prototypicality and Influence

Within any salient group there is a prototypicality gradient, with some members being more prototypical than others. In any given ingroup the prototypicality of a specific position in the group, and thus the person who occupies that position, can be expressed by a metacontrast ratio (the mean difference between the position and each outgroup position, divided by the mean difference between the position and each other ingroup position). Figure 13.1 shows the ingroup metacontrast distribution, on a single 17-point prototypical dimension, for a hypothetical intergroup context where individual ingroup positions are indicated by "A" through "G," outgroup positions by "O," and unoccupied positions by "-". There is a clear asymmetry within the group, with more prototypical members (higher metacontrast ratios) located towards the left. Person C is the most prototypical member but is not the average ingroup member, and marginal member A is far more prototypical than marginal member G.

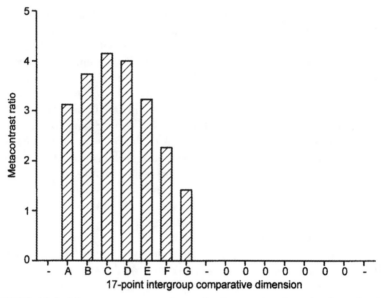

**FIGURE 13.1.** Metacontrast ratios for each of seven members (A through G) of an ingroup, in an intergroup context (17-point comparative dimension) where outgroup positions are indicated "O" and unoccupied positions "-". Comparative frame with the outgroup on the right.

Because depersonalization is based on prototypicality, group members are very sensitive to prototypicality. Prototypicality is the basis of perception and evaluation of self and other members, and thus people notice and respond to subtle differences in how prototypical fellow members are; that is, they are very aware not only of the prototype but also of who is most prototypical (e.g., Haslam, Oakes, McGarty, Turner, & Onorato, 1995; Hogg, 1993).

Within a salient group, then, people who are perceived to occupy the most prototypical position are perceived to best embody the behaviors to which other, less prototypical, members are conforming. There is a perception of differential influence within the group, with the most prototypical member appearing to exercise influence over less prototypical members. This "appearance" probably arises due to the human tendency to personify and give human agency to abstract forces—perhaps a manifestation of the fundamental attribution error (Ross, 1977) or correspondence bias (e.g., Gilbert & Malone, 1995). In new groups, this is only an "appearance" because the most prototypical person does not actively exercise influence; it is the prototype, which he or she happens to embody, that influences behavior. In established groups the appearance is reinforced by actual influence.

Where the social context is in flux, the prototype will likewise be in flux. As the prototype changes so will the person who appears to be most prototypical and thus most influential. Figure 13.2 illustrates this: it is the same ingroup distribution of people and positions as in Figure 13.1, but now the salient comparison outgroup (O) is located to the left, not the right of the ingroup. You will now see that C is no longer the most prototypical member; it is E. In addition, G who was originally the least prototypical ingrouper, is now significantly more prototypical. Under conditions of enduring contextual stability the same individual may occupy the most prototypical position over a long period and so appear to have enduring influence over the group. In new groups this person will be perceived to occupy an embryonic leadership role; although leadership has not been exercised. There is nascent role differentiation into "leader" and "followers."

So far, social identity processes ensure that as group membership becomes more salient and members identify more strongly with the group, prototypicality becomes an increasingly influential basis for leadership perceptions. However, it is important to keep this in perspective: prototypicality is not the only basis of leadership. People also rely on general and more task-specific schemas of leadership behaviors (what R. G. Lord and his colleagues call leader categories, e.g., Lord, Foti, & DeVader, 1984). However, either the importance of these schemas is unaffected by self-categorization or it diminishes as group prototypicality becomes more important. In either case, leadership schemas should become less influential *relative* to group prototypicality as group membership becomes psychologically more salient.

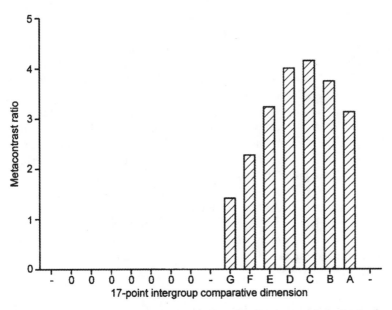

**FIGURE 13.2.** Metacontrast ratios for each of seven members (A through G) of an ingroup, in an intergroup context (17-point comparative dimension) where outgroup positions are indicated "O" and unoccupied positions "-". Comparative frame with the outgroup on the left.

## Social Attraction

Social categorization affects not only perceptions, but also feelings, about other people. Social identification transforms the basis of liking for others from idiosyncratic preference and personal relationship history (personal attraction) to prototypicality (social attraction); that is, ingroup members are liked more than outgroup members and more prototypical ingroupers are liked more than less prototypical ingroupers. Where there is a relatively consensual ingroup prototype, social categorization renders more prototypical members socially popular; that is, there is consensual and unilateral liking for more prototypical members. This depersonalized social attraction hypothesis (Hogg, 1992, 1993) is supported by a series of laboratory and field studies (e.g., Hogg et al., 1993; Hogg & Hains, 1996, 1998; Hogg & Hardie, 1991; Hogg, Hardie, & Reynolds, 1995).

From the point of view of leadership, the person occupying the most prototypical position may thus acquire in new groups, or possess in established groups, the ability to actively influence because he or she is socially attractive and thus able to secure compliance with suggestions and recommendations he or she makes. A well-researched consequence of liking is that it increases compliance with requests. If you like someone, you are more likely to agree with them and comply with requests and suggestions (e.g., Berscheid & Reis, 1998). In this way, the most prototypical person can actively exercise leadership by having his or her ideas accepted more readily and more widely than ideas suggested by others. This empowers the leader and publicly confirms his or her ability to influence. Consensual depersonalized liking, particularly over time, confirms differential popularity and public endorsement of the leader. It imbues the leader with prestige and status and begins to reify the nascent intragroup status differential between leader(s) and followers. It allows someone who is "merely" prototypical, a passive focus for influence, to take the initiative and become an active and innovative agent of influence.

Social attraction may also be enhanced by the behavior of highly prototypical members. More prototypical members tend to identify more strongly and thus display more pronounced group behaviors; they will be more normative, show greater ingroup loyalty and ethnocentrism, and generally behave in a more group-serving manner. These behaviors further confirm prototypicality and thus enhance social attraction. A leader who acts as "one of us" by showing ingroup favoritism and intragroup fairness not only is more socially attractive but is also furnished with legitimacy. According to the group value model of procedural justice, members feel more satisfied and more committed to the group if the leader is procedurally fair (Tyler, 1997; Tyler & Lind, 1992; see also Platow, Reid, & Andrew, 1998).

## Attribution and Information Processing

Prototypicality and social attraction work alongside attribution and information processing to translate perceived influence into active leadership. Attribution processes operate within groups to make sense of others' behavior. As elsewhere, attributions for others' behavior are prone to the fundamental attribution error (Ross, 1977) or correspondence bias (Gilbert & Jones, 1986; also see Gilbert & Malone, 1995; Trope & Liberman, 1993); a tendency to attribute behavior to underlying dispositions that reflect invariant properties, or essences, of the individual's personality. This effect is more pronounced for individuals who are perceptually distinctive (e.g., figural against a background) or cognitively salient (e.g., S. E. Taylor & Fiske, 1978).

We have seen that when group membership is salient, people are sensitive to prototypicality and attend to subtle differences in prototypicality of fellow members. Highly prototypical members are most informative about what is prototypical of group membership (see Turner, 1991), and so in a group context they attract most attention. They are subjectively important and are distinctive or figural against the background of other less informative members. Research in social cognition shows that people who are subjectively important and distinctive are seen to be disproportionately influential and have their behavior dispositionally attributed (e.g., Erber & Fiske, 1984; S. E. Taylor & Fiske, 1975). We have also seen how highly prototypical members may appear to have influence due to their relative prototypicality and may actively exercise influence and gain compliance as a consequence of consensual social attraction. Together, the leadership nature of this behavior and the relative prominence of prototypical members is likely to encourage an internal attribution to intrinsic leadership ability, or charisma.

In groups, then, the behavior of highly prototypical members is likely to be attributed, particularly in stable groups over time, to the person's personality rather than the prototypicality of the position occupied. The consequence is a tendency to construct a charismatic leadership personality for that person which, to some extent, separates that person from the rest of the group and reinforces the perception of status-based structural differentiation within the group into leader(s) and followers. This may make the leader stand out more starkly against the background of less prototypical followers, as well as draw attention to a potential power imbalance, thus further fueling the attributional effect.

There is some empirical support for the idea that followers tend to focus upon the leader and make dispositional attributions for that person's behavior. Fiske (1993; Fiske & Dépret, 1996) showed how followers pay close attention to leaders and seek dispositional information about leaders because detailed individualized knowledge helps redress the perceived power imbalance between leader and followers. Conger and Kanungo (1987, 1988) described how followers attributionally construct a charismatic leadership personality for organizational leaders who have a "vision" that involves substantial change to the group. Meindl, Ehrlich, and Dukerich (1985) showed that simplified dispositional attributions for leadership were more evident for distinctive leadership behaviors and under crisis conditions.

## Maintaining Leadership

Thus far we have seen how prototype-based depersonalization fairly automatically imbues the most prototypical member of a group with many attributes of leadership, for example, status, charisma, popular support, and the ability to influence. These attributes also allow the leader to actively maintain his or her leadership position. The longer an individual remains in a leadership position the more they will be socially "liked," the more consensual will social attraction be, and the more entrenched will be the fundamental attribution effect.

Social contextual changes impact prototypicality. Thus, over time and across contexts, the leader may decline in prototypicality while other members become more prototypical—opening the door, particularly under high salience conditions, to a redistribution of influence within the group. An established leader is well placed in terms of resources to combat this by redefining the prototype in a self-serving manner to prototypically marginalize contenders and prototypically centralize self. This can be done by accentuating the existing ingroup prototype, by pillorying ingroup deviants, or by demonizing an appropriate outgroup. Generally, all three tactics are used, and the very act of engaging in these tactics is often viewed as further evidence of effective leadership (e.g., Reicher, Drury, Hopkins, & Stott, in press; Reicher & Hopkins, 1996b).

Leadership endurance also benefits from consensual prototypicality because of the latter's effect on social attraction. In groups with less consensual prototypes, there is greater dissensus of perceptions of and feelings for the leader, and thus the leader may have less power and may occupy a less stable position. It is in the leaders's interest to maintain a consensual prototype. Simple and more clearly focused prototypes are less open to ambiguity and alternative interpretations and are thus better suited to consensuality. In addition, ingroup deviants serve an important function; by creating and rejecting such deviants the leader is well able to clarify the self-serving focus of the prototype (cf. Marques & Páez, 1994). Another strategy is to polarize or extremitize the ingroup relative to a specific "wicked" outgroup. These processes operate in extremist groups with all-powerful leaders.

# EMPIRICAL SUPPORT AND CONCEPTUAL EXTENSIONS

In this chapter my aim is to describe in some detail only the key components of a social identity analysis of leadership. The core idea is that as groups become more salient, leadership processes become more strongly influenced by perceptions of prototypicality that work in conjunction with social attraction and attribution processes. Concomitant extensions of this model focus on the way that prototype-based leadership in salient groups can evolve into power-based leadership, and on how social conditions of subjective self-conceptual uncertainty can produce highly focused consensual prototypes and cohesive extremist groups with hierarchical leadership structures (see Hogg, in press a, in press d; Hogg & Reid, in press).

Research is still underway to examine these extensions, as well as the attribution component. However, the central idea that group prototypicality can influence leadership in salient groups has been tested and supported. Direct tests have focused on the fundamental core prediction that as a group becomes more salient, emergent leadership processes and leadership effectiveness perceptions become less dependent on leader schema congruence and more dependent on group prototypicality. There is solid support for this idea from laboratory experiments (e.g., Duck & Fielding, 1999; Hains et al., 1997; Hogg et al., 1998; Platow & van Knippenberg, 1999) and a naturalistic field study of "outward bound" groups (Fielding & Hogg, 1997). There is also indirect support from a range of studies of leadership that are in the social identity tradition (de Cremer & van Vugt, in press; Foddy & Hogg, 1999; Haslam, McGarty, Brown, Eggins, Morrison, & Reynolds, 1998; Platow, Reid, & Andrew, 1998; Reicher & Hopkins, 1996b; van Vugt & de Cremer, 1999). There is also support for the idea that prototype-based depersonalized social attraction may facilitate leadership. There is some direct evidence from the studies by Fielding and Hogg (1997) and de Cremer and van Vugt (in press), whereas in other studies social attraction is a component of the leadership evaluation measure (e.g., Hains et al., 1997; Hogg et al., 1998).

## Limitations and Lacunae

There are a number of limitations of the proposed social identity analysis, which are currently being addressed. Most of the empirical studies have been conducted with short-lived laboratory groups under rigorously controlled experimental conditions. Although this research has been essential, there is a need to complement this research with investigations of naturally occurring groups. Organizational contexts provide an ideal opportunity for this. Another context that needs exploring is that of political and national leaders (but see Reicher & Hopkins, 1996a). One particular limitation of the laboratory studies is that they have, by necessity, focused on unidimensional prototypes (Figures 13.1 and 13.2 are a good example of this slimmed-down analog of prototypes). In reality, prototypes are, by definition, complex multidimensional representations. Leaders probably have much greater latitude to maintain power when they are located by a multidimensional prototype than a unidimensional prototype. It may be easier for leaders to acquire and maintain power by emphasizing different aspects of the prototype than by trying to keep unchanged a single group-defining attribute. Finally, the analysis proposed here is intended to apply to emergent leaders as well as to positional leadership; however, the empirical studies tend to focus on emergent leaders, and the analysis is admittedly slanted towards emergent leadership.

# SOME ORGANIZATIONAL CONTEXTS

In this final section, I want to sketch out one or two ways in which this social identity analysis may help address leadership phenomena in organizational contexts (also see Hogg & Terry, 2000). My aim is to be discursive and speculative—to raise questions and suggest directions, rather than to propose answers.

## Prototypical Leadership and Groupthink

Highly cohesive groups that are very salient may produce leaders who are prototypical but do not possess task-appropriate leadership skills. In organizational decision-making groups this may contribute to groupthink: suboptimal decision-making procedures in highly cohesive groups, leading to poor decisions with potentially damaging consequences (e.g., Janis, 1972). There is now some evidence that the critical component of "cohesiveness" associated with groupthink is social attraction rather than interpersonal attraction (Hogg & Hains, 1998; also see M. E. Turner, Pratkanis, Probasco, & Leve, 1992). If we assume that group-prototypes do not necessarily embody optimal procedures for group decision-making, then group prototypical leaders in cohesive groups may have less optimal decision making qualities than do leader schema–congruent leaders (i.e., leaders who, in this case, possess qualities that most people believe are appropriate for group decision making). This suggests that groupthink may arise because overly cohesive groups "choose" highly prototypical and thus perhaps task-inappropriate members as leaders. This implies that strong organizational identification may hinder endorsement of effective leaders, because leadership is based on group prototypicality and group prototypes may not embody effective leadership properties.

## Minorities as Organizational Leaders

Highly cohesive groups that are very salient may consolidate organizational prototypes that reflect dominant rather than minority cultural attributes and thus exclude minorities from top leadership positions. Research suggests that in Western societies, demographic minorities (e.g., people of color, ethnic minorities, women) can find it difficult to attain top leadership positions in organizations—there is a "glass ceiling" (e.g., Eagly, Karau, & Makhijani, 1995). If organizational prototypes (e.g., of speech, dress, attitudes, interaction styles) are societally cast so that minorities do not match them well, then minorities are unlikely to be endorsed as leaders under conditions where organizational prototypicality is more important than leadership stereotypicality, that is, when organizational identification and cohesion are very high. This might arise under conditions of uncertainty when, for example, organizations are under threat from competitors, a takeover is looming, or there is an economic crises, or situations where leaders, rather than mangers, may be badly needed. Thus, minorities may find it difficult to attain top leadership positions in organizations because they do not fit culturally prescribed organizational prototypes and thus are not endorsed under conditions where real leadership may be needed.

A direct test, adopting a computer-mediated laboratory analog, provides some preliminary support for this idea (Hogg, 2000a). We created ad hoc, noninteractive, virtual groups whose task was to make important decisions about undergraduate student resources. The groups were described as having a relatively agentic (male stereotypical) or a relatively communal (female stereotypical) prototype under conditions accentuating or diminishing group salience, and the male and female participants discovered that the randomly selected leader was either a male or a female. As predicted, on some measures of leader endorsement, participants with traditional sex-role attitudes (as measured by Glick & Fiske's, 1996, Ambivalent Sexism Inventory), endorsed, under high group salience, prototype-consistent leaders (male leaders in agentic groups, female leaders in communal groups) more strongly than prototype-inconsistent leaders.

## Leadership in the Context of Mergers and Acquisitions

Organizational mergers and acquisitions have a disappointingly low success rate: premerger loyalties can hinder smooth operation of the postmerger organization (e.g., S. Cartwright & Cooper, 1992a). Recent social psychological research offers an analysis in terms of social categorization processes, intergroup relations, and social identity theory (e.g., Terry & Callan, 1998; Terry, Carey, & Callan, in press; also see Gaertner, Bachman, Dovidio, & Banker, Chapter 17 of this volume; Terry, Chapter 15; van Knippenberg & van Leeuwen, Chapter 16). From a leadership perspective, merged organizations pose a particular problem, which is actually part of a broader leadership issue: Which organizational subgroup does the leader belong to (e.g., Duck & Fielding, 1999)?

From the social identity analysis presented here, we would expect that premerger organizational (subgroup) membership of the leader would be absolutely critical if premerger affiliations were highly charged, conditions that are likely to prevail given the assimilationist goal of mergers (see Hornsey & Hogg, 2000a). Organizational members would be focused on premerger (subgroup) organizational prototypes and would thus endorse a leader who was "one of us" (ingroup prototypical) and spurn a leader who was "one of them" (decidedly not ingroup prototypical). More specifically, leadership effectiveness in merged organizations would, among other things, depend on the relative levels of pre- and postorganizational identification, and the level of ingroup or outgroup prototypicality of the leader.

## Leadership and the Exercise of Power

Highly cohesive groups that are very salient may produce an organizational environment that is conducive to the exercise and perhaps abuse of power by leaders (see Hogg, in press a; Hogg & Reid, in press). Where leaders are merely prototypical they have influence over followers by virtue of being prototypical; followers automatically comply through self-categorization. It is unnecessary to exercise power to gain influence, and there are strong mutual bonds of liking and empathy between prototypically united leaders and followers that would inhibit the exercise of power in ways that might harm members of the group. However, once charisma and status-based structural differentiation gather pace, the leader becomes increasingly psychologically and materially separated from the group. This severs the empathic and social attraction bonds that previously guarded against abuse of power. A consensually endorsed status-based intergroup relationship between leader(s) (probably in the form of a power elite) and followers has effectively come into existence, and thus typical intergroup behaviors are made possible. The leader can discriminate against followers, favor self and the leadership elite, and express negative social attitudes against and develop negative stereotypes of followers

Under these conditions, leaders are likely to exercise power (in Yukl and Falbe's, 1991, sense of personal power; or Raven's, 1965, sense of reward power, coercive power, or legitimate power), and are able to abuse power, for example when they feel their position is under threat. This rigidly hierarchical leadership scenario is most likely to emerge when conditions cause groups to become cohesive and homogeneous, with extremitized and clearly delimited prototypes that are tightly consensual. In an organizational context, extreme societal or organizational uncertainty might produce these conditions (Hogg, in press d). Subjective uncertainty may produce a prototypically and demographically homogenous organization or work unit that has a hierarchical leadership structure with a powerful leader and has rigid, entrenched, and "extremist" attitudes and practices.

The progression from benign influence to the possibly destructive wielding of power is not inevitable. Conditions that inhibit the attribution of charisma and the process of structural differentiation and that reground leadership in prototypicality may curb the exercise of power. For example, if a group becomes less cohesive, more diverse, and less consensual about its prototype, followers are less likely to agree on and endorse the same person as the leader. The incumbent leader's power base is fragmented, and a variety of new "contenders" emerge. This limits the leader's ability to abuse power and renders the exercise of power less effective. Paradoxically, a rapid increase in cohesiveness, caused, for example, by imminent external threat to the group, may through a different process have a similar outcome. Cohesion may make the group so consensual that leader and group become temporarily re-fused. The empathic bond is reestablished so that the leader does not need to exercise power to gain influence, and any abuse of power would be akin to abuse of self. Emergent leaders may tend to abuse their power unless the organization is highly diverse or highly cohesive.

# CONCLUDING COMMENTS

My goal in this chapter has been to describe how the social identity approach may be able to contribute to an understanding of leadership processes. The key claim is that where group membership is psychologically salient as the basis of social categorization of self and others, ingroup prototypicality becomes the basis of leadership perceptions and endorsement, and thus leadership effectiveness. Under these circumstances, leadership schemas become relatively less important as a basis for leadership effectiveness. The processes linking social categorization to leadership are self-categorization, depersonalization, social attraction, and attribution: prototypicality lies at the heart of the analysis.

In salient groups, people are depersonalized in terms of the ingroup prototype, and thus those who are most prototypical appear to have exercised disproportionate influence. Highly prototypical members are consensually socially liked and are thus able actively to secure compliance. Highly prototypical members are figural against the background of the group, and thus their behavior (which includes popularity and perceived ability to influence) is likely to be internally attributed to stable attributes; that is, they appear charismatic. Together, these processes gradually instantiate a consensual status-based differentiation between the leader and the followers. Charisma, popularity, consensual status, and perceived ability to influence work in conjunction to provide a firm basis for effective leadership that involves other attributes such as innovation.

Stable social comparative contexts entrench prototype-based leadership, whereas changing comparative contexts provide a shifting prototype that moves the leadership spotlight onto different people as specific individuals wax and wane in prototypicality. People do not, however, bob about at the mercy of prototypicality. They can and do show agency and initiative: they can try to make themselves more like the prototype, they can redefine the prototype to look more like them, or they can accentuate or diminish the group membership salience of the followers to shift the basis of leadership perceptions towards or away from prototypicality.

Direct tests of this analysis have mostly been conducted with short-lived laboratory groups under tightly controlled experimental conditions and have mainly focused on the role of prototypicality, and to some extent social attraction. Other aspects of the analysis are currently being researched. Organizational contexts provide an ideal framework for an empirical extension to more naturalistic studies. Another context which needs exploring is that of political and national leaders. Conceptual extensions focus on the way that prototype-based leadership in salient groups can evolve into power-based leadership and on how social conditions of subjective self-conceptual uncertainty can produce highly focused consensual prototypes and cohesive extremist groups with hierarchical leadership structures. Finally, the analysis proposed here is intended to apply to emergent leaders as well as to positional leadership, however, the empirical studies tend to focus on emergent leaders, and the analysis is admittedly slanted towards emergent leadership.

There are many implications of this analysis of leadership for organizational contexts, implications which still need to be pursued conceptually and empirically. I simply sketched out one or two ideas, focusing on prototypical leadership and groupthink, minorities as organizational leaders, leadership in the context of mergers and acquisitions, and leadership and the exercise of power.

# 14

# Your Wish Is Our Command:
## The Role of Shared Social Identity in Translating a Leader's Vision into Followers' Action

S. ALEXANDER HASLAM
*University of Exeter*
MICHAEL J. PLATOW
*La Trobe University*

*A true leader is one who designs the cathedral and then shares the vision that inspires others to build it*
—Jan Carlzon, Former CEO,
Scandinavian Airline Systems

## INTRODUCTION: STATEMENT OF THE PROBLEM AND SOME TRADITIONAL SOLUTIONS

*E*xactly how the wishes of leaders get translated into the efforts of followers can be considered a master problem in the organizational field. How is it that the words and vision of an individual (or select individuals) become the wishes and actions of a multitude? What makes workers willing to "go the extra mile" in order to enact the commands of their bosses? And why do people sometimes set aside their own personal ambitions to ensure the success of someone else's?

At a practical level, the implications of solving these riddles would appear to be enormous, for they provide the key to a range of behaviors upon which organizational success depends. To name just three, these include *initiation of structure* (a leader's ability to move towards key organizational outcomes by clarifying subordinates' goals, roles, and tasks; Fleishman & Peters, 1962), *change responsiveness* (employees' willingness to embrace organizational change; King & Anderson, 1995), and *organizational citizenship* (employees' willingness to do more than is formally asked of them; Organ, 1988). These questions are important at a theoretical level, too, because they represent the nexus of the issues of leadership, power, and motivation which, despite being central organizational and social psychological topics, are rarely broached in the same theoretical or empirical treatment (Pfeffer, 1997).

Popular answers to the above questions often appeal to some special quality of a leader which allows a group to exceed expectations. These are most apparent in *personality approaches* which point to the ability of a leader's inherent *charisma* to energize and enthuse followers (e.g., Burns, 1978). According to this view, the inspirational capacity of people like Nelson Mandela, Norman Schwarzkopf, or Lee Iacocca can be traced back to their personality-based referent power. Allied with notions of *transformational leadership* (e.g., House, Spangler, & Woycke, 1991), these individuals are seen to achieve their impact through an ability to fundamentally redefine followers' goals, values, and aspirations.

Although this analysis captures important features of the leadership process, a core problem with such approaches is their lack of predictive power. Great leaders do indeed appear to transform the psychology of their followers and to be perceived by them as highly charismatic, but these phenomena appear to be *correlates* rather than *causes* of the leadership process. They are also highly contingent on social perspective and social context, so that charisma is never conferred by all of one's followers all of the time. Accordingly, Nadler and Tushman (1990) complained that "in real time, it is unclear who will be known as visionaries and who will be known as failures" (p. 80). The fact that a person's charisma can increase after their death is also highly problematic for arguments that its source lies in the individual alone (Haslam, 2001; J. C. Turner & Haslam, 2001).

Mindful of such problems, the most common way of dealing with the contextual basis of emergent charisma is to adopt a *contingency approach,* which sees leadership as the outcome of a "perfect match" between the leader's character and the situation that he or she confronts. Probably the most influential model of this form is that developed by Fiedler (e.g., 1978) in which effective leadership is seen to result from a happy marriage between the leader's style (relationship or task oriented) and the constellation of good or bad leader-member relations, high or low task structure, and the leader's strong or weak position power. Significantly, too, such models are usually favored by influential leaders themselves, so that effective management is seen as a question of having "the right person for the right job." In answer to the perennial question, "Are leaders born or made?" most commentators thus assume that the answer is "probably a combination of the two" (Sarros & Butchatsky, 1996, p. 210).

Yet while contingency models address matters of context, they still neglect those of perspective. If one were to argue, for example, that Martin Luther King Jr. was the right person to lead the civil rights movement in 1960s United

States, why did only a subset of the population respond to the dream of racial tolerance that he articulated? And why do some people in the contemporary United States continue to deny his claim to greatness?

To deal with these questions, a number of theorists have advocated a *transactional approach* to leadership which incorporates principles of social exchange. This approach is most associated with the work of Hollander (1985, 1995). His analysis focuses on the state of interdependence between leaders and followers and argues that leadership emerges from (a) the system of interpersonal relations between the two and (b) the capacity for that system to generate rewards for all those who are party to it. In Hollander's (1995) words, "Whether leadership is called transactional or transformational, the common persisting element is the significant relational nature of the intangible rewards provided to followers by leaders. This gets to the heart of motivations to follow" (p. 82).

This analysis deals with much of the subjectivity that surrounds attributions of leadership and it also highlights the role that followers play in conferring leadership on any given individual. Because it is followers who end up doing the work upon which any leader's success depends, the approach has also played an important role in recognizing *followership* as an essential component of the leadership equation. Nevertheless, as the above quotation reveals, the notions of cost and benefit upon which transactional principles depend are themselves intangible. Perceptions of mutual benefit do indeed appear to be central to leadership, but like judgments of charisma, they appear to be *outcomes* of the process that are much easier to specify after the event than before (Tyler, 1999). For example, if we look back on the events of 1978, it is possible to argue that the sense of enlightenment that Jim Jones offered the citizens of Jonestown before he orchestrated their mass suicide in the jungles of Guyana was beneficial, but it is hard a priori to see the benefits of his leadership outweighing its costs.

In short, leadership, and the organizational phenomena in which it is implicated, appears to be more than just a process of interpersonal exchange, a matter of "you scratch my back, I'll scratch yours." The key problem for social and organizational psychologists is therefore to explain what that "more" is, without resorting to some deus ex machina like charisma. Again, we are not arguing that charisma does not exist—it does. However, its explanatory potential is compromised by evidence that it is a context-dependent *consequence* of effective leadership rather than an invariant property of the individual that *causes* leader and group success (e.g., see Haslam, Platow, et al., in press; see also Hogg, Chapter 13 of this volume).

## THE SOCIAL IDENTITY APPROACH AND A THEORETICAL SOLUTION: LEADERSHIP AS THE CREATION, COORDINATION, AND CONTROL OF A SOCIAL SELF-CATEGORICAL RELATIONSHIP

As the introduction and other chapters in this book bear testament, the social identity approach offers a particularly fertile theoretical framework for examining a broad range of organizational issues (see also Haslam, 2001; Hogg & Terry, 2000; J. C. Turner & Haslam, in press). In large part, this is because the social identity and self-categorization theories that comprise the approach are both founded upon an assumption that people's group memberships (and the *psychological consequences* of those memberships) have a major role to play in shaping their reactions and contributions to social life, a role that cannot be reduced to their psychological status *as individuals* (Tajfel, 1972, 1978b). According to J. C. Turner (1982), this is because group behavior is underpinned not by people's personality or their sense of uniqueness (personal identity) but by an internalized sense of shared group membership (*social identity*).

As defined by Tajfel (1972), social identity refers to that part of individuals' self-concept associated with their membership in social groups. It is the social self (as defined by "we") rather than the personal self ("I"). Social identification reflects *depersonalized* self-categorization, such that individuals perceive their motivations and perspectives to be psychologically interchangeable with those of others who share the same social identity (J. C. Turner, 1982). Importantly, this leads to behavior that is qualitatively distinct from that which is predicated on personal identity because it is shaped by, and oriented towards, the interests of the group as a whole rather than those of the individual in isolation.

Building on these ideas, a major contribution of self-categorization theory has been to provide an analysis of *social identity salience* (Oakes, 1987; J. C. Turner, 1985; J. C. Turner et al., 1994). This specifies the processes that dictate whether people define themselves in terms of personal or social identity and, when social identity is salient, which particular group membership serves to guide behavior. In any given organization, when will employees see and act as individuals, rather than in terms of the department or team to which they belong, or in terms of the organization as a whole?

Oakes (1987) argued that social category salience is the product of an interaction between *perceiver readiness* and *fit*. One important factor that affects a perceiver's readiness to use a given social category to define themselves is *identification* with a group: the extent to which the group is valued and self-involving. Fit is the degree to which a social categorization matches subjectively relevant features of reality, so that the category appears to be a sensible way of organizing and making sense of the social world.

One component of fit is *comparative fit*. Following the principle of metacontrast (J. C. Turner, 1985), people should define themselves in terms of a particular self-category to the extent that the differences between members of that category on a given dimension are perceived to be smaller than the differences between members of that category and members of other categories that are salient in a particular context. Among other things, this implies that people will be more likely to categorize themselves as group members in intergroup than in intragroup contexts. For example, employees of Company X should be more likely to define themselves in terms of their membership of Company X if the company as a whole is focused on external rather than internal competition.

The second component of fit, normative fit, is determined by the *content* of the match between category specifications and the stimuli being represented. To represent sets of people (including the self) as members of distinct social categories, the differences between those sets must not only appear to be larger than the differences within them (comparative fit), but the *nature* of those differences must also be consistent with the perceiver's expectations about the categories. One general implication of this hypothesis is that because people are motivated to represent the self positively (Tajfel & Turner, 1979), the normative fit of a social self-category should generally be higher to the extent that it allows for *positive* self-definition. For example, employees of Company X should be more likely to define themselves as Company X members in situations where they might be proud of the company (perhaps because it has high status and is performing well) and where they feel respected by those who are representative of the organization. Support for this hypothesis is provided by Tyler (1999; in press a; H. J. Smith & Tyler, 1997; see also Haslam, Powell, & Turner, 2000).

Self-categorization theory also makes detailed predictions about the psychological and behavioral impact of social identity salience. Four of these are particularly relevant to the analysis of organizational behavior.

1. It leads individuals to see themselves as relatively interchangeable representatives of a particular social category, sharing self-defining norms, values, and goals with other members of that category (ingroup members).
2. It provides group members with a common perspective on reality that leads them (a) to expect to agree with each other on issues related to their group membership and (b) to actively seek agreement through processes of mutual influence.
3. It provides group members with motivation (and expectations of an ability) to coordinate their behavior with reference to emergent group norms (e.g., those that define the ingroup as different to and better than other groups).
4. It leads group members to work collaboratively to advance the interests of the group as a whole (their collective self-interest), even to the detriment of themselves as individuals (their personal self-interest).

Over the past two decades, self-categorization theorists have garnered extensive support for these various assertions (e.g., as broadly reviewed by Ellemers, Spears, & Doosje, 1999; Haslam, 2001; Hogg & Abrams, 1988; Oakes, Haslam, & Turner, 1994; Spears, Oakes, Ellemers, & Haslam, 1997; J. C. Turner, 1991; J. C. Turner et al., 1987). To illustrate them we can think of an individual soldier (Norman Schwarzkopf, say) who in different contexts may define himself in terms of personal identity (as an individual) or social identity (as a soldier in the U.S. Army). Now, to the extent that features of the prevailing context make Schwarzkopf's social rather than his personal identity salient (e.g., when America is at war with Iraq), he should be more likely (a) to perceive himself as having goals and values that are interchangeable with those of other American soldiers: (b) to expect to agree with those soldiers and to influence, and be influenced by; them, (c) to expect and be able to coordinate his actions with those soldiers, and finally (d) to act in a way that promotes the interests of the Army as a whole rather than fulfillment of his personal aspirations. In this last regard it is notable as a soldier on the battlefield Schwarzkopf might be prepared to lay down his life to help a comrade, while as a private citizen his activities (e.g., as a speaker on the international lecture circuit) would tend to be much less altruistic.

In this way, social identity salience can be seen to provide the psychological footing for a range of key organizational phenomena including information exchange, consensus seeking, cooperation, trust, empowerment, group productivity, and collective action (see Haslam, 2001, for a detailed elaboration of these ideas). Significantly too, these arguments also pave the way for a novel analysis of the process through which leaders and followers prove capable of mutual influence and enhancement. Applying the core lessons of the social identity approach, this suggests that for true leadership to emerge, that is, for followers to be motivated to contribute to the achievement of group goals, leaders and followers must define themselves in terms of a *shared social identity* such that the activities of each are understood in collective rather than personal terms. More specifically, we can assert that *leadership centers around the process of creating, coordinating, and controlling a social self-categorical relationship that defines what leader and follower have in common and that makes them "special."* In Reicher and Hopkins's (1996a, 1996b; Reicher, Drury, Hopkins, & Stott, in press, p. 8) terminology, leaders must be "entrepreneurs of identity." The success of their leadership hinges upon an ability to turn "me" and "you" into "us" and to define a social project that gives that sense of "usness" meaning and purpose.

## ELABORATION OF THE SOCIAL IDENTITY APPROACH: THREE PRACTICAL LESSONS

### Leaders Must Be "One of Us"

A key part of the above analysis is that leaders' capacity to evince leadership will depend upon their ability to embody those norms and values that the group they lead *shares* in any given context. One fairly straightforward implication of this analysis is that if group activities and interaction serve to emphasize what makes leaders *different* from other ingroup members in a way that undermines the collective meaning of the group, their leadership may be undermined and rendered less effective.

Paradoxically, perhaps, one process that might have exactly this effect is *leader selection*, at least if this gives rise to interpersonal competition among group members. Although it is customary to view this process as one that enhances group performance, it is possible that it might actually have the opposite effect to the extent that it invokes a state of heightened interpersonal rivalry. In part, this is because when group members vie competitively for the role of leader, consideration for the group as a whole (identified as a key determinant of leadership by Fleishman & Peters, 1962) may give way to consideration for the personal self.

This hypothesis was examined in two "random leader" studies reported by Haslam et al. (1998). In these, groups of three or four participants performed tasks that are customarily used to investigate leader effectiveness (the "winter survival task" or the "stranded in the desert task"). Groups were assigned leaders on either a formal or a random basis, or (in Experiment 2) had no leader at all. In both studies, formal leader selection involved participants completing a "leader skills inventory" in which individuals rated their own talents on a range of dimensions identified as predictors of long-term managerial success by Ritchie and Moses (1983). The appointed leader was the individual with the highest score on this measure. The impact of this manipulation was then assessed on two key indices of group productivity (after D. Cartwright & Zander, 1960): (a) the achievement of a specific group goal (in this case survival), and (b) the maintenance or strengthening of the group itself.

Our objective was not to demonstrate that the process of systematically selecting group leaders is generally counterproductive. Instead, we hypothesized that this might be the case in the particular conditions that prevailed in this study, where, in the absence of a leader being chosen, the group already had a salient social identity and was already oriented to a well-defined shared goal. This hypothesis was confirmed. In both studies the groups with random leaders outperformed those with formally selected leaders. As shown in Table 14.1, in the second study they also outperformed groups with no leaders and exhibited greater group maintenance (being more likely to adhere to a group decision when given an opportunity to defect).

These random leader studies suggest that shared social identity, and with it leaders' capacity to lead, can be eroded by activities and events that pit individuals against each other and that set leaders apart from the group they lead.

TABLE 14.1. Group performance and group maintenance as a function of leader selection strategy.

| Measure | Leader selection strategy | | |
| --- | --- | --- | --- |
| | Random | Formal | None |
| Group performance | 46.2 a | 51.7 b | 52.1 b |
| Group maintenance | 4.38 a | 6.09 b | 7.21 b |

*Note*: Different letters after means on the same measure indicate significantly different means ($p < .05$). On both measures a lower score is indicative of superior performance (less deviation from expert rankings, less deviation from group rankings).

Following on from this, we would expect that a sense of shared identity might be undermined where leaders are perceived to receive rewards (financial or otherwise) that unfairly differentiate them from their followers. In an attempt to provide some experimental evidence that would speak directly to this argument, Haslam, Brown, McGarty, and Reynolds (1998; as cited in Haslam, 2001) conducted a study that manipulated the role of individuals as leaders or followers and also the rewards that group members were led to expect as a result of their contribution to a group task.

Rewards were manipulated across three levels. Followers always received the same remuneration (3 points) but leaders were given either 3, 6, or 9 points (where each point was worth one ticket in a $100 lottery). Having been told about a particular reward structure, all participants were asked to indicate their feelings about the group and the upcoming task on a number of measures. In light of arguments derived from the social identity approach, our central prediction was that followers would be less favorably disposed to the group and less willing to exert effort on its behalf, to the extent that the reward structure differentiated (for no obvious or fair reason) between them and their leaders.

As Figure 14.1 indicates, this is what we found. Indeed, results indicated that although leaders' rewards varied across conditions, their motivation actually remained the same and that although followers received the same absolute reward in each condition, their motivation *declined* as the leader received more.

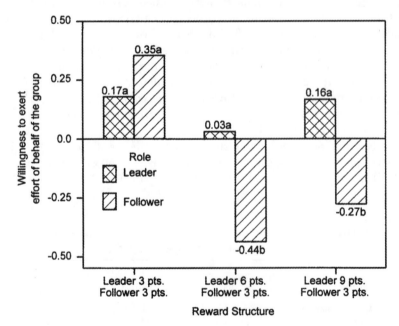

FIGURE 14.1. Willingness to exert effort on behalf of group as a function of role and reward structure (*z*-score). Note: Different letters after scores indicate significantly different means (*p* < .05).

Notwithstanding its continued appeal to senior executives, measured against Carlzon's criterion for true leadership (quoted at the start of this chapter), the strategy of increasing leader reward in order to increase group output appears to be highly problematic.

Further work elaborating the implications of these findings for actual group performance is underway, but it is worth noting that the above results are consistent with evidence that the correlation between organizational performance and the salaries of senior managers is typically very small, and in some cases negative (e.g., Hollander, 1995). Our findings also provide some empirical and theoretical support for J. P. Morgan's observation at the start of the 20th century that the only feature shared by his poorly performing clients was a tendency to overpay those at the top of the company. Moreover, Drucker's (1986, p. 14) explanation of this pattern sits comfortably with our social identity analysis:

> Very high salaries at the top, concluded Morgan—who was hardly contemptuous of big money or an "anticapitalist"—disrupt the team. They make even high-ranking people in the company see their own top management as adversaries rather than as colleagues. . . . And that quenches any willingness to say "we" and to exert oneself except in one's own immediate [personal] self-interest.

Our additional point is that when leadership *does* emerge it still taps into self-interest, but does so at a *collective* level by transforming the interests of the group into those of the self.

## Leaders Must Exemplify What Makes "Us" Better Than "Them"

The above research suggests that differences between leaders and followers can be problematic if they violate the sense of shared social identity that locks all its members into any collective enterprise. Nonetheless, it is also clear that for the most part leaders *do* differ from other group members in important ways, and that they need to. Indeed, J. C. Turner (1987b, p. 80; see also Hogg, 1996a, in press c; Reicher et al., in press; J. C. Turner, 1991) argued that in order to be the person who exerts most influence over other group members, the leader needs to be the *ingroup prototype*: the person who is most representative of the shared social identity and consensual position of the group as a whole. Following the principle of metacontrast, Turner suggested that this ingroup prototype will be the person who simultaneously exemplifies what ingroup members have in common (i.e., he or she should maximize intragroup similarity) *and* what makes them different from any comparison outgroup (maximizing intergroup difference). Principles of normative fit mean that the leader should not only make "us" feel different from "them," but he or she should make "us" feel *better than* "them" (a prediction that also follows from the general group motivation to achieve positive distinctiveness specified within social identity theory; Tajfel & Turner, 1979).

One important implication of these arguments is that the position which any leader needs to adopt in order to embody the ingroup prototype is not fixed but will vary with context (Hogg, in press c; Hogg, Hains, & Mason, 1998; J. C. Turner & Haslam, in press). In conflict with a left-wing group, leaders of middle-of-the-road political parties may have to be more right-wing (in order to maximize the interclass component of metacontrast), and in conflict with a right-wing group they may have to be more left-wing. Leaders may also need to encourage conflict with "appropriate" groups in order to shore up their own position. For example, right-wing leaders might seek to improve their leadership credentials by encouraging conflict with a left-wing group (Brown, 1988).

Support for these arguments has been provided by a large body of empirical research. In particular, it emerges from the experimental research of Hogg et al. (1998) showing, among other things, that support for a particular leader varies with manipulations of the group members' frame of reference. It emerges too from the field studies of Reicher and Hopkins (e.g., 1996a, 1996b) showing that would-be leaders tailor their political rhetoric so as to make their own views representative of a positively distinct social category. The analysis is also consistent with research by Rabbie and Bekkers (1978) and Platow and van Knippenberg (1999). In the former, leaders whose positions were insecure sought to improve their claim on leadership by engaging in conflict with an outgroup. In the latter, leaders who were nonprototypical actually gained their support only when they favored their own group over an outgroup.

Our recent work has also tested these arguments and serves to question the popular view that leader success is contingent upon possession of a particular set of attributes (in particular, leader intelligence; e.g., Stogdill, 1948; see J. C. Turner & Haslam, in press, for more detail). Haslam, Turner, & Oakes (1999; see also Haslam, 2001; J. C. Turner & Haslam, in press) reported a study in which participants had to vote for one of seven different types of business leader based on information contained in a personality profile which indicated that each leader had a different mix of dedication, intelligence, and consideration (attributes that R. G. Lord et al., 1984, identified as core to the business leader prototype). This task was completed either in a control condition or in one of six other conditions which suggested that the leader of a rival group had either an abundance or a lack of these three qualities.

Contrary to the view that followers are looking for leaders who embody a fixed constellation of traits (e.g., R. G. Lord & Maher, 1990, p. 132), the study revealed considerable variation in the pattern of voting as a function of the presumed qualities of the rival leader. Most significantly, though, when the outgroup leader was extremely intelligent, 68% of participants voted for a leader who was *un*intelligent (but dedicated and considerate), yet when the outgroup leader was also unintelligent, this same candidate was endorsed by only 20% of participants.

A more recent study replicated this pattern in a situation where students had to distribute three votes among seven potential candidates for the CEO of a company either in a control condition or one of three others in which the leader of a rival company was noted for his administrative efficiency (A), his dedication (D), or his easy-goingness (E). The seven prospective candidates had different combinations of these three attributes, having either a moderate level of all, or an abundance of one, a moderate level of another and a deficiency of the third. As the results presented in Figure 14.2 reveal, participants generally preferred the candidate who had moderate levels of all attributes—itself consistent with the argument that leaders should be more similar to other ingroup members than they are different from them (J. C. Turner, 1981). However, as predicted, in the study as a whole they were significantly more likely to vote for a candidate who had a profile that was different from that of the rival company's leader than for a candidate who had a similar profile. This pattern was particularly pronounced in followers' endorsement of a leader who was extremely dedicated, quite easy-going, but poor at administration (see the left-hand end of Figure 14.2). In the control condition this leader received at least one vote from 28% of participants, but when the rival leader was not at all dedicated this figure rose to 51% and when the rival was also extremely poor at administration it fell to 18%.

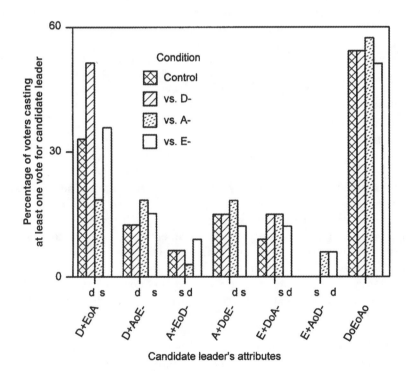

**FIGURE 14.2.** Followers' support for leader as a function of leader attributes and comparative context. Note: D = dedication, E = easy-going, A = good at administration, + = extremely, o = quite, - = not at all, d = leader has different profile from rival, s = leader has similar profile as rival.

Such findings support the general prediction that group members' preference for leaders is not a function of those leaders' qualities in the abstract. Instead, support is conditioned by followers' appreciation of a leader's qualities within a particular social comparative context. The attributes that "count" as good and worthy in a leader are partly determined by the normative expectations and theories that followers bring into any leadership situation (e.g., as suggested by R. G. Lord & Maher, 1990), but they are also contingent on their capacity to define the ingroup in a way that is comparatively and normatively fitting in the specific situation that the group confronts. Most particularly, what leaders stand for and what they do needs to contribute to a context-sensitive definition of the ingroup that allows "us" to be construed as different and better than "them"—whoever they might be.

## Leaders Must Stand Up for the Group

The previous two sections give some insight into the way in which structural features of organizations (e.g., selection processes, salary schemes, the nature of competitors) can impact upon a leader's effectiveness. It is obviously true, however, that leadership will be contingent upon what a leader actually *does*. In this regard, a major implication of the social identity approach is that leaders' capacity to marshal support for their plans and to ensure that followers act upon them will be enhanced to the extent that they are able to advance the collective interests and aspirations of the group. And because much of the demand for leadership emerges in intergroup contexts (Sherif, 1962), where an ingroup is in conflict or competition with an outgroup, it also follows that this will often involve promotion of the ingroup at the expense of an outgroup. Indeed, this prediction again follows from the motivation for positive distinctiveness and from principles of comparative and normative fit.

Initial support for these arguments was provided by Platow and colleagues, who examined the way in which group members respond to leaders who dispense justice in different ways (Platow, Hoar, Reid, Harley, & Morrison, 1997). In line with the social identity principles outlined above, the researchers argued that in intergroup contexts group members would be motivated by a desire for positive distinctiveness and hence would be more supportive of a leader who explicitly favored the ingroup over an outgroup. The research thus questioned the view that followers always respond most positively to leaders who are dispassionate and even-handed, asserting that followers may prefer leaders to be distributively *un*fair (in an ingroup-favoring way) when those leaders are charged with meting out justice to both "us" and "them."

In the first study that tested this idea, group members had to indicate their support for a leader who was observed distributing tasks to other people. Some of these tasks were easy and interesting (making word associations) and others were difficult and boring (counting vowels in a matrix of random letters). Fair allocations involved the leader giving two easy and two difficult tasks to two different people, and unfair allocation involved one person receiving four easy tasks and the other person receiving four dull tasks.

Following previous research by Tyler (e.g., 1994), Platow et al. (1997) predicted that when the two recipients were ingroup members, participants would be more likely to support the leader if she allocated tasks fairly rather than unfairly. However, this concern for fairness was expected to diminish when one of the recipients was an outgroup member. These predictions were supported (as they were in analogous research which examined procedural as well as distributive justice; Platow et al., 1998). So while even-handedness was much preferred when both recipients were ingroup members, there was no significant preference for fairness in the intergroup context. Here participants were as happy with a leader who gave all dull tasks to the outgroup and all interesting tasks to the ingroup as they were with one who assigned two dull and two interesting tasks to members of each group.

Haslam and Platow (in press) extended the above research by examining variation in followers' endorsement of a leader as a function of that leader's treatment of different members of his or her ingroup. In an initial study, participants were told about the student leader of a university student council, Chris. Chris had been given responsibility for deciding which council members to nominate for a prize from a selection of students who had adopted either a *normative* position (supporting gun control or opposing university funding cuts) or an *antinormative* position (supporting university funding cuts or opposing gun control). In different conditions participants were told that Chris had either rewarded more councilors who adopted a normative stance, more who had adopted an antinormative stance, or an equal number of normative and antinormative councilors.

In line with Platow et al.'s (1997) earlier findings, results indicated that participants perceived Chris as most fair when his reward policy had been evenhanded. But in addition, they also saw him as more fair when his policy favored ingroup members who had taken a normative line than when it favored ingroup members who had taken an antinormative line. However, support for the leader's decision was as high when he favored normative ingroup members as it was when he was fair, and in both these conditions, support was much greater than when Chris favored anti-normative ingroup members.

Both of the above studies show that followers' perceptions of leaders' behavior are conditioned by social identity concerns. Potentially more interesting, though, is the question of how knowledge of leaders' behavior shapes those followers' responses to *new* issues. A critical question here is not only whether followers express more support for a leader to the extent that he or she represents the interests of their group, but whether they show any willingness to translate that support into forms of action that help to achieve leader-defined goals. To use Carlzon's metaphor, followers may agree that a new cathedral is a good idea, but will they raise the money or lay the stones that help it to become a reality?

This line of enquiry was pursued in Platow et al.'s (1997) third experiment, which looked at the extent to which distributively fair and unfair leaders were capable of exerting *positive influence* over group members. The study's cover story suggested that a hospital CEO in New Zealand had been faced with a decision about how to allocate time on a kidney dialysis machine. He either had to allocate time to two ingroup members (long-time New Zealanders) or to an ingroup member and an outgroup member (a recent immigrant). A rationale for this decision was provided, but as well as this, in the course of indicating how the dialysis time would be allocated, the leader also stated his views about the appropriateness of internal memoranda as a means of informing employees about hospital policy.

Results on the leader endorsement measure replicated previous findings. Indeed, in the intergroup setting, participants actually favored a leader who was distributively unfair over one who was fair. Significantly though, there was also evidence that this pattern of leader endorsement extended to the internalization of the CEO's views about the appropriateness of internal memoranda. In the intergroup context, when the CEO had suggested that memoranda were a good method of communication, participants were more likely to express a similar view if he had allocated more dialysis time to the ingroup member. This pattern of influence has since been replicated by Platow, Mills, and Morrison (2000).

Similar issues were also addressed in a second study reported by Haslam and Platow (in press). In this, participants were told about Chris's reward of normative and antinormative student councilors but also that he had come up with a new plan to lobby the university to make it erect permanent billboard sites on campus. The study examined the perceived fairness of, and support for, Chris's reward policy as well as support for this new initiative. Moreover, participants were also asked to write down what they thought about Chris's decision to push for permanent billboard sites and to make open-ended comments and suggestions about the proposal. Independent coders examined the suggestions to record the number that discussed positive features of the proposal or that attempted to justify it in some way.

From the results summarized in Figure 14.2 it can be seen that, as predicted, Chris's reward policy had an impact that extended well beyond support for this initial decision. So while participants were again more supportive of a policy that was fair or that rewarded normative ingroup members than they were of one that rewarded antinormative ones, their support for Chris's new billboard campaign was also conditioned by the history of this behavior. Only when Chris had been fair or had stuck his neck out for their group in the past were followers willing to stick their hands up in support of his designs for the future.

As we have repeatedly observed, though, the key to leadership lies not in getting followers to say that they agree with your vision, it is in enjoining them to do the work that helps make that vision a reality. For this reason, the really interesting data from this study was provided by participants' open-ended reactions to Chris's billboard policy. Importantly, as the bottom panel of Figure 14.2 indicates, these provided evidence of a pattern that was quite different from

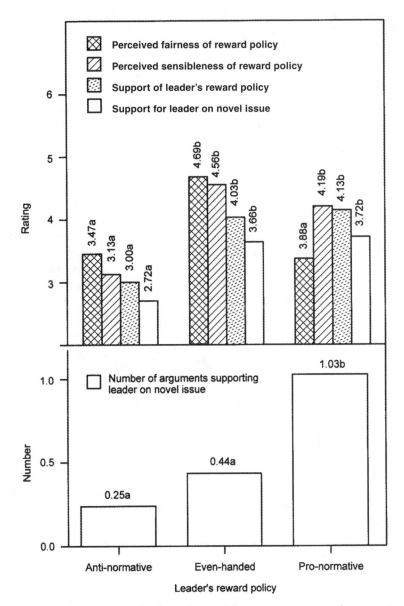

**FIGURE 14.3.** The impact of leader policy on follower perceptions and support. Note: Different letters after scores on the same measure indicated significantly different means ($p < .05$).

that observed on the measure of expressed support. Specifically, although Chris had elicited equal levels of support for his billboard policy when he had been fair or pronormative, students' willingness actually to generate arguments that supported or justified the proposal differed markedly across these two conditions. Where Chris had been pronormative, students on average generated at least one argument in support of the billboard scheme. However, when he had been antinormative *or fair*, the silence from his followers was deafening. In both conditions students provided virtually no supporting comments. Support for Chris the even-handed leader thus proved to be ephemeral and half-hearted, while support for Chris the pronormative leader was substantive and enduring. Only when he had a history of standing up for the group was the group prepared to stand up for him and *do the work* (in this case the intellectual justification and rationalization) necessary for his vision to be realized.

## CONCLUSION

The major theoretical point to emerge from the above research, and from other work conducted from a social identity perspective, is that the functioning of leaders and the emergence of leadership cannot be studied independently of the group-based social context that gives these roles and qualities expression. Our argument is not simply that the suitability of particular individuals for offices of leadership will change as a function of their circumstances (as contingency theories propose). Rather it is that *leaders and followers are transformed and energized as partners in an emerging social self-categorical relationship*. As we have attempted to show, leadership is all about the way in which this shared sense of "us" is created, coordinated, and controlled.

Accordingly, we would suggest that models that are founded solely upon an appreciation of individuals *in their individuality* (as most are) are necessarily limited. So, when we ask how it is that the vision of an individual gets translated into the actions of a group, established models allow us to appreciate the importance and size of the problem and of the explanatory gap that is to be breached, but few give us much confidence in making the leap. The primary attraction of the social identity approach is that it (a) predicts this gap as an aspect of the psychological discontinuity between interpersonal and intragroup processes (Tajfel, 1978b) and (b) explains how particular cognitive and motivational processes allow it to be traversed. Moreover, in doing this (c), it opens up a range of exciting prospects for the integrated study of leadership, motivation, and organizational behavior as a whole.

This last point appears to be particularly important in a field where it is possible to see much research (and most managerial fads) merely as "old wine in new bottles" (McGregor, 1960, p. 42; see also Chapter 11 in Haslam, 2001; Micklethwait & Wooldridge, 1997; P. Thompson & Warhurst, 1998) and where researchers like Pfeffer (1997) have continually lamented the lack of theoretical integration across topic domains. Indeed, for this reason, our analysis identifies a major leadership role for the social identity approach itself. This galvanizes the important insights of previous theorizing and urges us to explore new territory with renewed vigor and optimism.

# 15

# Intergroup Relations and Organizational Mergers

DEBORAH J. TERRY
*The University of Queensland*

*I*n an effort to become more competitive in an increasingly complex corporate environment (Dunphy & Staace, 1990; Nahavandi & Malekzadeh, 1988), mergers and acquisitions are rapidly becoming one of the most common means by which organizations seek to achieve growth and a diversification of their activity base. Cartwright and Cooper (1993) referred to the sharp increases in mergers and acquisitions that have been observed in recent years as an "unprecedented wave" of such activity (see also Shrivastava, 1986). Indeed, in 1999, Holson observed that the announced mergers involved $2.4 trillion U.S. dollars, which was the largest such value on record. However, although it is widely assumed that mergers are a potentially beneficial business practice, more than half of them fail to achieve their financial expectations (Cartwight & Cooper, 1993; Shivastava, 1986). Increasingly, the neglect of the "human" side of mergers and acquisitions has been cited as a possible explanation for many of these failures; in particular, the extent to which the merger partners can be integrated into the new organization has been recognized as a critical factor in determining the success of a merger (Cartwight & Cooper, 1993).

Despite the fact that there is a recognition that an analysis of merger failures needs to move beyond a consideration of financial and strategic fit (Cartwight & Cooper, 1993; Marks, 1988; Mirvis & Marks, 1986; Nahavandi & Malekzadeh, 1988), the extent to which the merger partners can be integrated into the new organization—a process that as been referred to as cultural fit—is not well understood. Much of the research in this area is essentially atheoretical (Nahavandi & Malekzadeh, 1988); moreover, until relatively recently, the intergroup nature of a merger situation has been neglected in research on mergers.

**229**

This is despite the clear relevance of this aspect of a merger on the extent to which the premerger organizations can be effectively integrated into the new organization. An organizational merger involves the imposition of a new organizational identity on employees (Haunschild, Moreland, & Murrell, 1994); however, embedded within this new superordinate category are the previously distinct premerger organizations. Such a situation is likely to engender competitive and antagonistic intergroup relations as a consequence of the fact that the employees of the two organizations will be motivated to establish an optimal position for their own group in the new organization. Indeed, as noted by Haunschild et al. (1994), case studies of mergers suggest that these negative intergroup behaviors and responses may jeopardize the success of the merger. There are many examples of mergers failing because of the "us" vs. "them" dynamics that occur if employees do not relinquish their old identities (e.g., Blake & Mouton, 1985; Buono & Bowditch, 1989).

This chapter considers employee responses to an organizational merger in terms of the intergroup nature of this type of organizational change, a consideration that is informed from the perspective of social identity theory (Hogg & Abrams, 1988; Tajfel & Turner, 1979; J. C. Turner, 1982—see also Gaertner, Bachman, Dovidio, & Banker, Chapter 17 of this volume; van Knippenberg & van Leeuwen, Chapter 16 of this volume). After outlining this perspective, the results of three studies examining the utility of the approach in the context of understanding employee responses to an organizational merger are briefly overviewed. The first aim of this research has been to demonstrate that intergroup rivalry does occur in the context of an organizational merger and that the nature and extent of this rivalry can be predicted from the social identity perspective. The second aim of the research has been to examine the effects of beliefs that employees hold about the intergroup relations in the new organization. From a social identity perspective, beliefs about the sociostructural characteristics of the relations between the two organizations should influence both the extent of intergroup rivalry and broader employee responses to the merger. In particular, the research has focused on perceptions relating to the permeability of the intergroup boundaries in the new organization and the role that judgments about the legitimacy of the status differences between the two organizations play in predicting employee responses to the merger situation.

## SOCIAL IDENTITY THEORY

Social identity theory (Tajfel & Turner, 1979; J. C. Turner, 1982; see also Hogg & Abrams, 1988) is a general social psychological theory of group processes and intergroup relations that addresses the social component of the self-concept, which is referred to as social identity. It derives from memberships in social groups and social categories, and contrasts with one's personal identity, which reflects one's characteristics as a unique individual. There are two underlying sociocognitive processes proposed to account for group and intergroup phenomena: social categorization and self-enhancement. Social categorization reflects the fact that when people define themselves as members of a self-inclusive social category (e.g., a sex, class, team, organization), distinctions between ingroup and outgroup members are accentuated, whereas differences among individual ingroup members are minimized (see J. C. Turner et al., 1987). Self-enhancement reflects the fact that, because the self is defined in terms of the group membership, people are motivated to favor the ingroup over the outgroup. Thus, the motivation to achieve and maintain a positive sense of self, or self-esteem, means that people tend to make intergroup comparisons that favor the ingroup, and they tend to perceive norms and stereotypes that achieve this same goal.

Central to social identity theory is the premise that, because people are motivated to enhance their feelings of self-worth, they seek to belong to groups that compare favorably with other groups or, in other words, they aspire to belong to high-status groups (Tajfel, 1974b, 1975; Tajfel & Turner, 1979). Membership in low-status groups—that is, groups that compare poorly to other groups—fails to provide members with a positive social identity, thus members of these groups should seek to gain membership in a high-status group. In contrast, members of high-status groups seek to maintain both their membership in the group and the existence of the social category. These behaviors are motivated by a desire to maintain and enhance the positive contribution that the identity makes to their self-concept (Ellemers et al, 1992; van Knippenberg, 1978; see also Zuckerman, 1979).

Laboratory studies have shown that participants assigned to a high-status group show pride in their group, identify strongly with the group, and seek to maintain their group membership (Ellemers, van Knippenberg, de Vries, & Wilke, 1988; Ellemers, van Knippenberg, & Wilke, 1990; Sachdev & Bourhis, 1987, 1991). Similar findings have been reported in field research (R. J. Brown, Condor, Mathews, Wade, & Williams, 1986). In contrast, there is evidence that memberships in low-status groups have a negative impact on strength of identification (Ellemers et al., 1990; Ellemers et al., 1993) and self-esteem (B. B. Brown & Lohr, 1987), and that members seek to disassociate themselves from such groups (Ellemers et al., 1988).

According to social identity theory, there are a number of strategies that members of low-status groups can use to improve or enhance their social identity (Hogg & Abrams, 1988; Tajfel & Turner, 1979; van Knippenberg & Ellemers, 1993). Low-status-group members may engage in individual mobility. The use of this strategy reflects efforts to seek membership in a relevant high-status comparison group. In contrast to this individualistic response, low-status-group members may engage in group-oriented or collective strategies. Social competition is one such response; it involves direct strategies to address the negative standing of the group, and to reverse the status differential that separates low- and high-status groups. Social creativity is a second collective-oriented strategy that is a cognitive response that involves making intergroup comparisons that favor the ingroup (also referred to as ingroup bias and ingroup favoritism). The aim of this strategy is to positively reevaluate the ingroup (Hogg & Abrams, 1988). To achieve this aim, intergroup comparisons may be made on new dimensions for comparison, a modification of values assigned to comparative dimensions, or the selection of a different comparison group (Hogg & Abrams, 1988; Lalonde, 1992).

There is some evidence that members of low-status groups engage in more ingroup bias than members of high-status groups (see Brewer, 1979; cf. Hinkle & R. J. Brown, 1990; Sachdev & Bourhis, 1987, 1991), a pattern of results that is consistent with Tajfel's (1974b) expectation that group differentiation is most marked when the classification is particularly salient or, in other words, personally relevant to group members. However, the status relevance of the dimensions or attributes on which ingroup and outgroup members can be judged needs to be taken into account when making predictions concerning the effects of group status on ingroup bias (see Mullen et al., 1992). As noted previously, low-status-group members may attain a positively valued group distinctiveness through the use of social creativity in their intergroup comparisons. One way in which this may be achieved involves the pursuit of positive ingroup differentiation on dimensions that do not form the basis for the status hierarchy, or which are only peripherally related to this hierarchy. Because the status-defining and status-relevant dimensions cannot be ignored (Lalonde, 1992), members of a low-status group may well acknowledge their relative inferior status on the status-relevant dimensions. However, on the status-irrelevant dimensions, that is, on those dimensions not directly related to the basis for the status hierarchy, members of low-status groups should show positive differentiation.

In contrast to members of low-status groups, high-status-group members should show ingroup bias on the status-defining dimensions (Mullen et al., 1992). This is because to do so serves to verify their dominant position in the intergroup context. Thus, among high-status-group members, ingroup bias should be more marked on status-relevant than status-irrelevant dimensions. In fact, on the latter type of dimension, a "magnanimous" outgroup bias or "reverse discrimination" effect may be evident (Mullen et al., 1992). In other words, high-status-group members may be willing to acknowledge that the outgroup is better than the ingroup on dimensions that are clearly irrelevant to the basis for the status differentiation (see also Sachdev & Bourhis, 1987; J. C. Turner & Brown, 1978).

## INGROUP BIAS IN RESPONSE TO AN ORGANIZATIONAL MERGER

The very nature of an organizational merger challenges employees' organizational identity, which serves to heighten not only the salience of the identity but also the likelihood of antagonistic intergroup perceptions and behaviors. The merger situation implies a direct confrontation between the two organizations as they both strive to optimize their position in the new organization. As noted, case studies of mergers have suggested that mergers engender "us" vs. "them" dynamics. In a laboratory study, Haunschild et al. (1994) found some further evidence of ingroup bias in the context of an organizational merger. Dyads who worked on a task together showed stronger ingroup bias when required to merge with other dyads than those dyads in the control group, who originally worked on the task alone, and hence were only nominal groups.

van Oudenhoven and de Boer (1995) observed that merger partners are unlikely to be equal in status. For this reason, the heightened salience of employees' premerger group memberships in the context of a merger is likely to mean that there is an accentuation of intergroup status differences (see Mullen et al., 1992). For employees of the lower status organization, their relative inferior status is likely to be highly salient. Thus, they should be particularly threatened by the merger situation and, for this reason, can be expected to engage in high levels of ingroup bias, particularly on the dimensions that are not central to the status differentiation. In contrast, levels of threat, particularly during the anticipatory phase of a merger situation, are likely to be lower for the employees of the high-status organization in comparison to the low-status employees. However, in an effort to verify their superior status in an unstable intergroup context, these employees are likely to engage in more ingroup bias than the low-status employees on dimensions that are central to the basis for the status differential.

For both the low-status and high-status employees, levels of threat associated with the merger should be positively related to ingroup bias. Among members of the low-status organization, high levels of threat are likely to be associated with efforts to attain a positive social identity through ingroup bias on status-irrelevant dimensions. A similar effect, but on the status-relevant rather than the status-irrelevant dimensions, should be evident for the members of the high-status organization. The more threatened high-status employees are about the merger situation, the more they should be motivated to reassert their superiority on status-relevant dimensions, an expectation that is predicated on the basis that a threatening intergroup context is likely to engender identity protection strategies among high-status-group members (Tajfel, 1975; van Knippenberg & Ellemers, 1993).

In a study of an organizational merger, Terry and Callan (1998) examined the interplay among premerger organizational status, perceived threat associated with the merger, and ingroup bias. Data were collected from 1,104 employees of two hospitals intending to merge—a high-status metropolitan teaching hospital and a relatively low-status local area hospital. To assess ingroup bias, participants indicated the extent to which they agreed that each of the two organizations (their own premerger organization and the other organization) could be described as possessing nine different characteristics. Preliminary discussions with healthcare workers indicated that three of the dimensions were status-relevant: high prestige in the community, challenging job opportunities, and high variety in patient type. In general, the other five dimensions were regarded as being peripheral to the basis of the status differential between hospitals. These dimensions included little industrial unrest, good relations among staff, good communication by management, relaxed work environment, and modern patient accommodation.

It was proposed that the employees of the low-status hospital would, overall, engage in more ingroup bias than the employees of the high-status hospital, particularly on the status-irrelevant dimensions. On the status-relevant dimensions, it was expected that the employees of the high-status hospital would engage in more ingroup bias than the employees of the low-status hospital. As expected, employees of the low-status hospital did engage in more ingroup bias, overall, than the employees of the high-status hospital. This result was qualified by a significant interaction between status and the type of dimension (status-relevant or irrelevant). As shown in Figure 15.1, ingroup bias among the low-status employees was evident only on the status-irrelevant dimensions. In contrast, on the status-relevant dimensions, they acknowledged the superiority of the high-status hospital. The opposite pattern of results was obtained for the high-status employees. Among these employees, there was evidence of ingroup bias on the status-relevant dimensions and bias in favor of the outgroup on the status-irrelevant dimensions.

The results of the research supported the expectation that the low-status employees would engage in more ingroup bias than the high-status employees, particularly on the status-irrelevant dimensions. Because of the possibility that the differences that emerged may have reflected accurate judgments of the

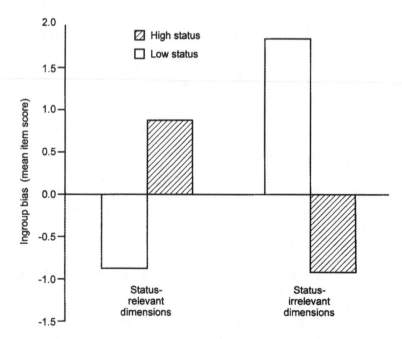

**Figure 15.1.** Ingroup bias on the status-relevant and status-irrelevant dimensions for employees of low-status and high-status organizations.

differences between the two hospitals, rather than actual bias, the absolute amount of differentiation exhibited by the high-status and low-status employees on the status-relevant and status-irrelevant dimensions was compared. This analysis showed that the amount of bias (in favor of the ingroup) exhibited by the low-status employees on the status-irrelevant dimensions exceeded the extent of differentiation (in favor of the outgroup) acknowledged by the high-status employees. On the status-relevant dimensions, there was no such difference: The amount of differentiation (in favor of the ingroup) exhibited by the high-status employees was the same as the amount of differentiation (in favor of the outgroup) acknowledged by the low-status employees. Thus, the difference between the groups in terms of levels of ingroup bias on the status-relevant dimensions appeared to reflect accurate (or at least agreed upon) differences between the groups and supported the identification of the larger hospital as the higher status hospital, whereas the difference observed on the status-irrelevant dimensions reflected ingroup bias among the low status employees.

As expected, employees from the low-status organization appraised the anticipated merger as more threatening than the employees of the high-status organization. Moreover, there was evidence, in line with predictions, of a positive relationship between appraised stress and intergroup differentiation on the status-irrelevant dimensions among the employees of the low-status organization, but not for the high-status employees. Thus, the more the employees of the low-status organization were threatened by the merger, the more likely they were to engage in ingroup bias on the status-irrelevant dimensions.

Adopting an intergroup perspective, Terry and Callan's (1998) study was designed to examine employee responses to an organizational merger. As predicted, and in line with results of case studies of organizational mergers, the research revealed clear evidence of intergroup differentiation in the context of an anticipated merger between two organizations. Although previous case studies have suggested that mergers between two previously independent organizations may fail because of the "us" vs. "them" dynamics that arise in such circumstances, such dynamics had not been documented in previous empirical research on employee responses to organizational mergers. In fact, the intergroup dimension of this type of organizational change has largely been neglected in previous research. Terry and Callan found clear evidence of ingroup bias, particularly among the low-status employees. Thus, the research provides quantitative support for the suggestion that intergroup rivalry is likely to be engendered in the context of an organizational merger.

As expected, there was more evidence of ingroup bias and heightened levels of threat among the low-status employees who should, as a consequence of the heightened salience of their relatively inferior status in the context of the impending merger, have been particularly motivated to differentiate themselves positively from the employees of the other organization. This pattern of results accords with the social identity perspective, as does the finding that organizational status interacted with type of dimension on which the two organizations were rated. For the high-status employees, there was a tendency to rate the ingroup as better than the outgroup on the status-relevant dimensions, whereas the low-status employees engaged in ingroup bias on the status-irrelevant dimensions. These results presumably reflected the motivation of the employees of the high-status organization to acknowledge their position of relative superiority in the new organization. In contrast, the low-status employees—presumably motivated by a desire to attain positive social identity—exhibited ingroup bias on the dimensions not centrally relevant to the basis for the status differences among hospitals.

On those items on which they did not show ingroup bias, the employees of both the low- and high-status hospital did not simply rate the two hospitals equally, they acknowledged the strengths of the other group. Thus, the low-status employees acknowledged the superior status of the high-status hospital, whereas the high-status employees exhibited a magnanimous outgroup bias on the status-irrelevant dimensions, an effect that has been demonstrated in previous research (Mullen et al., 1992). On the status-relevant dimensions, both groups of employees agreed that the high-status group was superior, and the extent to which this was acknowledged did not vary as a function of which employees provided the ratings. Thus, these results suggest that the employees of the high-status group were not engaging in any ingroup bias on the status-relevant dimensions. Instead, the evidence of ingroup bias among the high-status employees on these dimensions can be regarded as reflecting an accurate assessment of the superiority of their hospital, given that it was also acknowledged by the members of the low-status organization. There was, however, clear evidence of ingroup bias among the low-status employees. The amount of ingroup bias that the low-status employees exhibited on the status-irrelevant dimensions exceeded the extent to which the high-status employees were willing to acknowledge the strengths of the low-status employees on these dimensions. This pattern of results presumably reflects efforts by the low-status employees to achieve a positive group distinctiveness in the unstable context of an organizational merger.

## STATUS, PERMEABILITY, AND EMPLOYEE RESPONSES TO AN ORGANIZATIONAL MERGER

In addition to considering the role of group status on ingroup bias, subjective beliefs concerning the intergroup context are, according to social identity theory, critical to an understanding of intergroup relations. Fundamental to social identity theory is the distinction between social structures in which the strategy of individual mobility is possible and structures in which the predominant belief is that the boundaries between groups are impermeable, thus precluding individual mobility (Tajfel, 1974b; Tajfel & Turner, 1979). Group members' judgments concerning the extent to which social boundaries that separate their own group from another group can be crossed reflect perceptions of permeability. Impermeable group boundaries are those that are considered to be in a closed or a fixed state, whereas permeable boundaries are proposed to exist when group members feel that they can pass freely from one group to another. Permeable intergroup boundaries mean that group members perceive that they have access to the opportunities that are afforded to members of the other group.

According to social identity theory, the extent to which the boundaries that separate their own group from the high-status group are perceived to be permeable is a critical determinant of the strategy that members of low-status groups choose to adopt to improve their social identity (see also D. M. Taylor & McKirnan's, 1984, five-stage model of intergroup relations for a similar argument). When intergroup boundaries are perceived to be open or permeable, the dominant response of low-status-group members is likely to be one of individual mobility. In contrast, when intergroup boundaries are perceived to be relatively impermeable, low-status-group members should use collective strategies in order to satisfy their motivation to enhance their social identity. As noted above, one such strategy is social creativity or, in other words, ingroup-favoring intergroup differentiation on dimensions that are not related directly to the basis for the status differentiation (Tajfel, 1974b; see also Lalonde, 1992; Terry & Callan, 1998).

There is empirical evidence that the extent to which intergroup boundaries are perceived to be permeable influences the way in which members of low-status groups deal with their inferior social identity. S. Wright, Taylor, and Moghaddam (1990) found that the perceived intergroup permeability was negatively related to participants' willingness to engage in a collective protest (see also D. M. Taylor, Moghaddam, Gamble, & Zellerer, 1987, & Ellemers et al., 1993), a pattern of results that Lalonde and Silverman (1994) found was most marked when the social identity was made salient. There is also evidence for a link between perceived permeability and social creativity. Lalonde (1992) found that members of a team placed last in a competitive league (i.e., a low-status group in a low permeability situation) engaged in ingroup bias on the attributes not related to performance.

Members of low-status groups—attuned to opportunities to enhance their identity—are likely to respond favorably to conditions of high permeability (see also Zuckerman, 1979). Thus, low-status-group members are driven by identity enhancement motives. In contrast, high-status-group members are driven by identity protection motives (Tajfel, 1975; van Knippenberg & Ellemers, 1993). Thus, members of high-status groups are likely to respond negatively to such a situation because of the threat that open group boundaries poses to their high-status-group membership. In support of this supposition, Ellemers et al. (1988) found that permeable group boundaries reduced ingroup identification among low-status-group members, but there was some evidence of an associated increase in identification among members of the high-status group. In a subsequent study, Ellemers et al. (1992) found evidence of status protection strategies among high-status-group members, but only if the group was a minority group.

In an effort to examine the role that perceptions of intergroup permeability plays in the context of an organizational merger, Terry, Carey, and Callan (in press) conducted a study of pilots involved in an airline merger. It was proposed that employees of the low status premerger organization who perceived the intergroup boundaries to be highly permeable would be better adjusted to the merger (on both person- and job-related outcome measures), less likely to engage in ingroup bias (a collective response), and be more likely to identify with the new organization (reflecting the opportunity for individual mobility) than low-status employees who perceived the intergroup boundaries to be relatively impermeable. For the employees of the high-status premerger organization, motivated by a need for social identity protection, an opposite pattern of results was predicted. The high-status group membership should be regarded positively; however, it was proposed that the salience of the intergroup context engendered by the merger situation would mean that the situation would be a source of threat if the group boundaries were perceived to be permeable. Specifically, it was proposed that, when intergroup boundaries were perceived to be relatively open, employees of the high-status premerger organization would exhibit poor adjustment to the merger, high levels of ingroup bias, and weak identification with the new organization.

The merger involved two previously independent airline companies, one of relatively high status (an international carrier) and one of relatively low status (a domestic carrier). Respondents were 465 employees of the fleet staff (pilots and flight engineers) from the newly merged airline who ranged in age from 25 to 60 years old. Ingroup bias was assessed by asking participants to indicate the extent to which they agreed that each of the two premerger organizations (their own premerger organization and the other organization) could be described as having eight different characteristics. A measure of ingroup bias was obtained by averaging the difference scores (ingroup rating minus outgroup rating) obtained for each item. Preliminary pilot work distinguished between dimensions only peripherally related to the basis for the status differentiation between an international and a domestic airline (good communication skills, administrative efficiency, capable and hard-working employees, providers of quality services, helpful and cooperative, and friendly attitude) and those that are centrally relevant to this status differential (technical expertise and professional attitudes). Commitment to the new organization and job satisfaction were assessed as job-related outcomes, whereas emotional well-being and self-esteem were assessed as person-related outcomes. Strength of identification with the new organization was also assessed. Perceptions of the permeability or openness of the intergroup boundaries in the new organization were assessed using three items developed for use in the research, e.g., "If you wanted to, how easy would it be for you to become involved in the activities and work previously done by members of the other premerger organization?"

As expected, employees of the low-status premerger organization were less strongly identified with the new organization than the high-status employees. There was also evidence that employees of the low-status premerger organization were less committed to the new organization and were less satisfied with their job than employees of the high status premerger organization. There were, however, no differences in scores on the person-related outcomes (self-esteem and emotional well-being). As in the study of the planned hospital merger, ingroup bias among the low-status employees was more marked on the status-irrelevant dimensions than on the status-relevant dimensions, whereas the opposite pattern of results was evident for the high-status employees (see Figure 15.2). However, in contrast to Study 1, both groups favored the ingroup over the outgroup on both types of dimensions. In other words, there was no evidence of a magnanimous outgroup bias among the high-status group on the status-relevant dimensions, nor was there evidence that the low-status group members acknowledged the superiority of the high-status group on the status-defining dimensions. Given that relations between merger partners are likely to be more competitive and antagonistic after the merger has formally taken place than during the anticipatory phase, it is not surprising that there was stronger evidence of ingroup bias in the airline merger than in the hospital merger (Terry & Callan, 1998).

As expected, perceptions of permeability influenced employees' responses to the merger. In relation to identification, organizational commitment, and job satisfaction, there was a positive relationship between perceived permeability

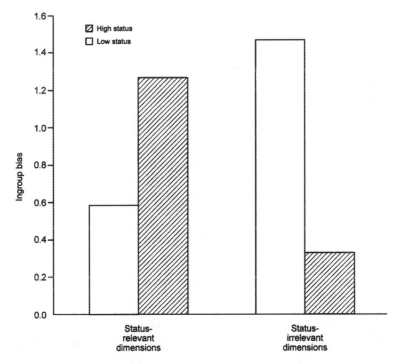

**Figure 15.2.** Ingroup bias on status-relevant and status-irrelevant dimensions for employees of low-status and high-status premerger organizations.

and scores on each of these outcome variables for low-status-group members but not for the high-status-group members. Similar results were found on the person-related outcomes: For the employees of the low status group, the perception that the intergroup boundaries in the new organization were relatively permeable was associated with higher self-esteem and better emotional well-being. There was also, as expected, evidence that high levels of perceived permeability were associated with poorer emotional well-being and lower self-esteem for members of the high-status premerger organization (the findings for self-esteem are shown in Figure 15.3).

Overall, the findings are in accord with social identity theory in that they show that an inferior group membership—a comparison that is likely to be heightened in a merger situation—has a negative impact on a person's social identity and means that affective responses to the group in terms of such variables as pride or commitment to the group and satisfaction with the group are reduced (see also R. J. Brown et al., 1986; Ellemers et al., 1993; Sachdev & Bourhis, 1991). Overall, employees of the low-status organization identified less strongly with the new organization than the high-status employees, engaged in more ingroup bias, had lower levels of job satisfaction, and were less committed to the new organization.

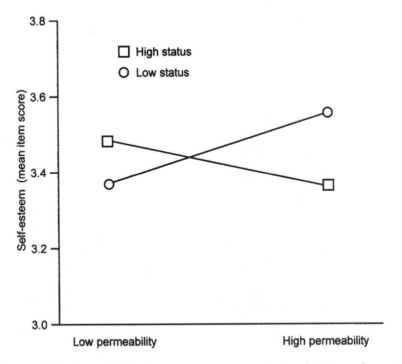

Figure 15.3. Interaction between premerger organizational status and perceived permeability on self-esteem.

The fact that the evidence of ingroup bias among the low-status employees was most evident on the dimensions of comparison only peripherally related to the basis for the status differentiation provides further support for social identity theory and is in accord with the findings reported by Terry and Callan (1998) in the context of a planned merger between two hospitals. According to social identity theory, the need for low-status group members to establish a positively valued group distinctiveness can be met through the use of social creativity, such as the pursuit of positive ingroup differentiation on dimensions other than those that form the basis for the status hierarchy. Because it is difficult to ignore their relative inferiority on the latter dimensions (Lalonde, 1992), members of a low-status group are not likely to exhibit positive differentiation on such dimensions. For the employees of the high-status premerger organization, the difference in levels of ingroup bias between status-relevant and status-irrelevant dimensions is also consistent with social identity theory. By exhibiting bias on the status-defining dimensions, members of high-status groups are able to verify their dominant position. In the study of the airline merger, members of the high-status premerger organization showed weakened ingroup bias on the status-irrelevant dimensions rather than a magnanimous outgroup bias (see Mullen et al., 1992), which presumably reflects the operation of a status-protection motive engendered as a consequence of the threat associated with the organizational merger.

On a range of empirically distinct measures of employee responses to an organizational merger, there was consistent evidence that the effects of premerger organizational status were moderated by the perceived permeability of the intergroup boundaries in the new organization. In accord with social identity theory, there was clear evidence that the perception that the intergroup boundaries in the new organization were permeable was positively associated with more favorable responses to the merger among employees of the low-status but not the high-status premerger organization. Consistent with the basic premise of social identity theory, these findings indicate that the dominant strategy of members of low-status-group members faced with a clearly superior group is one of individual mobility if the intergroup boundaries are perceived to be relatively open. In the pursuit of identity enhancement, low-status employees, who perceived that the intergroup boundaries in the new organization would be permeable, appeared to transfer their allegiance to the new organization, presumably reflecting a disidentification with their premerger organization.

On the person-related outcomes, there was, in addition to the proposed positive relationship between permeability and adjustment among the low-status employees, some support for the prediction that, among the employees of the high-status premerger organization, perceptions of group permeability would be negatively associated with employee adjustment. In accord with social identity theory, these findings indicate that members of high-status groups are motivated by identity protection and, as a consequence, are threatened by permeable intergroup boundaries. Research in laboratory settings has provided only weak evidence of status protection motives among members of high-status groups (Ellemers et al., 1988; Ellemers et al., 1992), possibly because the transient group memberships typically invoked in such settings do not engender such motives. The fact that the negative relationship between perceived permeability and adjustment among the high-status employees was evident only on the person-related outcome variables suggests that the detrimental effects of a perceived threat on high-status group memberships is evident only on person-related outcomes. This pattern of results is not inconsistent with the central premise of social identity theory, namely, that people derive a positive sense of self-worth, and presumably also emotional well-being, from high-status-group memberships.

## STATUS, LEGITIMACY, AND EMPLOYEE RESPONSES TO AN ORGANIZATIONAL MERGER

According to Tajfel (1974b, 1975), the extent to which group members perceive their status position to be legitimately attained is an additional sociostructural belief that should be an important determinant of group members' identity management strategies. Specifically, high-status group members who perceive their status position to be legitimate, that is, as a deserved outcome of a just procedure, are likely to react to the threat of a merger more negatively than those who view their status position as less legitimate (R. Brown, 1995). Dominant group members who feel that their status position is legitimate are likely to react in a negative manner to the possibility that the intergroup status relations may change as a consequence of the merger, presumably because they believe their superior status position to be deserved (see Tajfel & Turner, 1979).

In contrast, low-status-group members who perceive their status position to be a legitimate outcome of a just procedure are likely to be more accepting of a merger situation than those who perceive that it is an illegitimate reflection of the group's relative standing. The perception that their low-status position is legitimate is undesirable, and hence employees who feel this way are likely to react more positively to the merger because of the possibility that the situation may facilitate individual mobility attempts. On the other hand, the perception of an illegitimately low-status position may engender the behavior and responses that are more typically observed in members of high-status groups. In other words, an illegitimately low-group status is likely to give rise to mutual solidarity (i.e., strong ingroup identification) and hence a negative reaction to the threat of an organizational merger

Research has shown that members of groups perceiving an illegitimately low-status position do display behavior that is usually observed among high-status group members, such as relatively strong ingroup identification and ingroup-favoring discrimination in reward allocation (R. J. Brown & Ross, 1982; Caddick, 1982; Ellemers et. al., 1993; J. C. Turner & Brown, 1978). There is also evidence that low-status-group members are more likely to engage in collective status improvement when the situation is perceived to be illegitimate, whereas individual action is more likely when the status differential is perceived to be legitimate (Lemaine, 1974; Moghaddam & Perreault, 1991; Taylor et al., 1987). Thus, there is some support for the proposal that low-status-group members who perceive their status position to be a legitimate outcome of a just procedure are likely to be more accepting of a merger situation than those who perceive that it is an illegitimate reflection of the group's relative standing. In contrast, little empirical attention has focused on the effects of perceptions of legitimacy on the intergroup behavior and responses of members of high-status groups; however, J. C. Turner and Brown (1978) did find that members of high-status groups were most biased towards low-status groups when the status hierarchy was perceived to be unstable (which is relevant to an organizational merger) but legitimate.

To examine the interplay between relative group status and judgments about the legitimacy of the group's status position in the context of an organizational merger, a study of the merger between two previously independent scientific organizations—one of relatively high status, in terms of research performance, budget, and viability, and one of relatively low status—was undertaken (Terry & O'Brien, in press). First, it was proposed, once again, that members of the low-status group would show the most negative responses to the merger. Both individual outcomes (perceived threat and job satisfaction) and group-related outcomes (identification with the merged organization, common ingroup identity, and intergroup anxiety) were assessed. Second, it was proposed that the employees of the low-status group would exhibit higher levels of ingroup bias on dimensions not directly relevant to the basis for the status differentiation than the employees of the high-status organization, but that employees of the high-status group would exhibit the most ingroup bias on the status-relevant dimensions. Third, it was proposed that the effects of premerger group status would be moderated by employees' perceptions of the legitimacy of the status differential between the two groups. Specifically, it was anticipated that for members of the low status premerger group, high levels of perceived legitimacy would be related to low levels of status-irrelevant ingroup bias and more positive responses to the merger, whereas the opposite was proposed for the high-status employees; for these employees, it was anticipated that high levels of legitimacy would be associated with high levels of status-relevant ingroup bias and more negative responses to the merger.

Respondents were 120 employees of the newly merged organization who ranged in age from 20 to 64 years old. The sample comprised approximately equal numbers of employees from the two premerger organizations. A single item measure was used to assess the legitimacy of their group's status position: Participants indicated on a 7-point scale whether their perceptions of their group's status reflected the way things should be. To assess ingroup bias, participants indicated the extent to which they agreed that each of the two premerger organizations (their own premerger organization and the other organization) could be described as having 10 different characteristics. Six items reflected dimensions that are relevant to the status differential between scientific organizations (e.g., scientific excellence, scientific diversity, project accountability), whereas the three items focused on dimensions not related directly to the basis for the status differentiation (administrative efficiency, good communication skills, professional attitudes). Subscales based on these results were used to examine levels of bias across status-relevant and status-irrelevant dimensions.

The outcome measures included measures of strength of identification with the merged organization (e.g., "How much do you identify with the new organization") and common ingroup identity (e.g., "At work, despite the different divisional backgrounds, it usually feels as though we are all just one group"; see Gaertner, Dovidio, & Bachman, 1996). Anxiety in response to intergroup contact was also assessed (see Stephan & Stephan, 1985), as was job satisfaction and perceived threat associated with the merger. As expected, participants from the high-status premerger organization identified more strongly with the new organization than the employees of the low-status organization. Employees of the low-status premerger organization were also less likely to perceive a common ingroup identity than employees of the high-status premerger organization and they appraised the merger as more stressful. There was also a weak tendency for employees of the high-status organization to be more satisfied with their job than the employees of the low status organization. Thus, the third study replicated the finding that, overall, employees of the low status premerger organization are likely to react most negatively to the merger situation.

As in the previous studies, ingroup bias varied as a function of whether or not the dimension was central to the basis of the status differentiation (status-relevant) between scientific organizations or more peripheral (status-irrelevant). Ingroup bias among the low-status employees was more marked on the status-irrelevant dimensions than on the status-relevant dimensions, whereas the opposite pattern of results was evident for the high-status employees. These results were in accord with predictions; however, in accord with the findings of the airline study, both groups engaged in significant bias on both types of dimensions, presumably because of the fact that the intergroup relations in the context of an organizational merger are likely to be more antagonistic after the merger has formally taken place than in the anticipatory phase of the merger (see Terry & Callan, 1998). It was expected that threat would relate to differentiation on the status-relevant dimensions for the high-status employees and to differentiation on the status-irrelevant dimensions for the low-status employees. In line with predictions, the positive relationship between perceived threat and ingroup bias on the status-relevant dimensions was significant for the employees of the high-status organization but not for the low status employees. In contrast, perceived threat was positively related to ingroup bias on the status-irrelevant dimensions for the employees of the low-status premerger organization, but not for employees of the high-status organization.

As expected, there was consistent evidence—on a range of empirically distinct measures of employee responses to an organizational merger—that the effect of premerger organizational status was moderated by the perceived legitimacy of the status differentiation in the new organization. There were significant status by legitimacy interactions on each of the measures of employee responses to the merger, but not on the measures of ingroup bias. In accord with social identity theory, the perception that the basis for the status differentiation was legitimate was associated with positive responses to the merger (in terms of scores on the measures of identification, common ingroup identity, job satisfaction, and weakly on the measure of threat) among the employees of the low-status organization, but with negative responses to the merger among the employees of the high-status group. This result was evident on the measures of ingroup anxiety, common ingroup identity, and perceived threat (the latter two results were relatively weak). The fact that the status by legitimacy interaction was not evident on the measures of ingroup bias was unexpected. It is possible that the unstable nature of relations in the merged organization, combined with the fact that negotiations concerning the nature of the new organization were still being conducted, meant that the extent of ingroup bias was not influenced by perceptions of legitimacy.

The consistent link between perceptions of legitimacy and acceptance of the merger among the employees of the low-status premerger organization accords with previous research (e.g., R. J. Brown & Ross, 1982; Ellemers et. al., 1993; Moghaddam & Perreault, 1991; J. C. Turner & Brown, 1978). Because the perception of an illegitimately low-group status is likely to give rise to mutual solidarity and collective attempts to change the status quo, it should be associated with low acceptance of the merger. In contrast, the perception that a low-status position accurately reflects the group's lack of capacities (Ellemers et al., 1993) is likely to give rise to acceptance of the new organizational structure, given that it may offer options for individual mobility. For the high-status premerger group, the observed results are consistent with the expectation that dominant group members who feel that their status position is legitimate are likely to react in a negative manner to the possibility that the intergroup status relations may change, presumably because they believe their superior status position to be deserved (Tajfel & Turner, 1979; see also J. C. Turner & Brown, 1978). The fact that the evidence linking perceptions of legitimacy to responses to the merger among the employees of the high-status organization was relatively weak is not surprising, given that the threat associated with the merger was most marked for members of the low-status group, and hence their responses to the situation are particularly likely to be influenced by perceptions of the sociostructural characteristics of the intergroup context.

## CONCLUSIONS

Taken together, the research reviewed in the present chapter provides strong support for the assertion that employee responses to an organizational merger can be usefully understood from an intergroup perspective and, more specifically, from the perspective of social identity theory. As such, the results extend the laboratory work of Haunschild et al. (1994) by showing the relevance of this perspective in the context of a number of actual organizational mergers. More specifically, the research reveals clear evidence that the nature and extent of intergroup rivalry in the context of an organizational merger can be predicted from the social identity perspective, and that, in line with this perspective, the relative status position of an employee's premerger organization and his or her beliefs concerning the nature of the relations between the two groups have an important role to play in predicting employees' responses to a merger situation.

Overall, the results of the present research add to a growing body of literature that has supported the importance of adopting an intergroup perspective and, more specifically, a social identity perspective, in research on employee responses to an organizational merger (see Haunschild et al., 1994; Mottola et al., 1997; Terry & Callan, 1998; see also Gaertner et al., Chapter 17 of this volume; van Knippenberg & van Leeuwen, Chapter 16 of this volume). Theoretically, the results of the research are important to the extent that they help to clarify the effects of group status, perceived permeability, and perceptions of the legitimacy of the status differential on responses to an unstable intergroup context, an area that, to date, has been limited by its reliance on laboratory studies—a focus that may have mitigated against revealing evidence of status protection motives among high-status group members. The present results also have implications for the understanding of the interplay among group status, perceived threat, and ingroup bias. Despite the large amount of empirical attention that has been conducted on ingroup bias, the relations among these variables are not well understood (see Mullen et al., 1992).

The applied significance of the present research derives from the social significance of protecting the well-being of employees and the effectiveness of organizations involved in mergers. Increasingly, it is being recognized that employee responses to a merger may account for the frequent failure of this type of organizational change (e.g., Mirvis & Marks, 1986). Indeed, recent commentators have pointed to the need to move beyond a consideration of financial and strategic fit in the implementation of a merger to a focus on the extent to which the two organizations can achieve "cultural fit" in the new organization (e.g., Mirvis & Marks, 1996; Nahavandi & Malekzadeh, 1988). Central to whether the new partners can be effectively integrated into the new organization or, in other words, whether cultural fit can be attained, is a consideration of the intergroup dynamics that are likely to be engendered in the context of an organizational merger. The results of the present research point to the fact that intergroup rivalry is likely to be observed in this context, presumably as a consequence of the motivation of both groups of employees to optimize the position of their new group in the newly merged organization. In order to reduce the intergroup rivalry and the other negative employee responses observed in the present research, newly merged organizations should engage in efforts to encourage the development of common ingroup identity. Facilitating intergroup contact in a supportive normative environment that emphasizes cooperative interdependence is one way in which this may be achieved (Gaertner et al., 1993), as may efforts to increase the salience of a relevant outgroup or competitor, such that "us" reflects the superordinate identity of the new organization rather than the self-inclusive premerger organization and "them" resides outside rather than within the new organization (Haunschild et al., 1994).

# 16

# Organizational Identity After a Merger:
## Sense of Continuity as the Key to Postmerger Identification

DAAN VAN KNIPPENBERG
*University of Amsterdam*
ESTHER VAN LEEUWEN
*Leiden University*

*T*he great psychological impact of mergers and acquisitions on the people involved has long been recognized. A loss of psychological attachment to the organization is often cited as one of the major psychological consequences of mergers (e.g., Buono, Bowditch, & Lewis, 1985; Cartwright & Cooper, 1992b; Dutton et al., 1994; Schweiger & Walsh, 1990; Schweiger & Weber, 1989). In this chapter, we focus on the social identity processes affecting postmerger organizational identification, to address among other things the *why* of this lowered attachment (see also Gaertner et al., Chapter 17 of this volume; Terry, Chapter 15 of this volume). We present a model of postmerger identification that highlights the intergroup dynamics that may affect identification in organizational mergers, and discuss empirical findings in support of the model. First, however, we briefly discuss the theoretical framework on which our analysis is based.

## SOCIAL IDENTITY, SELF-CATEGORIZATION, AND ORGANIZATIONAL MEMBERSHIP

The social identity approach embodied by social identity theory (Hogg & Abrams, 1988; Tajfel, 1978a; Tajfel & Turner, 1986) and self-categorization theory (J. C.

Turner, 1985; J. C. Turner et al., 1987) may be described as a theory of intergroup relations (Tajfel & Turner, 1986), a theory of the self (J. C. Turner et al., 1994), but perhaps best as a theory of psychological group membership. The social identity approach outlines how through self-categorization, individuals define themselves as members of social categories and ascribe characteristics that are typical of these categories to the self. Self-categorization leads individuals to perceive themselves in terms of the characteristics they share with other members of their ingroups. This conception of the self as a group member provides a basis for the perceptual, attitudinal, and behavioral effects of group membership. The more an individual conceives of the self in terms of the membership of a group, that is, the more the individual identifies with the group, the more the individual's attitudes and behavior are governed by this group membership (Hogg & Abrams, 1988; Tajfel & Turner, 1986; J. C. Turner et al., 1987).

Applying this approach to membership in organizations, Ashforth and Mael (1989) proposed that through organizational identification organizational membership reflects on the self-concept just as (other) social group memberships do (see also Dutton et al., 1994; Haslam, 2001; Hogg & Terry, 2000; Pratt, 1998; A. van Knippenberg, van Knippenberg, van Knippenberg, & van Knippenberg, 2000). Organizational identification thus reflects "the perception of oneness with or belongingness to an organization, where the individual *defines* him or herself in terms of the organization(s) in which he or she is a member" (Mael & Ashforth, 1992; p. 104). Because identification with a social category engenders a tendency to think in terms of that category membership, identification leads to activities that are congruent with that identity. As a consequence, higher levels of organizational identification are associated with a higher likelihood that employees will take the organization's perspective and will act in the organization's best interest (Ashforth & Mael, 1989; Dutton et al., 1994; D. van Knippenberg, 2000). Identification has, for instance, been proposed to lead to ingroup cooperation (R. M. Kramer, 1991; Tyler, 1999), organizational citizenship behavior (Dutton et al., 1994), support for the organization (Mael & Ashforth, 1992), increased task performance (van Leeuwen & van Knippenberg, 1999), and lower likelihood of turnover (Abrams et al., 1998; Mael & Ashforth, 1995). Therefore, the ability to elicit a certain level of identification can be considered to be important to an organization's functioning.

## IDENTIFICATION AFTER A MERGER

In view of the suggestion that employee identification is often at stake in mergers and acquisitions and the proposed importance of organizational identification, it seems a highly relevant question what factors affect postmerger identification. Obviously, we may expect factors that have been shown to more generally affect organizational identification to also be related to identification after a merger (for a discussion of these factors, see, e.g., Ashforth & Mael, 1989; Dutton et al., 1994; Pratt, 1998), but their influence is not unique to mergers. In this chapter, in contrast, we present a social identity analysis of mergers that focuses on factors that are unique to the context of mergers and acquisitions.

We are definitely not the first to analyze mergers from a social identity (or "social categorization" or "intergroup") perspective (e.g., Blake & Mouton, 1985). Prior analyses have, however, focused on intergroup relations between the merger partners and not on postmerger identification. Thus, even though it is not the first social identity analysis of mergers and acquisitions, our analysis makes a unique contribution by its focus on postmerger identification. However, because research on intergroup relations in mergers and acquisitions yields insights that may be relevant to the study of postmerger identification, we first review this line of research before we present our analysis of postmerger identification.

## MERGERS AS ARENAS FOR INTERGROUP CONFLICT: THE PROBLEM OF CREATING A NEW GROUP

Mergers inevitably entail the confrontation of two social groups, the employees of the merger partners. Every intergroup encounter has the potential to elicit intergroup biases, prejudice, and stereotyping (e.g., Brewer & Miller, 1996; Tajfel, 1978a; Tajfel & Turner, 1986). Mergers are no exception. Indeed, a social identity analysis suggests that mergers may be especially likely to elicit intergroup biases and intergroup conflict. The merger itself is likely to make the membership in the own premerger organization salient, and may thus bolster the link between the self and the premerger identity (cf. Haslam, 2001; J. C. Turner et al., 1987). Moreover, mergers and acquisitions are likely to be perceived as a threat to the group's way of life (Buono et al., 1985), and identity threats have been associated with an increase in intergroup discrimination and hostility (e.g., Branscombe & Wann, 1994). It is therefore not surprising that case studies of mergers show that mergers are often arenas for intergroup conflict. Several researchers have noted that merged organizations are often faced with an "us versus them" mentality among their employees (e.g., Blake & Mouton, 1985; Buono et al., 1985; Haunschild et al., 1994; Terry & Callan, 1998). Buono et al. (1985), for example, described a bank merger in which the employees of both merger partners regarded the other organization as an "invading enemy" that took over their organization. Employees tended to attribute difficulties arising within the merged organization to the other bank, negative stories about the merger partner circulated in each organization prior to the official coming together, and each group was defensive about "their way" of doing things and considered their way superior to that of the merger partner.

In social identity terms, these findings show that employees of merged organizations tend to act on the basis of their premerger identity (i.e., their membership in their premerger organization) rather than on the basis of the identity implied by the merger (i.e., their membership in the merged organization). This conclusion is corroborated by Graves (1981), who concluded in a study of a merger of two firms of brokers that the main problem of the merger seemed to be to replace the old organizational boundaries by new organizational boundaries, that is, to establish a shift from perceptions in premerger terms to perceptions in terms of the new, unified entity. This tendency to hold on to the old organizational identity is likely to fuel the "us versus them" mentality so often quoted to cause problems in mergers. Arguably, if employees acted on the basis of their new organizational identity, they would not display hostility towards the merger partner: the merger partner would not be perceived as another group that threatened the own way of life, but as part of the own group. More recent work by Gaertner and colleagues (e.g., Gaertner et al., 1993) yielded direct evidence in support of this proposition. In a series of experiments, Gaertner et al. demonstrated that the perception of two merged groups as one single entity rather than as two distinct entities (i.e., the merger partners) is associated with reduced bias towards the other group. Later studies have shown that this conclusion extends to the perception of the aggregate as two groups within a larger whole (for a review, see Gaertner & Dovidio, 2000), suggesting that the crucial factor here is the perception of the larger whole as an entity rather than not perceiving two groups. These perceptual representations of the situation have been shown to be contingent on conditions of contact such as equal status, cooperative intergroup interaction, opportunities for personal acquaintance, and egalitarian norms (Gaertner et al., 1993; Gaertner & Dovidio, 2000).

This body of research suggests that the extent to which a merged organization is perceived as a single entity is of crucial importance for intergroup relations within the merged organizations. The higher the organization's *entitativity* ("the degree of having the nature of an entity, of having real existence," Campbell, 1958, p. 17; for recent discussions of entitativity, see Brewer & Harasty, 1996; Hamilton & Sherman, 1996), the lower the intergroup biases between the merger partners. Indeed, Gaertner, Dovidio, and Bachman (1996) reported a study in which perceptions of the organization as one single group were found to attenuate intergroup biases in evaluations of the merger partners.

Although Gaertner et al.'s (1996) findings and the more general framework Gaertner and colleagues present are highly relevant to mergers and acquisitions, they concern intergroup relations and not identification with the superordinate entity (e.g., the merged organization). From the perspective of the present discussion, the most interesting question is how all this relates to postmerger identification. Is there a link between perceptual representations of the merged organization (i.e., organizational entitavity) and identification? Self-categorization theory posits that people do not need to interact or be in each other's presence to be a psychological group, that is, to perceive themselves as a group (e.g., you may perceive organizational behavior researchers as a group without knowing all the people in this group). Conversely, being in each other's presence, interacting, and even being interdependent, does not automatically turn an aggregate of people into a psychological group (J. C. Turner et al., 1987). This implies that it is the psychological reality and not the physical reality of a group that is essential for its ability to elicit identification. In other words, organizational entitativity (i.e., its psychological reality) should be positively related to organizational identification. Indirect evidence for this proposition may be found in a scenario study by Mottola et al. (1997). When presented with a merger scenario, participants' anticipated commitment to the merged organization (i.e., they were to suppose that they would be involved in the merger) was contingent on the extent to which they anticipated that they would see the merged organization as a single entity (the effect of entitativity was mediated by perceived threat). Although this is a study of commitment and not of identification (cf. Ashforth & Mael, 1989) and involves a hypothetical rather than an actual merger, these results do corroborate the proposition that postmerger identification is contingent on organizational entitativity. Below, we discuss more direct evidence for this proposition. First, however, we discuss what is probably the central concern in postmerger identification: the relationship between premerger and postmerger organizational identities.

## IS IT STILL MY GROUP?:
## THE IMPORTANCE OF A SENSE OF CONTINUITY

Organizational entitativity may be an important precondition for organizational identification, but that does not mean that people will identify with an organization when it is perceived as a single entity. Other factors are required as well (for a discussion of the antecedents of organizational identification, see Ashforth & Mael, 1989; Dutton et al., 1994; Pratt, 1998). Most of these are not specific to mergers and should not have a greater effect on members of merging organizations than of other organizations. A factor that is of special concern in mergers, is a *sense of continuity*.

From a social identity perspective, a merger can be construed as a recategorization of two social groups as one new group. On the one hand, this new group (i.e., the merged organization) is not entirely new, because it incorporates the organization where the individual worked before the merger. From this perspective, one might expect a transfer of identification with the premerger organization to identification with the merged organization (i.e., a positive relationship between premerger and postmerger organizational identification). On the other hand, it is new, because the merged organization incorporates another, "new," group, the merger partner. From this perspective, there is no compelling reason to expect a strong relationship between premerger and postmerger identification. A merger thus implies a change of group membership, because the group's organization is combined with another organization, but at the same time implies a continuation of an existing group membership, because the premerger organization is part of the merged organization. This continuity suggests that identification may transfer from premerger to postmerger situation, that is, that postmerger identification might to a large extent be a function of premerger identification. Yet, anecdotal evidence suggests that after a merger, employees often feel that the organization has changed so much that "it is no longer their company," and that it sometimes seems to employees as if they in fact have switched jobs and moved to another organization rather than gone through a phase of transition and change with their own organization. Change seems not to be the issue here. Rather, what employees seem to miss is the feeling that, despite all the changes, they are still working for essentially the same organization they worked for before the merger. As Rousseau (1998) put it in her discussion of organizational identification in times of change:

> Sameness is not a required feature of identity; rather, what is required is a sense of continuity. Because identification entails the expansion of psychological boundaries in mental models of self, the very formation of identity implies the capacity to change and adjust, both throughout the life cycle and throughout the course of one's relationship with a firm. (p. 227)

A sense of continuity may in fact be the crucial moderating variable in the process of transferring from premerger to postmerger situation, and thus in the relationship between premerger and postmerger organizational identification. The more the individual feels that the merged organization is a continuation of the premerger organization, the more the basis for identification with the organization remains unchanged, and the more identification may be unaffected by the merger.

## ORGANIZATIONAL DOMINANCE AND SENSE OF CONTINUITY

As Rousseau's (1998) discussion suggested, change per se may not be the issue here. Even though organizational change may affect the sense of continuity, employees are generally aware of the fact that organizations need to change and that the work itself and the way the work is structured cannot remain unchanged forever. Rather, mergers may imply discontinuity because they may carry with them the suggestion that the merged organization is predominantly a continuation of the *other* organization. Even though mergers as opposed to acquisitions in principal involve equal partners, the distinction between mergers and acquisition is in practice primarily a legal one. Most mergers are, from a psychological perspective (i.e., as opposed to a legal perspective), to a certain extent takeovers (Cartwright & Cooper, 1992b). Although the merger partners may pay lip service to the notion of equality, one partner generally dominates the other because it is larger, richer, more viable, or otherwise more powerful and influential than its partner (cf. Rentsch & Schneider, 1991). Indeed, several researchers make a distinction between mergers (of equal partners) and acquisitions (where one partner dominates the other) within what are legally speaking mergers (e.g., Hogan & Overmyer-Day, 1994). These differences in *organizational dominance* may play in important role in determining how the merger is experienced.

Because of its "acquiring" role, the dominant organization is likely to be more influential in determining the shape of the merged organization than the dominated organization. Thus, the merged organization is more likely to be shaped in the image of the dominant organization than of the dominated organization. This makes the change from premerger to postmerger situation smaller for employees of the dominant partner, who find themselves a member of an organization that is very similar to their premerger organization, than for employees of the dominated partner, who are more likely to find themselves in an organization that is quite different from their own premerger organization. Perhaps of even more importance, and possibly irrespective of the size of the changes, is the notion that the dominance asymmetry may work to communicate to the employees of the dominant organization that the merged organization is "their" organization, whereas it may communicate to the employees of the dominated partner that "they are now a member of the other organization." As a consequence, employees of a more dominant partner are more likely to have a sense of continuity than employees of a more dominated partner. Thus, for employees of the dominant organization, there is a clear link between premerger and postmerger organizational membership. For employees of the dominated organization, on the other hand, premerger and postmerger organizational membership are not so closely related, because they are more likely to have experienced the merger as an actual change of group membership. This suggests that premerger identification is more likely to transfer to postmerger identification for members of more dominant organizations than for members of more dominated organizations.

## DIFFERENCES BETWEEN THE MERGER PARTNERS AS A THREAT TO CONTINUITY

Differences between the merger partners may also play an important role in post-merger identification. Differences between the merger partners, especially cultural differences, are among the factors most often cited as causing problems on the "psychological side" of a merger (e.g., Buono et al., 1985; Cartwright & Cooper, 1992b; Hogan & Overmyer-Day, 1994; Nahavandi & Malekzadeh, 1988). Partners may differ in the way they do the work (or, indeed, in the work they do), in styles of leadership or interpersonal interaction, in beliefs and values, etc. To the extent that merging forms a threat to identity because one (believes one) has to adjust to the merger partner's ways (cf. Buono et al., 1985), interorganizational differences may exacerbate this threat, because they suggest a greater discontinuity between premerger and postmerger identity. As argued above, this greater discontinuity should be associated with lower levels of identification. According to the same reasoning, interorganizational differences should primarily introduce discontinuity for members of dominated as opposed to dominant organizations, because dominant partners should be more able to maintain their identity-defining features. As a consequence, differences between the merger partners should be related to postmerger identification primarily for members of dominated as opposed to dominant organizations.

## A SOCIAL IDENTITY MODEL
## OF POSTMERGER IDENTIFICATION

We may summarize our theoretical analysis in a model of postmerger identification that reflects the core concern with continuity (i.e., the relationship between old and new organizational identities) and relates this concern to two key aspects of the relationship between the merger partners: organizational dominance and perceived interorganizational differences. This model is displayed in Figure 16.1. Organizational dominance plays a key role in determining postmerger organizational identification, because it is associated with a sense of continuity. This should be evident both in a stronger relationship between premerger and postmerger organizational identification for members of the dominant as opposed to the dominated partner and in a stronger relationship between perceived differences between the merger partners and postmerger identification for members of the dominated as opposed to the dominant partner. In the following, we present results from our research on postmerger identification that provides a test of the proposed relationships.

## EMPIRICAL SUPPORT FOR THE MODEL: FIELD STUDIES

We studied the proposed moderating role of organizational dominance in the relationships between premerger and postmerger identification and perceived

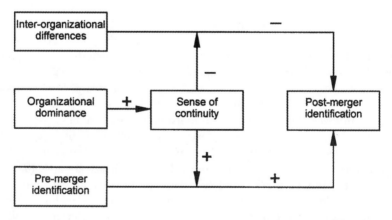

FIGURE 16.1. A social identity model of postmerger identification.

interorganizational differences and postmerger identification in two surveys of merged organizations (D. van Knippenberg, van Knippenberg, Monden, & de Lima, in press). For the first study, we conducted a survey of the employees of the administrative organization of a recently merged town government (i.e., two towns merged to form one new town and, as a consequence, the organizations representing the town governments were also merged). We assessed perceived differences between the merger partners and premerger and postmerger identification with a questionnaire. One of the merger partners clearly dominated the other (e.g., this organization was approximately 10 times as large as the other, and gave its own name to the newly formed organization), allowing us to examine the role of organizational dominance (i.e., former membership of the dominant vs. dominated organization). The second study aimed to replicate the results of the first study, but with a different type of organization (a merged institute for secondary education) and a different basis for organizational dominance (the merger partners were of equal size, but the one partner needed the merger for its survival, while the other could take the role of savior, and thus take a dominant position; Rentsch & Schneider, 1991). The second survey incorporated the same measures as the first.

In both studies, we observed important differences between members of the dominant and members of the dominated organization. First, in Study 1, postmerger identification was lower than premerger identification, but only for members of the dominated organization, whereas in Study 2 postmerger identification was lower than premerger identification for members of both organizations, but more so for members of the dominated organization. This corroborates the proposition that identification is at stake for members of dominated organizations in particular, presumably because they experience a greater discontinuity. Second, premerger organizational membership (i.e., dominant vs. dominated partner) moderated the relationships of premerger identification and perceived interorganizational differences with postmerger identification, as our model predicts. For members of the dominant partner, premerger and postmerger identification were positively related in both studies, suggesting that identification was transferred from premerger to postmerger organization. For members of the dominated partner, premerger and postmerger identification were unrelated (Figure 16.2 provides a graphic representation of this interaction from one of the studies). Perceived differences were negatively related to postmerger identification, but only for members of the dominated organization (Figure 16.3 provides a graphic representation of this interaction from one of the studies). These findings corroborate the model's proposition that organizational dominance affects postmerger identification (i.e., through its influence on sense of continuity), because it moderates the transfer of premerger to postmerger organizational identification and the impact of perceived differences between the merger partners.

The finding that organizational dominance moderates the relationships of perceived differences and premerger identification with postmerger identification supports our proposition that differences in sense of continuity foster stron-

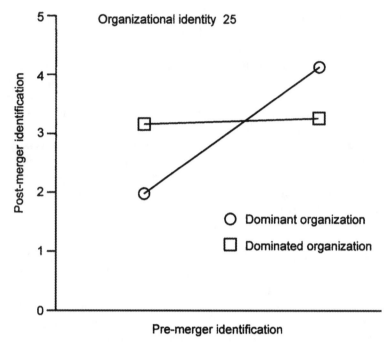

**FIGURE 16.2.** Postmerger identification as a function of premerger identification and organizational dominance; van Knippenberg et al. (in press), Study 1.

ger identification of employees of more dominant as compared with more dominated organizations. Sense of continuity was, however, not measured, but inferred from premerger organizational membership. In a follow-up study (van Knippenberg & Groeneveld, 1999) we did assess sense of continuity directly. In this study, we focused on work-group identification rather than organizational identification, because the work group is the primary setting where organizational life takes place and therefore likely to be the more important target of identification (D. van Knippenberg & van Schie, 2000; cf. Ashforth & Mael, 1989; Moreland & Levine, 12000). We focused on the prediction that postmerger identification with the work group is contingent on the extent to which one feels that the postmerger work group is a continuation of one's premerger work group. Because we did not assess premerger identification in this study, we predicted a main effect of sense of continuity rather than the moderating effect predicted earlier (i.e., at a given level of premerger identification, postmerger identification should be stronger, the stronger the sense of continuity).

In a survey of the employees of recently merged health care organizations, we assessed the extent to which employees felt that their own premerger work group was continued in the postmerger work group (with items like "the work group I now work in really is a continuation of the work group I worked in

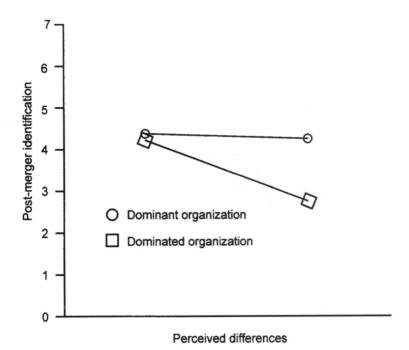

**FIGURE 16.3.** Postmerger identification as a function of perceived interorganizational differences and organizational dominance; van Knippenberg et al. (in press), Study 2.

before the merger" and "I have the feeling that with the creation of [new organization] the work group in which I worked ceased to exist"). Although the merger could be considered to be a merger of equals, we anticipated that there would be differences between work groups in the extent to which the work group was seen as a continuation of the premerger work group (i.e., even in a merger of equals, one of the merger partners may be "locally dominant," being more powerful and influential within a given division, department, or work unit).

Because sense of continuity should at least to some extent have an objective basis (i.e., be based on "real" continuity and discontinuity between premerger and postmerger situation), it should to some extent be shared by all members of the same premerger organization within a work group. That is, sense of continuation is not statistically independent for individuals from the same premerger organization within the same work group. As a consequence, analysis at the individual level is inappropriate. Therefore, we treated within–work group subgroup (i.e., members from the same premerger organization within the work group) as the unit of analysis rather than the individual respondent. Subgroup means of sense of continuity were entered in a regression analysis, together with three control variables (premerger organizational membership, department, and percentage of employees from premerger organization in the work group), as predictors of work-group identification (measured with the van Knippenberg et al., in press, identification scale adapted to the work-group level; cf. van Knippenberg & van Schie, 2000). Results of this analysis indicated that sense of continuity ($\beta = .30, p < .01$) was significantly related to work-group identification. These findings are important for two reasons. First, they yield direct evidence for the role of sense of continuity rather than the indirect evidence from the D. van Knippenberg et al. (in press) study. Second, they demonstrate that our conceptual framework extends to work-group identification after a merger.

We also argued that postmerger identification is related to organizational entitativity. To test this prediction, we also assessed entitativity in the three studies reported above (at the organizational level in the first two studies, at the work group level in the third). As predicted, entitativity was related to identification in all three samples (cf. Mottola et al., 1997). Because one might argue that differences between the merger partners render the premerger categorization salient and are therefore detrimental to organizational entitativity, we also explored the possibility that perceived differences were related to entitativity and that entitativity mediated the relationship of perceived differences with identification. Perceived differences were negatively related to entitativity, as expected, but entitativity did not mediate the relationship of perceived differences with postmerger identification. Entitativity was also unrelated to organizational dominance (i.e., there was no indication that entitativity mediated the effects of dominance). Finally, principal components analysis in the third study indicated that the sense of continuity and entitativity measures represented separate constructs, and regression analysis indicated that the two construct had independent relationships with identification. Thus, although entitativity is related to identification as predicted (corroborating the importance of perceptual representations as proposed by Gaertner and colleagues), entitativity plays no role in our proposed model of the relationship between premerger and postmerger organizational identities (i.e., our model is distinct from the model proposed by Gaertner and associates).

## ELIMINATING AMBIGUITY: EXPERIMENTAL EVIDENCE

Even though the field studies support our model of postmerger organizational identification, these studies have two important drawbacks. First, as they are all correlational, they are by necessity mute regarding causality. Second, causality set aside, because of the richness and uncontrollability of the field settings, there may be explanations other than self-categorization and social identity processes for the observed relationships (e.g., relative standing rather than a continuation of one's organizational identity might cause the effect of organizational dominance; cf. Hambrick & Cannella, 1993). To resolve these issues, we need findings from controlled experiments in which the social categorization variables of interest are manipulated and other influences are placed under experimental control.

Because the social identity analysis suggests that the relationships discussed here hold even for minimal groups (cf. Tajfel, 1978a; J. C. Turner et al., 1987), and studying intergroup processes in a minimal group setting is the obvious way to exclude the influence of other group membership–related variables (Tajfel, 1970), we (van Leeuwen, van Knippenberg, & Ellemers, 2000a) designed two experiments along the lines of the minimal group paradigm (Tajfel, 1970, 1978). We suggested to our participants that they were a member of one of two four-person teams (a red team and a blue team) that would work on a computer-mediated group task (a brainstorming task). In reality, all participants were assigned to the blue team. These teams were symbolically represented on the computer screens of all participants during the premerger phase of the experiment. In addition, participants were told that for each team a computer file was created that would be used to store the ideas generated during the brainstorm task. After participants had worked on the group task in separate cubicles, we measured identification with the premerger team.

In Experiment 1, half of the participants were told after the first task that they would proceed to a second brainstorming task with their four-person group (no merger condition). The other half of the participants were informed that the next brainstorm task required a larger team and that for that purpose the two teams would be combined into one eight-person team (merger condition). After participants were led to believe either that they continued to work in the team from the first task or that they now worked in a newly merged team, participants performed the second task. At the end of the task, identification was again assessed (i.e., with the four-person team in the no merger condition and with the merged team in the merger condition). This first experiment aimed to establish that merging indeed introduces a discontinuity of identity. Predictions were straighforward: In the no-merger condition, Time 1 identification and Time 2 identification were expected to be strongly related, whereas in the merger condition both identifications were expected to show a weaker relationship. As displayed in Figure 16.4, this is exactly what we found.

The aim of Experiment 2 was to extend these findings in two ways. First, we aimed to show that an experimental manipulation of the extent to which the own premerger group was represented (i.e., continued) in the merger group would affect the relationship between premerger and postmerger identification. Second, we expected to establish that this effect would be mediated by the extent to which the merged group was perceived to be a continuation of the premerger group. We focused on merger conditions only and created three conditions that varied in the extent to which participants' premerger team was represented in the postmerger team. In the low-representation condition, participants were told that the computer had randomly selected their blue team to be dissolved and the members to be added to the red team. This postmerger red team, now existing of eight persons, was symbolically represented on participants' computer screens during this postmerger phase of the experiment. In addition, participants were now given access to the red team's file on the laboratory server. In the high-representation condition, members of the red team were added to participants' blue team in a similar vein. In the equal representa-

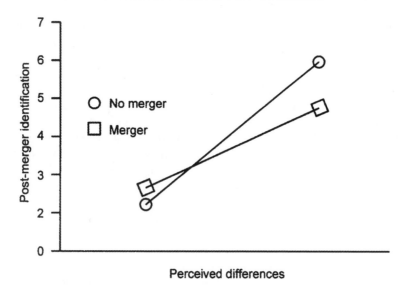

FIGURE 16.4. Time 2 identification as a function of Time 1 identification and merging; van Leeuwen et al. (2000a), Experiment 1.

tion condition, a new team was created out of the members of the red and blue premerger teams. This team was referred to as the purple team, and a new file was created for this team to which all participants were given access. As in Experiment 1, identification was assessed before and after the merger. As predicted, the relationship between premerger and postmerger identification was contingent on representation within the merger group. High and equal representation yielded strong relationships between premerger and postmerger identification, whereas these two identifications were unrelated in the low-representation condition (see Figure 16.5). In addition, perceptions of the extent to which the merger group was a continuation of the own premerger group were found to mediate this effect.

These experimental findings support the conclusion that merging introduces a discontinuity of identity and that the magnitude of this discontinuity is the *cause* of the stronger or weaker relationship between premerger and postmerger identification. In addition, the minimal group setting of the study excludes alternative explanations for the effects of the continuation of one's group identity and thus provides a firm basis for our proposed model.

## CONCLUSION

To the extent that the social identity approach has been applied to organizational mergers, analyses have focused on intergroup relations. Without challenging the value of these studies, our analysis introduces a different emphasis

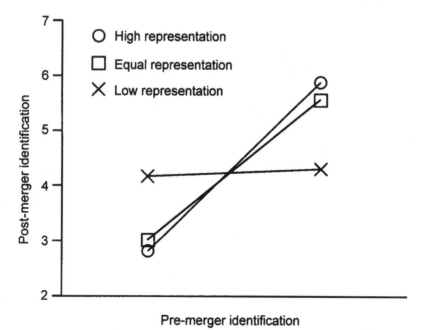

**FIGURE 16.5.** Post-merger identification as a function of premerger identification and representation; van Leeuwen et al. (2000a), Experiment 2.

by focusing not on the subgroup level (i.e., relations between subgroups) but on the superordinate level (i.e., identification with the superordinate category). This shift in emphasis is of interest from a practical point of view, because organizational identification may often be at stake in mergers, as well as from a theoretical point of view, because identification has typically not been studied in the context of fundamental changes in the membership group itself. Taken together, the findings discussed in this chapter lend support to our social identity model of postmerger identification. Central to this model is the interplay between the new and the old organizational (or group) identities, reflected in the concept of sense of continuity. An important aspect of our model is that it links this concept to the two aspects of the relationship between the merger partners that have probably been most frequently cited as major influences in the merger process, organizational dominance and interorganizational differences.

Yet, even though support for the model is promising, we should realize that it is a very broad, general model. Future research should clarify and qualify the relationships proposed in the model. For instance, it seems likely that the nature of the interorganizational differences will greatly affect their impact. Differences on dimensions that are central to an organization's identity (e.g., cultural differences) may exert a far greater influence on postmerger identification than differences on dimensions that are only peripheral in, or even unrelated to, the organization's identity. In the same vein, future research should unravel what aspects of organizational dominance, and of mergers in general, are most important in maintaining a sense of continuity. Which merger partner is perceived to be in control seems to be important in this respect, but possibly of equal importance is that, whatever the magnitude of the changes made, what is seen as the core of the organization's identity (i.e., the characteristics that are most defining of the organization's "personality") is preserved. A more in-depth exploration of the factors that contribute to a sense of continuity is of special interest where the position of the *dominated* group is concerned. The present analysis links a sense of continuity to holding a dominant position, and this leaves the question of what factors would contribute to a sense of continuity for the dominated group unanswered. Identifying the factors that underlie dominance's presumed effect on sense of continuity may help uncover factors that may work to the same end for dominated groups.

In this respect, it is also important to note that case studies of mergers show that dominant organizations often aim to assert their dominance. It is, for instance, not uncommon for an acquiring organization to fire the (top) management of an acquired organization in an attempt to make it easier to impose the own organizational culture (cf. identity) on the acquired organization (Cartwright & Cooper, 1992b). Our analysis suggests that, even though this may ensure a sense of continuity for the dominant group, such attempts to establish the dominance of own culture are conducive to loss of identification on the part of the dominated group. Not trying to force their culture on the merger partner, possibly even fostering distinct subcultures within the merged organization, which may be counterintuitive at first sight, might turn out to work better in the end for the organization as a whole. It would ensure a greater sense of continuity for the dominated group without necessarily introducing an similar discontinuity for the dominant group (although this latter proposition, especially, should be carefully evaluated in future research). Moreover, as work by Hornsey and Hogg (2000a) has shown, the recognition of distinct subgroups is unproblematic for intergroup relations as long as the superordinate identity is also recognized. Future research will have to determine how subgroup distinctiveness impacts the sense of continuity and identification, and particularly whether the proposed benefits for the dominated partner do not go at the expense of the dominant partner. Research along these lines seems particularly valuable, as uncovering ways to ensure a sense of continuity for both dominant and dominated partners seems to be one of the real challenges for both theory and practice.

# 17

# Corporate Mergers and Stepfamily Marriages:
## Identity, Harmony, and Commitment

SAMUEL L. GAERTNER
*University of Delaware*
BETTY A. BACHMAN
*Siena University*
JACK DOVIDIO
*Colgate University*
BRENDA S. BANKER
*University of Delaware*

C orporate mergers and stepfamily marriages are two examples of a ubiquitous social phenomenon: the merger of formerly separate groups into a single organizational structure. In each case, members of two groups are asked to extend their boundaries to include another group that has its own history, a different identity, and a previously established set of relationships among its members. Each group comes with a leadership structure and a set of norms, often peculiar to that group, that regulated members' behavior prior to the merger. Mergers in corporate and family contexts also frequently require that the members of at least one group forsake their previous identity as symbolized, for example, by a change in name, in venue, and, more generally, in their culture. The present chapter examines the role of group identity in establishing harmony and commitment in corporate mergers and stepfamilies and considers the factors that may inhibit or promote the achievement of a common ingroup identity (see also Terry, Chapter 15 of this volume & van Knippenberg & van Leeuwen, Chapter 16 of this volume).

The merger of two companies or families into a single structure is complex and potentially discordant. Whereas the initial development of each participating group normally involved the interaction and socialization of *individuals* who arrived without previous connection to other group members, corporate and stepfamily mergers primarily represent a collision between *groups*. Mergers, therefore, are primarily an intergroup phenomenon. Moreover, companies and families are particularly influential groups in their members' lives. They are fundamentally linked to one's social, economic, and psychological well-being and to personal and collective identity. Allport (1954), for example, stated that the biological family "constitutes the smallest and firmest of one's ingroups" (p. 43).

Although interpersonal relations are not always smooth and harmonious, intergroup relations are usually even more conflictual. Group members who are interdependent with other groups are more distrusting and less likely to be concerned with maximizing joint outcomes compared to individuals who share interdependence (Schopler & Insko, 1992). As a consequence, the potential for conflict and failure in merged organizations is likely to be higher than in the formation of each original group (Haunschild et al., 1994). In addition, conflict between groups in merged organizations is generally more intractable than conflict between individuals because disputants arrive with a network of social support for their respective positions. Ironically, in an atmosphere of distrust and propensity for conflict, members of merging groups are expected to identify with the merged entity and to become committed to its well-being, with the hopes of possibly living together "happily ever after."

We certainly are not the first to note the similarities between corporate mergers and family marriages. Indeed, "a marriage" is frequently used as an analogy for the wedding of corporate entities through merger or acquisition (Cartwright & Cooper, 1994). "Divorce" and "marital discord," however, are also terms equally well suited to both contexts. Unfortunately, corporate and stepfamily marriages share an extraordinarily high failure rate. For corporate mergers and acquisitions, the estimates of failure range from 50% (Cartwright & Cooper, 1992a; M. Porter, 1987) to 80% (Ellis & Pekar, 1978; Kitching, 1967; M. L. Marks, 1988). Likewise, for second marriages the divorce rate is estimated at 60% (Norton & Miller, 1992; L. K. White & Booth, 1985). the divorce rate for second marriages is even higher when children are involved (Furstenberg & Spanier, 1984): The divorce rate in complex stepfamilies composed of mother and father with biological children from previous marriages approximates the failure rate of corporate mergers.

Apparently, something very frequently goes awry that threatens the success and longevity of these intergroup marriages. Given the substantial economic and emotional consequences that result from failures in these domains, it is important to understand some of the fundamental causes of these intergroup catastrophes as well as factors that are related to successful marriages between groups in these domains. Indeed, there are reasons to believe that the intergroup nature of these relationships, in part, places the success of these ventures in jeopardy, and it is the purpose of this chapter to examine group mergers from the perspective of intergroup theory and research. In particular, we focus on the implications of the *common ingroup identity model* (Gaertner et al., 1993; see also Gaertner & Dovidio, 2000), a theoretical framework we developed to conceptualize factors that are instrumental to the creation and reduction of intergroup bias, for addressing intergroup conflict in these settings.

Although we have identified similarities between corporate mergers and stepfamily marriages, we also acknowledge that there are important differences that could impact intergroup and intragroup relations as well as the success of these merged ventures. Corporations and families differ greatly in size, which can influence how information about members is processed, dynamics involving leadership and social influence, and the frequency and nature of interactions within and across groups. Corporate mergers, for example, generally involve relations between very large entities that are subdivided into different divisions and departments. This structure limits interaction among members of the organization and contact between groups, which often occurs between appointed representatives. In contrast, stepfamilies involve intergroup relations between much smaller, more intimate groups with frequent opportunity for communication among all members. In addition, membership in stepfamilies may have greater salience, historical significance, and personal value than membership in corporations. The boundaries of corporations and stepfamilies also differ in permeability. For example, it is mutually understood that an individual may choose to leave a company for a more interesting or lucrative opportunity and, also, that a company may terminate an individual's membership if so desired. However, a person's membership in a stepfamily is presumed to be more permanent and irrevocable, at least with regard to the status of any single member. While it is debatable how much the study of stepfamilies can directly inform the recipe for successful corporate mergers, or vice versa, mergers in both domains share ingredients at a theoretical level to permit multiple tests of our theoretical perspective, which is our major objective.

## MERGERS, SOCIAL CATEGORIZATION, AND INTERGROUP BIAS

Group mergers are likely to heighten the salience of group boundaries because, by definition, group boundaries are targeted to be transformed and broadened, and thereby threatened. Perceptions of people, including the self, can vary from individuated and personalized to categorized and group based in which there is little differentiation among the members (Brewer, 1988; Fiske & Neuberg, 1990; Tajfel & Turner, 1979; J. C. Turner et al., 1987). As the salience of group boundaries increase, impressions slide toward the group end of this continuum. As a consequence, people are regarded simply as members of a social category rather than distinctive individuals. Thus, when social categories are salient primarily, cognitive and motivational processes are activated that produce intergroup biases and stereotyping.

Because of the centrality of the self in social perception (Kihlstrom, Cantor, Albright, Chew, Klein, & Niedenthal, 1988), social categorization involves most fundamentally a distinction between the group containing the self, "the ingroup," and other groups, "the outgroups"—the "we's" and "they's" (J. C. Turner et al., 1987). The insertion of the self into the social categorization process has a profound influence on evaluations, cognitions, and behavior. Tajfel and Turner's (1979) social identity theory hypothesizes that a person's need for positive self-identity motivates social comparisons that favorably differentiate ingroup from outgroup members. In addition, J. C. Turner's (1985) self-categorization theory proposes that "the attractiveness of an individual is not constant, but varies with the ingroup membership" (p. 60).

Another important contextual dynamic that is quite prevalent in mergers is competition. Sherif and Sherif (1969) proposed that the functional relation between groups is the critical factor determining intergroup attitudes (see also realistic conflict theory: Bobo, 1999; Campbell, 1965; LeVine & Campbell, 1972). In corporate mergers there is competition for jobs, status, and influence; in stepfamilies, there is competition for privileges, space in the home, financial resources, and attention from the biological parent and the stepparent. Win-lose, zero-sum competitive relations between groups, in particular, enhance the salience of group boundaries and produce negative feelings toward and stereotypes about the other group. Also, competition increases cohesion within premerger groups and thus helps to polarize the perceived differences between the groups (Blake & Mouton, 1979).

During corporate or stepfamily mergers, the combination of realistic competition between groups and implicit threats to social identity can produce feelings of ingroup favoritism, hostility for members of the other group, and significant emotional discomfort, often associated with suspicion and distrust of the other group (Schopler & Insko, 1993). This distrust can be particularly threatening if the other group possesses greater power or status in the merged entity. These feelings of threat and discomfort, in turn, can lower members' commitment to the newly merged entity and their willingness to cooperate with the members of the other constituent group (Buono et al., 1985; Sales & Mirvis, 1984). Of course, such consequences are counterproductive to the achievement of the goals and rewards that were anticipated by the architects of the merger. Nevertheless, understanding the intergroup nature of mergers can help to facilitate successful organizational transitions and transformations.

## THE COMMON INGROUP IDENTITY MODEL

Whereas social categorization provides a perspective for understanding the origins of intergroup bias and conflict, this perspective also has implications for minimizing these biases. One category-based strategy, recategorization, encourages the members of both groups to regard themselves as belonging to a common, superordinate group—*one group* that is inclusive of both memberships (see Gaertner et al., 1993; Gaertner & Dovidio, 2000).

Theoretically, the rationale for the recategorization strategy for reducing intergroup bias rests on two related conclusions from Brewer's (1979) analysis that fit nicely with social identity theory (Tajfel & Turner, 1979) and self-categorization theory (J. C. Turner, 1985). First, intergroup bias often takes the form of ingroup enhancement rather than outgroup devaluation. Second, the formation of a group brings ingroup members closer to the self, whereas the distance between the self and non-ingroup members remains relatively unchanged. Thus, upon ingroup formation or when an individual assumes a group-level identification, the egocentric biases that favor the self are transferred to other ingroup members. Increasing the inclusiveness of group boundaries enables some of those cognitive and motivational processes that contributed initially to intergroup bias to be redirected or transferred to former outgroup members (Gaertner, Mann, Murrell, & Dovidio, 1989).

Because the major intent of a merger is to unite two groups into one and to encourage members to adopt the new common ingroup identity, we believe that the common ingroup identity model may offer a useful perspective for understanding the problems associated with the merger process. Specifically, we hypothesize that if members of different groups are induced to conceive of themselves as a single group rather than as completely separate groups, attitudes toward former outgroup members will become more positive through processes involving pro-ingroup bias (Gaertner & Dovidio, 2000; Gaertner et al., 1993). If, however, contextual factors perpetuate the impression that the groups are separate and not unified, intergroup interactions will be discordant, which could thereby undermine the productivity and success of the merged organization.

This recategorization approach also offers an explanation for how the apparently loosely connected, diverse features specified by the contact hypothesis may operate psychologically to reduce bias. Allport's (1954) revised contact hypothesis proposed that to reduce bias successfully, certain qualities of contact were required: equal status between the groups, cooperative (rather than competitive) intergroup interaction, opportunities for personal acquaintance between the members, and supportive norms by authorities within and outside of the contact situation. In terms of the common ingroup identity model, these contact conditions facilitate a reduction in bias, in part because they share the capacity to transform members' representations from separate groups to a more inclusive social entity.

The common ingroup identity model identifies antecedents and outcomes of recategorization and considers the critical mediating role of group cognitive representations (i.e., as one group, two subgroups within one group, two separate groups, or separate individuals; see Gaertner & Dovidio, 2000). Antecedent factors, such as those specified by the contact hypothesis (e.g., cooperation; see Gaertner et al., 1999), can alter individuals' cognitive representations of the aggregate and facilitate the development of a one-group representation. Alternatively, common ingroup identity may be achieved by increasing the salience of existing common superordinate memberships (e.g., a school, a company, a family) or by introducing factors (e.g., common goals or fate) that are perceived to be shared by the memberships. The development of a one-group representation then mediates the relationship between the antecedent factors and the cognitive, affective, and behavioral consequences. These consequences include reduced bias in evaluations and greater intergroup self-disclosure and helping (see Dovidio et al., 1997).

The development of a common ingroup identity can also have implications for the effectiveness and productivity of a merged organization. For example, in a military context, Manning and Ingraham (1987) obtained a correlation between battalion cohesion and measures of performance effectiveness, including operations readiness. Similarly, we have found that the extent to which members of two groups perceived of themselves as one superordinate group correlated with the actual effectiveness of their task solution ($r = .28$, $p < .02$). This relationship is also consistent with the meta-analytic conclusions of Mullen and Copper (1994), who found that group cohesiveness significantly predicts group productivity ($r = .25$). Moreover, Mullen and Copper suggested that the relationship between cohesiveness and productivity may be bidirectional and thus iterative: cohesiveness may enhance productivity, and successful accomplishment, in turn, further increases cohesiveness. Indeed, the relationship between successful performance and subsequent productivity is even stronger ($r = .51$) than the relationship between initial cohesiveness and productivity. Thus, the development of a common ingroup identity can help form a basis for more harmonious intergroup relations to develop through mutual success and achievement, which reinforces the common bond and identity between the groups.

It is important to note that in some domains the development of a common ingroup identity does not necessarily require each group to forsake its less inclusive group identity completely. As depicted by the "subgroups within one group" (i.e., a dual identity) representation, we believe that it is possible for members to conceive of two groups (for example, parents and children) as distinct units within the context of a superordinate (i.e., family) identity. Sometimes it would be undesirable or impossible for people to relinquish these group identities or, as perceivers, to be oblivious to them. If, however, people continued to regard themselves as members of different groups but all playing on the same team or as part of the same superordinate entity, intergroup relations between these "subgroups" which are convergent with prior group boundaries would be more positive than if members only considered themselves as "separate groups" (see Brewer & Schneider, 1990). In this chapter, we explore the generalizability of this proposition in a different context, in business mergers and stepfamily marriages in which the very purpose of the intergroup relationship is to forge a single, common identity. In the next section, we examine two initial empirical tests of the common ingroup identity model before turning to evidence directly addressing corporate mergers and stepfamilies.

# INITIAL TESTS OF THE COMMON INGROUP IDENTITY MODEL

Early tests of our model involved structural aspects of the situation, such as integrated seating, and social features that have been identified in the contact hypothesis as necessary for intergroup contact to reduce bias successfully, such as cooperation (see Gaertner & Dovidio, 2000). For instance, we conducted one experiment that brought two 3-person laboratory groups together under conditions designed to vary independently (a) the members' representations of the aggregate as one group or two groups through manipulation of the contact situation and (b) the presence or absence of intergroup cooperative interaction (Gaertner et al., 1990). The interventions designed to emphasize common group membership through structural changes in the contact situation (e.g., integrated vs. segregated seating; a new group name for all six participants vs. the original group names) and the presence or absence of cooperative interaction both reduced intergroup bias. Moreover, they did so through the same mechanism. Contextual features emphasizing common "same groupness" and intergroup cooperation each increased one-group representations (and reduced separate-group representations), which in turn mediated lower levels of bias. The experimental studies helped establish the chain of causality among the variables as hypothesized by the model.

To explore external validity, we supplemented the experimental work with a series of survey studies of relations between groups, often with histories of conflict, under more naturalistic circumstances. One of these studies involved a survey of Black, White, Hispanic, and Asian high school students (see Gaertner, Rust, Dovidio, Bachman, & Anastasio, 1996). The primary theoretical question we pursued in this study was whether students' perceptions of the student body as one group, different groups "playing on the same team" (a dual identity in which subgroup identities are maintained within the context of a superordinate entity), or separate groups would mediate the proposed relation between their perceptions of the favorableness of the conditions of contact (e.g., cooperative interaction, equal status) and their levels of affective bias (i.e., positive feelings induced by members of their own ethnic groups relative to the other groups).

The findings were consistent with the processes we hypothesized in the common ingroup identity model. Across all of the racial and ethnic groups in this study, more favorable perceptions of the conditions of intergroup contact predicted stronger representations of the student body as one group and as different groups on the same team (the dual identity item), and this, in turn, predicted less bias in affective reactions. The beneficial effects of a dual identity was further revealed by students who identified themselves on the survey as members of a minority group and also American. These students had lower bias in affective reactions than minority students who did not use a superordinate American identity.

Further analyses of these data examined the moderating role of status, defined in terms of majority or minority group status (see Gaertner et al., 1996). Consistent with Islam and Hewstone's (1993) research and the idea that social-contextual factors influence intergroup attitudes, majority (i.e., Caucasian) students relative to the minority group students (disregarding whether they used a dual identity) perceived the conditions of contact more favorably. They also had stronger representations of the student body as "all playing on the same team" and had lower degrees of bias in affective reactions, primarily because their attitudes toward outgroup members were more favorable. Thus, status (in this case majority and minority racial or ethnic group membership) is a critical moderating factor determining the results of group contact.

The next sections of this chapter explore the implications of the common ingroup identity model and the empirical findings associated with intergroup status and contact for two specific types of organizational mergers, first corporate mergers and then stepfamily marriages.

### Corporate Mergers

Our tests of the how the common ingroup identity model relates to corporate mergers initially considered perceptions of intergroup relations and intergroup attitudes within organizations, measures most directly comparable to those in our previous work on intergroup, interracial, and interethnic evaluations. Further research that has extended our model and examined other mediating factors, however, has considered an additional measure that is critical to organizational effectiveness: organizational commitment. The results reported in this section primarily reflect various aspects of a dataset of detailed surveys by Bachman (1993) of the experiences and responses of 416 banking executives from a variety of banking institutions across the United States.

**Intergroup attitudes.**   In a study of intergroup attitudes in corporate mergers, Bachman (1993) examined questionnaire responses from 229 banking executives who had participated in corporate mergers and 187 banking executives who had not. Many of the primary measures in our earlier laboratory and field studies were also included. These measures were (a) perceptions of the conditions of contact; (b) representations of the memberships as one group or as separate groups (e.g., us vs. them); and (c) intergroup bias. Factor analyses revealed two types of bias. One type involved perceptions of work-related characteristics (intelligent, hard-working, reliable, organized, skilled, and creative). The other type of bias involved sociability (including the traits of sociable, helpful, and cliquish). In addition to the other measures, an index measuring pragmatic and social identity threat was examined, as was merger participants' status as a member of the acquiring or acquired organization.

Comparisons of identical items on the merger and nonmerger surveys suggested that corporate mergers were indeed regarded as an intergroup event. Moreover employees' status regarding their association with either the acquiring or the acquired organization moderated the degree to which a one-group or separate-group orientation characterized perceptions of the merged organization (see also Terry, Carey, & Callan, Chapter 15 of in press; and Terry, this volume). Overall, separate-group representations and threat were significantly stronger among members of the acquired organization relative to those of the acquiring organization, which in turn were stronger than those for respondents whose companies had not had a merger. In addition, conditions of contact between groups in the organization were perceived to be least favorable among employees associated with an acquired organization. Perceptions of respondents belonging to an acquiring company in a merger and respondents who had not experienced a merger were more favorable and, interestingly, did not differ from one another.

In general, comparisons of the perceptions of acquired and acquiring organizations' employees appear to be similar to the impressions of minority and majority students, respectively, in the multiethnic high school study (Gaertner et al., 1996) described earlier in this chapter. Just as minority students had less favorable impressions of contact in their high school than did majority students (see also Islam & Hewstone, 1993), employees of the lower status, acquired organization had less favorable impressions of the relations between groups within the merged organization than those employees associated with the higher status, acquiring organization.

In addition, as it did in the multiethnic high school, intergroup bias among the banking executives who experienced a merger varied as a function of status. This effect, however, was not a simple one, and it was different depending on the type of bias (sociability or work-related) considered. Supportive of the processes hypothesized in the common ingroup identity model, across members of both the acquired and acquiring companies, more favorable perceptions of the conditions of contact and the associated more inclusive representations of the merged organization corresponded with lower levels of sociability bias. When bias is measured in terms of work competence, however, a different pattern emerges. In contrast to the results for sociability bias, members of acquiring organizations exhibited significantly higher levels of ingroup favoritism on the work-competence index than did members of acquired organizations. Thus, higher work-related status, in terms of organizational role in a merger, was related to lower sociability bias but to greater ingroup bias in their perceptions of work competence (see also Terry & Callan, 1998).

Although not intuitively obvious at first glance, the effects of status on our bias measures are consistent with other studies that have found that high-status groups tend to emphasize their superiority on power and competence dimensions (e.g., "We are more clever, richer, and stronger"), whereas low-status groups tend to show "social creativity" in the terms of social identity theory by emphasizing the importance of alternative social dimensions (e.g., "We are nicer"; see Doojse & Ellemers, 1997; Mummendey & Schreiber, 1983; Spears & Manstead, 1989). These effects of status suggest the importance of considering the relevance and centrality of the dimensions on which bias is assessed; that is, the social context of the dependent measures as well as the social context of the intergroup contact and the relative status of the groups. It is possible, for instance, that members of acquired organizations, recognizing their disadvantage in the work situation, were particularly motivated to seek positive distinctiveness on an alternative dimension, manifested in this case as higher levels of sociability bias than exhibited by members of acquiring organizations (see also, Brewer, Manzi, & Shaw, 1993; Mullen et al., 1992; Sachdev & Bourhis, 1991).

Despite the parallels in the results between the high school and corporate merger studies of intergroup bias, there are potential differences between these contexts that are important to consider. For instance, a dual identity in terms of racial or ethnic identity among students (e.g., African American) may be valued and reflect an integrative orientation within a multicultural school environment. However, vestiges of one's former organizational identity within a merged company may indicate resistance to the merger and signal intergroup disharmony. Consistent with this reasoning, Gaertner, Dovidio, and Bachman (1996) found in the data from the banking executives that, as in the high school study, more favorable perceptions of intergroup contact related to stronger one-group representations but, in contrast to the results of the high school study, *less* favorable perceptions of contact related to stronger dual-identity representations. Moreover, whereas stronger dual identities predicted lower levels of intergroup bias in the high school study, they predicted higher levels of work-related bias within merged companies. Thus the nature of the context and the goals of organizations and individuals may critically determine how different representations mediate intergroup attitudes.

Whereas the previous work focused on the attitudes toward different groups within an organization, the research in the next section extends the common ingroup identity model to investigate employees' relation to the merged organization itself.

### Organizational commitment and the intergroup merger model.

Bachman's (1993) research also elaborated upon the common ingroup identity model by including variables specifically relevant to corporate mergers. In this expanded version of the model, designated the *intergroup merger model* (see Figure 17.1), threat induced by the merger plays a central role in determining employee perceptions of the new organization and their commitment to its well-being. As in the original model, the extent to which the merged organization is perceived to be a single entity rather than fractionalized along premerger group lines (i.e., an us vs. them orientation) also plays a central role in the expanded model. The intergroup merger model includes outcome variables critical to the well-being of the merged organization, such as employees' commitment to the organization and their intention to remain with the organization (i.e., turnover intentions), are also included. Therefore, to the extent that employee commitment to contribute to the merged organization's survival and growth is critical to the merged organization, the intergroup merger model has implications for understanding the high degree of failure of these merged ventures.

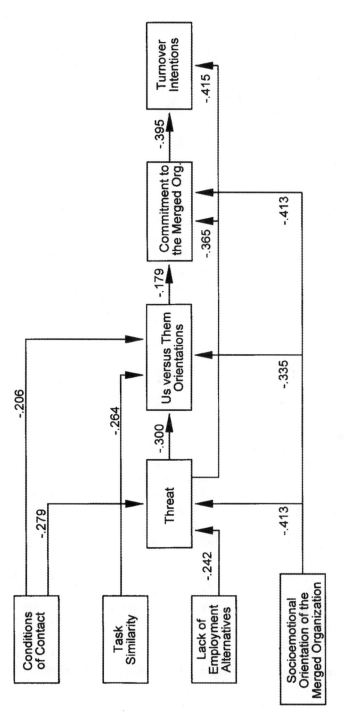

FIGURE 17.1. The intergroup merger model.

As illustrated in Figure 17.1, perceptions of favorable conditions of contact are predicted to influence employees' representations of the memberships as a single entity. In addition, favorable contact conditions facilitate intergroup interactions by making them less threatening and anxiety arousing (see Stephan & Stephan, 1984). For example, perceptions of egalitarian norms and equal status between the merged groups are proposed to reduce threats to social identity as well as threats about being discriminated against within the organization, a consequence that would further exacerbate an us versus them orientation between the members of the merging units.

The intergroup merger model also considers the role of the similarity between the premerger partners' products or services. Consistent with the principles of social identity theory, high similarity between these groups is expected to increase the need for employees to perceive their respective premerger organizations in a distinctive and positively differentiated manner vis a vis one another (see Hewstone & Brown, 1986). Thus, high levels of similarity between the merging groups is expected to increase employees' perceptions of an us versus them orientation. The functional overlap between the groups further drives a competitive wedge between the premerger groups given the high likelihood that subsequent downsizing could be used to reduce unnecessary redundancy (Caves, 1992).

In the intergroup merger model, the extent to which employees perceive fewer available alternative employment opportunities increases the degree of threat associated with the merger. Another influence on threat is the perceived socioemotional orientation of the merged organization. The socioemotional orientation of the organization includes perceptions that the organization appreciates and cares about the employee's well-being (i.e., perceived organizational support, see Eisbenberger et al., 1986), that it communicates in ways that reduce ambiguities about the merger, and the degree to which the organization allows employees to have some voice or influence. When organizations demonstrate an active involvement with and concern for employees, threat is reduced and employees are more likely to reciprocate by enhancing their commitment to the organization, which in turn reduces the likelihood of employee turnover (Eisenberger et al., 1986). Nevertheless, the manner in which two organizations are integrated may critically influence employees' reactions to the merged organization.

This test of the intergroup merger model relied on the relevant items in Bachman's (1993) survey of the 229 banking executives who had participated in corporate mergers. Thirty-eight percent of the participants were female and the average age of all participants was 40 years old. Approximately 5% of the respondents were bank presidents, 16% were senior vice presidents, 45% were vice presidents, 8% were assistant vice presidents. Other positions included chief executive officer, bank director, chief financial officer, controller, and operations officer, among others. The average amount of time since the merger took place was 3.25 years.

Many of the survey items were adapted from those used in our earlier laboratory and multiethnic high school studies. For example, the conditions of contact included employees' perceptions of the degree to which the merger partners held equal status within the merged organization; the degree to which there were egalitarian norms with regard to salary, benefits, evaluations, and promotions; the degree to which both merger partners were necessary to achieve corporate goals (i.e., positive interdependence); and the degree to which inter-group interactions were intimate, frequent, and pleasant (alpha = .77). The us versus them orientation measure included questions relating to group repre-sentations used previously in our laboratory studies (e.g., the extent to which the merged organization felt like one group) and also perceived cohesiveness and similarity between the memberships. Threat was measured using items selected from related scales: role ambiguity (Rizzo, House, & Lirtzman, 1970), intergroup anxiety (Stephan & Stephan, 1985), self-esteem at work (Quinn & Shepard, 1974), as well as items pertaining to anxiety about job and benefit loss, uncertainty about the personal ramifications of the merger, status change as a result of the merger, and loss of authority as a result of the merger (alpha = .83). Commitment to the merged organization was assessed by combining items from the Organizational Commitment Questionnaire (Mowday, Steers, & Porter, 1979) and the Identification with Psychological Group Scale (Mael, 1988).

Path analysis (LISREL) tested the assumed causal chain proposed among the variables in the model. The model fit the data well ($X^2$ [10df] = 12.47, $p$ = .255; goodness of fit index [GFI] = .983; adjusted goodness of fit index [AGFI] = .938, RMSR = .028). Figure 17.1 provides a representation of the model with path coefficients estimated from the LISREL analysis. All of the proposed paths were statistically significant. As illustrated in Figure 17.1, members of merged organizations experienced greater threat when conditions of contact were less favorable, when employment opportunities were perceived to be lower, and when socioemotional orientation of the merged organization was weaker. As expected, threat seemed to exacerbate us versus them orientations, reduce com-mitment to the merged organization, and increase turnover intentions. Sup-portive of the hypothesized central mediating role of cognitive representations of the groups, stronger us versus them orientations were associated with lower levels of commitment to the merged organization, which in turn were related to higher turnover intentions. Although task similarity was associated with us ver-sus them orientations, the direction of the relationship was in a direction oppo-site to what we expected. Higher levels of task similarity between the merging companies was associated with lower levels of us versus them orientations. Nev-ertheless, overall, the proposed model explained 55% of the variance in threat, 62% of the variance in us versus them orientations, 73% of the variance in com-mitment to the merged organization, and 58% of the variance in turnover in-tentions.

In general, the results of this study extend support for the basic principles of the common ingroup identity model into a new realm, corporate mergers, and to different consequences, organizational commitment. The version of the model devised especially for this context, the intergroup merger model

(Bachman, 1993), demonstrates how basic intergroup perceptions (in this case, an us vs. them orientation) play a central role in developing connections to others in the organization and to the organization itself—and ultimately to organizational commitment. The findings also indicate the importance of potential factors that can directly operate on perceived threats, such as status change within the organization as a result of the merger. In the next section, we consider how one such factor, the structure of a merger, can shape intergroup perceptions and organizational commitment.

**Patterns of integration during a merger.** To examine the role of structural integration patterns on expectations regarding the likely contact conditions between two groups and members' commitment to a superordinate entity, we executed an experiment involving a corporate merger simulation with college students (Mottola, Bachman, Gaertner, & Dovidio, 1997). In this study we manipulated the merger integration pattern utilized to bring two companies together in terms of whether the culture (policies and norms) of the merged organization reflected either just one of the premerger companies (an absorb pattern, a type of assimilation in which one group is expected to forsake its cultural identity), aspects of both companies (a blend pattern, analogous to pluralism), or an entirely new culture (a combined pattern that reflected a more egalitarian form of assimilation). Supportive of our expectations, perceptions of the conditions of contact, us versus them orientation, and commitment to the merged organization were most favorable with the combine pattern (which has the strongest potential to reduce the salience of premerger group boundaries), followed in turn by the blend pattern and then the absorb pattern. Also, conceptually similar to our high school and bank merger studies, the relationship between favorable conditions of contact and increased commitment to the merged organization in this laboratory study was mediated by participants' perceptions of organizational unity (i.e., an inclusive "we" rather than an us versus them orientation). In the next study, we explore the merger process and the role of perceiving unity in a different intergroup context, a merger that is intensely personal and increasingly common: the stepfamily.

### Stepfamily Marriages

As we noted at the beginning of this chapter, families involve a primary form of group membership. Beyond genetic relatedness, there is a profound social connection among family members. Biological, or first-married families, generally share memories, ancestral histories, traditions, daily rituals, and a common family name that contribute to a strong sense of family group identity (see Settles, 1993).

Given the importance of family group identity, stepfamilies represent an interesting domain to examine the utility of the common ingroup identity model. When the first-married family is fragmented by divorce or death and remarriage to a new partner occurs, the biological parents and children from the two families come together under new circumstances. Through remarriage, members of two separate "ingroups" with no common memories, histories, daily rituals, or even family name find themselves in an intensive intergroup context.

Relative to biologically related, first-married families, stepfamilies have generally been described as more stressful and less cohesive. Stepfathers, for example, not only report being less satisfied with their own lives than do first-married fathers, but they also indicate that the lives of their stepchildren are less than satisfactory as well (Fine, McKenry, Donnelly, & Voydanoff, 1992). Bray and Berger (1993) found that, in couples remarried for 5 to 7 years, there were less positive wife-to-husband and biological parent–child interactions in stepfamilies than in their first-married counterparts. And, several studies have found that stepparent–stepchild relationships are more conflict-ridden than are those between biological parents and children in first-married families (J. Z. Anderson & White, 1986; Furstenberg, 1987; Sauer & Fine, 1988).

One reason why stepfamilies may experience less harmony is less than satisfactory contact among the stepfamily members. S. D. James and Johnson (1987) reported that competitiveness in stepfamilies is related to marital dissatisfaction and psychological pathology in both husbands and wives. Cooperativeness, however, relates to marital satisfaction for both partners and to the husbands' positive psychological adjustment. Furthermore, the failure of stepchildren to respond in kind to their stepparents' positive behaviors toward them has been found to be associated with stepfamily dysfunction (J. Z. Anderson & White, 1986; A. C. Brown, Green, & Druckman, 1990). A more positive relationship between the stepparent and stepchild, in contrast, is associated with more positive stepfamily functioning (J. Z. Anderson & White, 1986) and happiness (Crosbie-Burnett, 1984).

This study (Banker & Gaertner, 1998) examined, within the context of the common ingroup identity model, how those factors involved in positive contact among stepfamily members (e.g., cooperativeness) influence stepfamily functioning and harmony. Specifically, it was predicted that more favorable conditions of contact in the stepfamily home would relate to increased perceptions of the family as one group and to increased stepfamily harmony. The relationship between favorable conditions of contact and increased harmony were expected to be mediated by the one-group representation.

Eighty-six undergraduate stepfamily members completed a questionnaire for this study. During pretesting, participants who were selected for this study reported that they lived at home with a married biological parent and stepparent and had at least one stepsibling. Each of these stepfamiles was therefore composed of at least four people who could view themselves initially as two separate groups (Aa and Bb). The average age of the participants was 19.2 years, and the average length of their custodial parent's current marriage to the stepparent was 7 years. Most of the participants (86%) lived with the biological mother and stepfather. A measure of favorability of the contact conditions within the stepfamily was created by averaging together measures of cooperation, opportunities for self-revealing interaction, and equal status. Participants also rated the extent to which the stepfamily unit felt like one group, two subgroups within one (a measure of dual identity), two groups, and separate individuals. The measure of stepfamily harmony represented the average of four items, such as "Generally, there is a feeling of contentment in my house," and "I would characterize the environment in my house as 'harmonious.'"

Of central importance to the model was the relationships among the variables for predicting stepfamily harmony (see Figure 17.2). As hypothesized, more favorable conditions of contact predicted higher one-group ratings (*beta* = .52) and lower two-groups (*beta* = −.61) and two-groups-within-one-group (*beta* = −.65) ratings. Consistent with our mediation hypothesis, one-group representations, in turn, significantly predicted higher levels of stepfamily harmony (*beta* = .37). However, it is important to note that the "dual identity" (two groups in one) item correlated *negatively* with favorable conditions of contact. The less favorable the conditions of contact were perceived to be between stepfamily units, the more participants perceived their family as two smaller families in one family, and additional analyses revealed that this dual-identity item also correlated negatively with stepfamily harmony (*r* = −.44).

Similar to the corporate merger research in which we compared executives who experienced a merger with those who have not, Banker and Gaertner (1998) also administered a questionnaire to students from first-married families (*n* = 65) whose biological families are intact. The results revealed that, com-

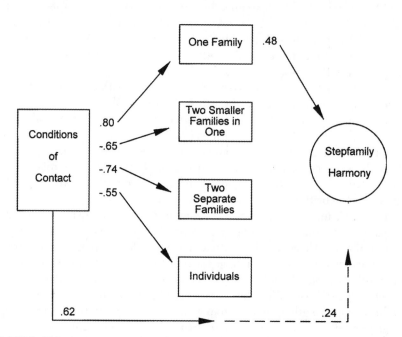

**FIGURE 17.2.** Perceptions of conditions of contact and stepfamily harmony. Adapted from Banker, B. S., & Gaertner, S. L. (1998). Achieiving stepfamily harmony: An intergroup relations approach. *Journal of Family Psychology, 12,* 310–325.

pared to the undergraduates from first-married families, participants from stepfamilies reported less favorable conditions of contact and representations of their families which were less like one group and more like two, mirroring the reactions of employees affiliated with the acquired organization in the bank merger study. Family harmony, however, was only nonsignificantly lower for students in stepfamilies than for those in first-married families. Nevertheless, the results from a subsequent study (Banker & Gaertner, 2000) that included a stepmother and stepfather from the same complex stepfamily indicated that stepmothers relative to stepfathers perceive more conflict in their stepfamilies, experience more stress in their homes, have less marital satisfaction, and find the relationship with their stepchildren to be less positive. These results may be due to stepmothers having a more difficult time due to their primary caregiving role in the stepfamily (Quick, McKenry, & Newman, 1994) or to their greater dissatisfaction with their role (Ahrons & Wallisch, 1987). Overall, our findings are consistent with the view that gender inequality may disadvantage stepmothers such that their perceptions of family life are comparable to those of the lower status employees of an acquired company during a corporate merger.

## SUMMARY AND CONCLUSION

The results of our research offer support for the common ingroup identity model and its utility for studying problems across the very different domains of corporate mergers and stepfamily marriages. Moreover, the findings support and extend previous work in business and family research and suggest ways that intergroup harmony, and consequently the success of the merged venture, can be achieved within these settings. The process of recategorization from two separate groups to one, single, inclusive group and the development of identification and commitment to the merged entity is central to facilitating successful mergers (see D. van Knippenberg, van Knippenberg, Monden, & de Lima, in press). The relationships between the conditions of contact and commitment and identification to a merged corporation and harmony within stepfamiles were mediated by the extent to which the aggregate felt like one group. Supportive of the model, the more it felt like one group, the greater the organizational commitment among the banking executives, and the greater the amount of stepfamily harmony.

In contrast to the consistent, significant effect for the one-group representation within our studies, we also observed that the role of the "dual identity" measure functioned differently across the high school, corporate merger, and stepfamily studies. In the high school setting, the better the conditions of contact, the more students regarded the aggregate as "different groups on the same team." In contrast, in the corporate merger and stepfamily settings, the more favorable the conditions of contact, the less participants indicated that the aggregate felt like two subgroups or two smaller families within a larger group. Also, in the corporate merger context, the more the merged organization felt like two subgroups within a group, the greater the amount of ingroup bias these executives had in their perceptions of the work-related characteristics among the members of the two formerly separate organizations. Thus, in this context, the more strongly both subgroup and superordinate group identities were salient simultaneously, the greater the extent to which ingroup members were regarded as more intelligent, hard-working, skilled, and creative than were outgroup members. In the multiethnic high school context, however, the more students felt that the aggregate felt like "different groups all playing on the same team" (the dual identity item), the lower their bias in affective reactions.

We suspect that contextual differences among these intergroup settings may alter the relative desirability and utility of maintaining a dual identity in lieu of a more inclusive one-group representation (see Gaertner, Dovidio, & Bachman, 1996). For example, maintaining strong identification with the earlier subgroup identities following a corporate merger may threaten the primary goal of the merger. Similarly, in stepfamilies, the salience of the former family identities, even with the simultaneous recognition of a more inclusive family identity, may violate members' expectations about what their ideal family should be like. Consequently, the salience of these subgroup identities may be diagnostic of serious problems, reflected, in part, by the fact that these "dual identities" become stronger in the merger and stepfamily contexts as the conditions of contact are more unfavorable. However, the relationship is quite different than in the high school context, in which the salience of subgroup and superordinate identities would not be incompatible with the goals of the superordinate organization. Here, the salience of the subgroup identities, within the context of a superordinate entity that provides connection between the subgroups, may signal the prospects for good intergroup relations without undermining the goals of the school or those of the different ethnic or racial groups.

In conclusion, the merger of two organizations, whether corporations or families, is a complex task with a substantial risk of failure. Companies and families are primary groups, closely connected to one's identity and social and physical well-being. As a consequence, successful mergers require managing intergroup as well as interpersonal processes in constructive and productive ways. Of central importance is the development of a common ingroup identity: changing perceptions from "us" and "them" to a collective "we." Although strategic, financial, and operational issues frequently receive primary attention in the merger process and are obviously important factors, mergers are also fundamentally social events. How people respond personally and socially is also a critical determinant of whether a merger will succeed or fail. Understanding the nature of the social processes involved in mergers can thus be an important, although often overlooked element, for facilitating successful mergers.

## ACKNOWLEDGMENT

Preparation of this manuscript was supported by National Institute of Mental Health grant MH 48721.

# References

Abrams, D. (1985). Focus of attention in the minimal group paradigm. *British Journal of Social Psychology, 24,* 65–74.

Abrams, D. (1990). *National Health Authority Report.* University of Kent, UK.

Abrams, D. (1992). Processes of social identification. In G. M. Breakwell (Ed.), *Social psychology of identity and the self-concept* (pp. 57–100). San Diego, Academic Press.

Abrams, D. (1994). Social self-regulation. *Personality and Social Psychology Bulletin, 20,* 273–283.

Abrams, D. (1999). Social identity, social cognition, and the self: The flexibility and stability of self-categorization. In D. Abrams (Ed.), *Social identity and social cognition* (pp. 197–229). Malden, MA: Blackwell.

Abrams, D. (2000, July). *Is social identity an organizational asset?* Paper preseted at the EAESP Small Group Meeting on Social Identity Processes in Organizations, Amsterdam.

Abrams, D., Ando, K., & Hinkle, S. (1998). Psychological attachment to the group: Cross-cultural differences in organizational identification and subjective norms as predictors of workers' turnover intentions. *Personality and Social Psychology Bulletin, 24,* 1027–1039.

Abrams, D., & Emler, N. P. (1992). Self-denial as a paradox of political and regional identity: Findings from a study of 16- and 18-year olds. *European Journal of Social Psychology, 22,* 279–295.

Abrams, D., Hinkle, S., & Tomlins, M. (1997, July) *Social identity in transition: Implications for commitment to Hong Kong.* Paper presented at the International Conference on the Transition to Hong Kong Special Administrative Region of the People's Republic of China, Hong Kong.

Abrams, D., Hinkle, S., & Tomlins, M. (1999). Leaving Hong Kong? The roles of attitudes, subjective norm, perceived control, social identity and relative deprivation. *International Journal of Intercultural Relations, 23,* 319–338.

Abrams, D., & Hogg, M. (1988). Comments on the motivational status of self-esteem in social identity and intergroup discrimination. *European Journal of Social Psychology, 18,* 317–334.

Abrams, D., & Hogg, M. A. (1990a). Social identification, self-categorization and social influence. *European Review of Social Psychology, 1,* 195–228.

Abrams, D., & Hogg, M. A. (Eds.). (1990b). *Social identity theory: Constructive and critical advances.* London: Harvester Wheatsheaf.

Abrams, D., & Hogg, M. A. (1998). Prospects for research in group processes and intergroup relations. *Group Processes and Intergroup Relations, 1,* 7–20.

Abrams, D., & Hogg, M. A. (Eds.) (1999). *Social identity and social cognition.* Oxford, UK: Blackwell.

Abrams, D., & Hogg, M. A. (2001). Collective identity: Group membership and self-conception. In M. A. Hogg & R. S. Tindale, (Eds.), *Blackwell handbook of social psychology: Group processes* (pp. 425–460). Oxford, UK: Blackwell.

Abrams, D., Marques, J. M., Bown, N., &

Henson, M. (2000). Pro-norm and anti-norm deviance within and between groups. *Journal of Personality and Social Psychology, 78*, 906-912.

Abrams, D., Randsley de Moura, G., Vaughan, C., Gunnarsdottir, S., & Ando, K. (2000). *The role of organizational identification and job satisfaction in predicting turnover intentions.* Manuscript submitted for publication.

Adler, N. J. (1997). *International dimensions of organizational behavior* (3rd ed.). Cincinatti, OH: South-Western College Publishing.

Ahrons, C. R., & Wallisch, K. (1987). Parenting in the binuclear family: Relationships between biological and stepparents. In K. Pasley & M. Ihinger-Tallman (Eds.), *Remarriage and stepparenting: Current research and theory* (pp. 225–256). New York: Guilford.

Ajzen, I. (1991). The theory of planned behavior. *Organizational Behavior and Human Decision Processes, 50*, 179–211.

Ajzen, I., & Fishbein, M. (1980). *Understanding attitudes and predicting social behavior.* Englewood Cliffs, NJ: Prentice-Hall

Albert, S., & Whetten, D. A. (1985). Organizational identity. In L. L. Cummings & B. M. Staw (Eds.), *Research in organizational behavior* (Vol. 7, pp. 263–295). Greenwich, CT: JAI Press.

Alderfer, C.P. (1987). An intergroup perspective on group dynamics. In J.W. Lorsch (Ed.), *Handbook of organizational behavior* (pp.190–222). Englewood Cliffs, NJ: Prentice-Hall.

Alexander, V.D., & Thoits, P.A. (1985). Token achievement: An examination of proportional representation and performance outcomes. *Social Forces, 64*, 332–340.

Allen, N. J., & Meyer, J. P. (1990). The measurement and antecedents of affective, continuance and normative commitment to the organization. *Journal of Occupational Psychology, 63*, 1–18.

Allen, N. J., & Meyer, J. P. (1996). Affective, continuance, and normative commitment to the organization: An examination of construct validity. *Journal of Vocational Behavior, 49*, 252-276.

Allmendinger, J., & Hackman, J. R. (1995). The more the better? A four-nation study of the inclusion of women in symphony orchestras. *Social Forces, 74*, 423–460.

Allport, G. W. (1954). *The nature of prejudice.* Cambridge, MA: Addison-Wesley.

Alutto, J. A., Hrebiniak, L. G., & Alonso, R. C. (1973). On operationalizing the concept of commitment. *Social Forces, 51*, 448–454.

Amir, Y. (1976). The role of intergroup contact in change of prejudice and ethnic relations. In P. A. Katz (Ed.), *Towards the elimination of racism* (pp. 245–308). New York: Pergamon.

Ancona, D. G. (1990). Outward bound: Strategies for team survival in an organization. *Academy of Management Journal, 33*, 334–365.

Ancona, D. G., & Caldwell, D. F. (1988). Beyond task and maintenance: Defining external functions in groups. *Group and Organization Studies, 13*, 468–494.

Ancona, D. G., & Caldwell, D. F. (1992a). Bridging the boundary: External activity and performance in organizational teams. *Administrative Science Quarterly, 37*, 634–665.

Ancona, D. G., & Caldwell, D. F. (1992b). Demography and design: Predictors of new product team performance. *Organizational Science, 3*, 321–331.

Anderson, J. Z., & White, G. D. (1986). An empirical investigation of interaction and relationship patterns in functional and dysfunctional nuclear families and stepfamilies. *Family Process, Inc. 25*, 407–422.

Anderson, N., & Thomas, H. D. C. (1996). Work group socialization. In M. A. West (Ed.), *Handbook of work group psychology* (pp. 423-450). Chichester, UK: Wiley.

Arcuri, L. (1982). Three patterns of social categorization in attribution memory. *European Journal of Social Psychology, 12*, 271–282.

Aron, A., & McLaughlin-Volpe, T. (in press). Including others in the self: Extensions to own and partner's group memberships. In C. Sedikides & M. Brewer (Eds.), *Individual self, relational self, and collective self.* Philadelphia: Psychology Press.

Arrow, K. (1974). *The limits of organization.* New York: Norton.

Arthur, M. B., & Rousseau, D. M. (1996a). A new career lexicon for the 21st century. *Academy of Management Executive, 10*, 28–39.

Arthur, M.B., & Rousseau, D.M. (Eds.). (1996b). *The boundaryless career: A new employment principle for a new organizational era.* New York: Oxford University Press.

Asch, S. E. (1951). Effects of group pressure upon the modification and distortion of judgments. In H. Guetzkow (Ed.), *Groups, leadership, and men* (pp. 177–190). Pittsburgh, PA: Carnegie Press.

Ashford, S. J. (1988). Individual strategies for coping with stress during organisational transitions. *The Journal of Applied Behavioral Science, 24,* 19–36.

Ashford, S. J., & Cummings, L. L. (1985). Proactive feedback seeking: The instrumental use of the information environment. *Journal of Occupational Psychology, 58,* 67–79.

Ashforth, B. E. (2001). *Role transitions in organizational life: An identity-based perspective.* Mahwah, NJ: Erlbaum.

Ashforth, B., & Humphrey, R. (1993). Emotional labor in service roles: The influence of identity. *Academy of Management Review, 18,* 88–115.

Ashforth, B.E., & Humphrey, R.H. (1995). Labeling processes in the organization: Constructing the individual. *Research in Organizational Behavior, 17,* 413–461.

Ashforth, B. E., & Kreiner, G. (1999). "How can you do it?": Dirty work and the dilemma of identity. *Academy of Management Review, 24,* 413–434.

Ashforth, B. E., Kreiner, G. E., Fugate, M., & Johnson, S. A. (2001). Micro role transitions. In B. E. Ashforth (Ed.), *Role transitions in organizational life: An identity-based perspective.* Mahwah, NJ: Erlbaum.

Ashforth, B. E., & Mael, F. (1989). Social identity theory and the organization. *Academy of Management Review, 14,* 20–39.

Ashforth, B. E., & Mael, F. A. (1996). Organizational identity and strategy as a context for the individual. *Advances in Strategic Management, 13,* 17–62.

Ashforth, B. E., & Mael, F. A. (1998). The power of resistance: Sustaining valued identities. In R. M. Kramer & M. A. Neele (Eds.), *Power and influence in organizations* (pp. 89–119). Thousand Oaks, CA: Sage.

Ashmore, R. D. (1970). Solving the problem of prejudice. In B. E. Collins (Ed.), *Social psychology, social influence, attitude change, group processes, and prejudice* (pp. 246–296). Reading, MA: Addison-Wesley.

Baba, M. L. (1995). The cultural ecology of the corporation: Explaining diversity in work group responses to organizational transformation. *Journal of Applied Behavioral Science, 31,* 202–233.

Bachman, B. A. (1993). *An intergroup model of organizational mergers.* Unpublished doctoral. dissertation, University of Delaware, Newark.

Bales, R. F. (1950). *Interaction process analysis: A method for the study of small groups.* Reading, MA: Addison-Wesley.

Banaji, M. R., & Hardin, C. T. (1996). Automatic stereotyping. *Psychological Science, 7*(3), 136–141.

Banker, B. S., & Gaertner, S. L. (1998). Achieving stepfamily harmony: An intergroup relations approach. *Journal of Family Psychology, 12,* 310–325.

Banker, B. S., & Gaertner, S. L. (2000). Unpublished data. Department of Psychology, University of Delaware, Newark.

Bantel, K. A., & Jackson, S. E. (1989). Top management and innovations in banking: Does the composition of the top team make a difference? *Strategic Management Journal, 10,* 107–124.

Baratta, J. E., & McManus, M. A. (1992). The effect of contextual factors on individuals' job performance. *Journal of Applied Social Psychology, 22,* 1702–1710.

Barber, B. (1983). *The logic and limits of trust.* New Brunswick, NJ: Rutgers University Press.

Barker, J. R., & Tompkins, P. K. (1994). Identification in the self-managing organization: Characteristics of target and tenure. *Human Communication Research, 21,* 223–240.

Barnett, W. P., & Miner, A. S. (1992). Standing on the shoulders of others: Career interdependence in job mobility. *Administrative Science Quarterly, 37,* 262–281.

Baron, J., & Pfeffer, J. (1994). The social psychology of organizations and inequality. *Social Psychology Quarterly, 57,* 190–209.

Baron, R. M., & Kenny, D.A. (1996) The moderator-mediator distinction in social psychological research: Conceptual, strategic and statistical considerations. *Journal of Personality and Social Psycohlogy, 51,* 1173–1182.

Barreto, M., & Ellemers, N. (2000). You can't always do what you want: Social identity and self-presentational determinants of the choice to work for a low status group. *Personality and Social Psychology Bulletin, 26,* 891–906.

Bartel, C. A. (2001). *Strengthening organizational identification through community ser-*

vice: When "giving back" generates psychological and behavioral outcomes. Manuscript submitted for publication.

Bass, B. M. (1985). *Leadership and performance beyond expectations.* New York: Free Press.

Bass, B. M. (1990a). *Bass and Stogdill's handbook of leadership: Theory, research and managerial applications.* New York: Free Press.

Bass, B. M. (1990b). From transactional to transformational leadership: Learning to share the vision. *Organizational Dynamics, 18,* 19–31.

Bass, B. M. (1998). *Transformational leadership: Industrial, military, and educational impact.* Mahwah, NJ: Erlbaum.

Bass, B. M., & Avolio, B. J. (1993). Transformational leadership: A response to critiques. In M. M. Chemers & R. A. Ayman (Eds.), *Leadership theory and research: Perspectives and directions* (pp. 49–80). London: Academic Press.

Batson, C. D., Turk, C. L., Shaw, L. L., & Klein, T. R. (1995). Information function of empathic emotion: Learning that we value the other's welfare. *Journal of Personality and Social Psychology, 68,* 300–313.

Bauer, T. N., Morrison, E. W., & Callister, R. R. (1998). Organizational socialization: A review and directions for research. In G. R. Ferris (Ed.), *Research in personnel and human resources management* (Vol. 16, pp. 149–170). Stamford, CT: JAI Press.

Baumeister, R. F. (1998). The self. In D. T. Gilbert, S. T. Fiske, & G. Lindzey (Eds.), *The handbook of social psychology* (4th ed., Vol. 2, pp. 680–740). Boston: McGraw-Hill.

Baumeister, R. F., & Leary, M. R. (1995). The need to belong: Desire for interpersonal attachments as a fundamental human motivation. *Psychological Bulletin, 117,* 497–529.

Baumeister, R. F., & Tice, D. M. (1990). Anxiety and social exclusion. *Journal of Social and Clinical Psychology, 9,* 165–195.

Beaton, A. M., & Tougas, F. (1997). The representation of women in management: The more, the merrier? *Personality and Social Psychology Bulletin, 23,* 773–782.

Becker, T. E. (1992). Foci and bases of commitment: Are they distinctions worth making? *Academy of Management Journal, 35,* 232–244.

Becker, T. E., & Billings, R. S. (1993). Profiles of commitment: An empirical test. *Journal of Organizational Behavior, 14,* 177–190.

Becker, T. E., Randall, D. M., & Riegel, C. D. (1995). The multidimensional view of commitment and the theory of reasoned action: A comparative evaluation. *Journal of Management, 21,* 617–638.

Ben-Bakr, K. A., Al-Shammari, I. S., Jefri, O. A., & Prasad, J. N. (1994). Organizational commitment, satisfaction, and turnover in Saudi organizations: A predictive study. *Journal of Socio Economics, 23,* 449–456.

Berscheid, E., & Reis, H. T. (1998). Attraction and close relationships. In D. T. Gilbert, S. T. Fiske, & G. Lindzey (Eds.), *The handbook of social psychology* (4th ed., Vol. 2, pp.193–281). New York: McGraw-Hill.

Besser, T. L. (1993). The commitment of Japanese workers and U.S. workers: A reassessment of the literature. *American Sociological Review, 58,* 873–881.

Bettencourt, B. A., Brewer, M. B., Croak, M., & Miller, N. (1992). Cooperation and the reduction of intergroup bias: The role of reward structure and social orientation. *Journal of Experimental Social Psychology, 28,* 301–319.

Bettencourt, B. A., Charlton, K., & Kernahan, C. (1997). Numerical representation of groups in co-operative settings: Social orientation effects on ingroup bias. *Journal of Experimental Social Psychology, 33,* 630–659.

Bettman, J. R., & Weitz, B. A. (1983). Attributions in the board room: Causal reasoning in corporate annual reports. *Administrative Science Quarterly, 28,* 165–183.

Bhappu, A., Griffith, T.L., and Northcraft, G. B. (1997). Media effects and communication bias in diverse groups. *Organizational Behavior and Human Decision Processes, 70*(3), 199–205.

Bielby, W. T., & Baron, J. N. (1986). Men and women at work: Sex segregation and statistical discrimination. *American Journal of Sociology, 91,* 759–799.

Blake, R. R., & Mouton, J. S. (1979). Intergroup problem solving in organizations: From theory to practice. In W. Austin & S. Worchel (Eds.), *The social psychology of intergroup relations* (pp. 19–31). Monterey, CA: Brooks/Cole.

Blake, R. R., & Mouton, J. S. (1984). *Solving costly organizational conflicts.* San Francisco: Jossey-Bass.

Blake, R. R., & Mouton, J. S. (1985). How to achieve integration on the human side of the merger. *Organizational Dynamics, 13,* 41–56.

Blalock, H. M. (1967). *Toward a theory of minority group relations.* New York: Wiley.

Blau, G. (1995). Influence of group lateness on individual lateness: A cross-level examination. *Academy of Management Journal, 38,* 1483–1496.

Blumer, H. (1966). Sociological implications of the thought of George Herbert Mead. *American Journal of Sociology, 71,* 535–548

Bobo, L. (1999). Prejudice as group position: Micro-foundations of a sociological approach to racism and race relations. *Journal of Social Issues, 55,* 445–472.

Boldry, J. G., & Kashy, D. A. (1999). Intergroup perception in naturally occurring groups of differential status: A social relations perspective. *Journal of Personality and Social Psychology, 77,* 1200–1212.

Bouas, K., & Arrow, H. (1996). The development of group identity in computer and face-to-face groups with membership change. *Computer Supported Cooperative Work, 4,* 153–178.

Bourhis, R. Y. (1994). Power, gender, and intergroup discrimination: Some minimal group experiments. In M. P. Zanna & J. M. Olson (Eds.), *The psychology of prejudice: The Ontario Symposium* (Vol. 7, pp. 171–208). Hillsdale, NJ: Erlbaum.

Brandon, D., & Pratt, M.G. (1999). Managing the formation of virtual team categories and prototypes by managing information: A SIT/SCT perspective. *Best Paper Proceedings for the Academy of Management.*

Brann, P., & Foddy, M. (1988). Trust and consumption of a deteriorating common resource. *Journal of Conflict Resolution, 31,* 615–630.

Branscombe, N. R., & Ellemers, N. (1998). Coping with group-based discrimination: Individualistic versus group level strategies. In J. K. Swim & C. Stangor (Eds.), *Prejudice: The target's perspective* (pp. 243–266). New York: Academic Press.

Branscombe, N. R., & Wann, D. L. (1994). Collective self-esteem consequences of outgroup derogation when a valued social identity is on trial. *European Journal of Social Psychology, 24,* 641–657.

Bray, J. H., & Berger, S. H. (1993). Developmental issues in stepfamilies research project: Family relationships and parent-child interactions. *Journal of Family Psychology, 7,* 76–90.

Brenner, L. (1995). The myth of incentive pay. *CFO,* July, 26–34.

Brewer, M. B. (1979). Ingroup bias in the minimal intergroup situatuion: A cognitive motivational analysis. *Psychological Bulletin, 86,* 307–324.

Brewer, M. B. (1981). Ethnocentrism and its role in interpersonal trust. In M. B. Brewer & B. E. Collins (Eds.), *Scientific inquiry and the social sciences* (pp. 345–360). New York: Jossey-Bass.

Brewer, M. B. (1988). A dual process model of impression formation. In T. S. Srull & R. S. Wyer (Eds.), *Advances in social cognition: Vol. I. A dual process model of impression formation* (pp. 1–36). Hillsdale, NJ: Erlbaum.

Brewer, M. B. (1991). The social self: On being the same and different at the same time. *Personality and Social Psychology Bulletin, 17,* 475–482.

Brewer, M. (1993a). The role of distinctiveness in social identity and group behavior. In M. A. Hogg & D. Abrams (Eds.), *Group motivation: Social psychological perspectives* (pp. 1–16). New York: Harvester Wheatsheaf.

Brewer, M. B. (1993b). Social identity, distinctiveness, and in-group homogeneity. *Social Cognition, 11,* 150–164.

Brewer, M.B. (1995). Managing diversity: The role of social identities. In S. E. Jackson & M. N. Ruderman (Eds.), *Diversity in work teams: Research paradigms for a changing workplace* (pp. 47–68). Washington, DC: American Psychological Association.

Brewer, M. B. (1996). In-group favoritism: The subtle side of intergroup discrimination. In D. M. Messick & A. Tenbrunsel (Eds.), *Behavioral research and business ethics.* New York: Russell Sage.

Brewer, M. B. (2000). Reducing prejudice through cross-categorization: The effects of multiple social identities. In S. Oskamp (Ed.), *Reducing prejudice and discrimination* (pp. 165–183). Mahwah, NJ: Erlbaum.

Brewer, M. B., & Brown, R. J. (1998). Intergroup relations. In D. T. Gilbert, S. T. Fiske, & G. Lindzey (Eds.), *Handbook of social psychology* (4th ed., pp. 554–594). Boston, MA: McGraw-Hill.

Brewer, M. B., & Campbell, D. T. (1976). *Eth-

*nocentrism and intergroup attitudes: East African evidence.* New York: Halstead Press.

Brewer, M. B., & Feinstein, A. H. (1999). Dual processes in the cognitive representation of persons and social categories. In S. Chaiken & Y. Trope (Eds.), *Dual-process theories in social psychology* (pp. 255–270). New York: Guilford.

Brewer, M. B., & Gardner, W. (1996). Who is this 'we'?: Levels of collective identity and self-representations. *Journal of Personality and Social Psychology, 71,* 83–93.

Brewer, M. B., & Gaertner, S. L. (2000). Toward reduction of prejudice: Intergroup contact and social categorization. In R. Brown & S. Gaertner (Eds.), *Blackwell handbook of social psychology: Intergroup processes* (pp. 451–472). Oxford: Blackwell.

Brewer, M. B., & Harasty, A. S. (1996). Seeing groups as entities: The role of perceiver motivation. In E. T. Higgins & R. M. Sorrentino (Eds.), *Handbook of motivation and cognition: Vol. 3. The interpersonal context* (pp. 347–370). New York: Guilford.

Brewer, M. B., Ho, H., Lee, J., & Miller, N. (1987). Social identity and social distance among Hong Kong school children. *Personality and Social Psychology Bulletin, 13,* 156–165.

Brewer, M. B., & Kramer, R. M. (1985). The psychology of intergroup attitudes and behavior. *Annual Review of Psychology, 36,* 219–243.

Brewer, M. B., & Kramer, R. M. (1986). Choice behavior in social dilemmas: Effects of social identity, group size, and decision framing. *Journal of Personality and Social Psychology, 50,* 543–549.

Brewer, M. B., Manzi, J. M., & Shaw, J. S. (1993). In-group identification as a function of depersonalization, distinctiveness, and status. *Psychological Science, 4,* 88–92.

Brewer, M. B., & Miller, N. (1984). Beyond the contact hypothesis: Theoretical perspectives on desegregation. In N. Miller & M. B. Brewer (Eds.), *Groups in contact: The psychology of desegregation* (pp. 281–302). Orlando, Florida: Academic Press.

Brewer, M. B., & Miller, N. (1988). Contact and cooperation: When do they work? in P. Katz & D. Taylor (Eds.), *Eliminating racism: Means and controversies* (pp. 315–326). New York: Plenum

Brewer, M. B., & Miller, N. (1996). *Intergroup*

*relations.* Buckingham, UK: Open University Press.

Brewer, M. B., & Schneider, S. (1990). Social identity and social dilemmas: A double-edged sword. In D. Abrams & M. Hogg (Eds.), *Social identity theory: Constructive and critical advances* (pp. 169–184). London: Harvester Wheatsheaf.

Brickson, S. L. (1999). *The impact of relational and collective identity orientations on prejudice toward nontraditional workers.* Unpublished manuscript, Harvard University.

Brickson, S. L. (2000). The impact of identity orientation on individual and organizational outcomes in demographically diverse settings. *Academy of Management Review, 25,* 82–101.

Brickson, S. L. (in press). Re-assessing the standard: How understanding identity orientation informs—and improves—intergroup relations interventions. *Academy of Management Best Paper Proceedings.*

Brief, A. P., & Motowidlo, S. J. (1986). Prosocial organizational behaviors. *Academy of Management Review, 11,* 710–725.

Brothers, D. (1995). *Falling backwards: An exploration of trust and self-experience.* New York: Norton.

Brown, A. C., Green, R. J., & Druckman, J. (1990). A comparison of stepfamilies with and without child-focused problems. *American Orthopsychiatric Association, Inc., 60,* 556–566.

Brown, B. B., & Lohr, M. J. (1987). Peer-group affiliation and adolescent self-esteem: An integration of ego-identity and symbolic-interaction theories. *Journal of Personality and Social Psychology, 52,* 47–55.

Brown, M. E. (1969). Identification and some conditions of organizational involvement. *Administrative Science Quarterly, 14,* 346–355.

Brown, R. J. (1978). Divided we fall: An analysis of relations between sections of a factory workforce. In H. Tajfel (Ed.) *Differentiation between social groups: Studies in the social psychology of intergroup relations* (pp. 395–430). London: Academic Press.

Brown, R. J. (1988). *Group processes: Dynamics within and between groups.* Oxford, UK: Blackwell.

Brown, R. (1995). *Prejudice. Its social psychology.* Oxford, UK: Blackwell.

Brown, R. J., Condor, S., Mathews, A., Wade, G., & Williams, J. A . (1986). Explaining intergroup differentiation in an industrial organisation. *Journal of Occupational Psychology, 59,* 273–286.

Brown, R. J, & Ross, G. F. (1982). The battle for acceptance: An exploration into the dynamics of intergroup behaviour. In H. Tajfel (Ed.), *Social Identity and Intergroup Relations* (pp. 155–178). London: Cambridge University Press.

Brown, R., & Smith, A. (1989). Perceptions of and by minority groups: The case of women in academia. *European Journal of Social Psychology, 19,* 61–75.

Brown, R., Vivian, J., & Hewstone, M. (1999). Changing attitudes through intergroup contact: The effects of group membership salience. *European Journal of Social Psychology, 29,* 741–764.

Bruins, J., Ellemers, N., & De Gilder, D. (1999). Power use and differential competence as determinants of subordinates' evaluative and behavioural responses in simulated organizations. *European Journal of Social Psychology, 29,* 843–870.

Bryman, A. (1992). *Charisma and leadership in organizations.* London: Sage.

Bullis, C. A., & Tompkins, P. K. (1989). The forest ranger revisited: A study of control practices and identification. *Communication Monographs, 56,* 287–306.

Buono, A. F., & Bowditch, J. L. (1989). *The human side of mergers and acquisitions: Managing collisions between people, cultures, and organizations.* San Francisco: Jossey-Bass.

Buono, A. F., Bowditch, J. L., & Lewis, III, J. W. (1985). When cultures collide: The anatomy of a merger. *Human Relations, 38,* 477–500.

Burke, R. J., & Bolf, C. (1986). Learning within organizations: Sources and content. *Psychological Reports, 59,* 1187–1198.

Burns, J. M. (1978). *Leadership.* New York: Harper & Row.

Burt, R. S., & Knez, M. (1995). Kinds of third-party effects on trust. *Rationality and Society, 7,* 255–292.

Buss, D. M., & Scheier, M. F. (1976). Self-consciousness, self-awareness, and self-attribution. *Journal of Research in Personality, 10,* 463–468.

Caddick, B. (1982). Perceived illegitimacy and intergroup relations. In H. Tajfel (Ed.), *Social Identity and Intergroup Relations* (pp. 137–154). London: Cambridge University Press.

Callan, V. J., Terry, D. J., & Schweitzer, R. J. (1995). Coping resources, coping strategies and adjustment to organizational change: Direct or buffering effects. *Work and Stress, 8,* 372–383.

Campbell, D. T. (1958). Common fate, similarity, and other indices of the status of aggregates of persons as social entities. *Behavioral Science, 3,* 14–25.

Campbell, D. T. (1965). Ethnocentric and other altruistic motives. In D. Levine (Ed.), *Nebraska symposium on motivation* (Vol. 13, pp. 283–311). Lincoln, NE: University of Nebraska Press.

Caporael, L. R. (1997). The evolution of truly social cognition: The core configurations model. *Personality and Social Psychology Review, 1,* 276–298.

Cartwright, D., & Zander, A. (1960). Leadership and group performance: Introduction. In D. Cartwright & A. Zander (Eds.) *Group dynamics: Research and theory* (3rd ed., pp. 487–510). Evanston, IL: Row Peterson.

Cartwright, D., & Zander, A. (Eds.) (1968). *Group dynamics: Research and theory* (3rd ed.). London: Tavistock.

Cartwright, S., & Cooper, C. L. (1992a). The impact of mergers and acquisitions on people at work: Existing research and issues. *British Journal of Management, 1,* 65–76.

Cartwright, S., & Cooper, C. L. (1992b). *Mergers and acquisitions: The human factor.* Oxford: Butterworth-Heinemann.

Cartwright, S., & Cooper, C. L. (1993) The role of culture compatibility in successful organizational marriage. *Academy of Management Executive, 7,* 57–70.

Cartwright, S., & Cooper, C. L. (1994). The human effects of mergers and acquisitions. In C. L. Cooper & D. M. Rousseau (Eds.), *Trends in organizational behavior* (Vol. 1, pp. 47–61). Chichester, UK: John Wiley & Sons.

Cascio, W. F. (1995). Whither industrial and organizational psychology in a changing world of work? *American Psychologist, 50,* 928–939.

Cassidy, J. (1999, September 13). Wall Street follies: A new study shows America's fat cats getting fatter. *The New Yorker,* p. 32.

Caves, R. (1992). *American industry: Structure, conduct, performance.* Englewood Cliffs, NJ: Prentice-Hall.

Chao, G. T. (1988). The socialization process:

Building newcomer commitment. In M. London & E. Mone (Eds.), *Career growth and human resource strategies* (pp. 31–47). Westport, CT: Quorum Press.

Chatman, J. A. (1991). Matching people and organizations: Selection and socialization in public accounting firms. *Administrative Science Quarterly, 36,* 459–484.

Chatman, J. A., Polzer, J. T., Barsade, S. G., & Neale, M. A. (1999). Being different yet feeling similar: The influence of demographic composition and organizational culture on work processes and outcomes. *Administrative Science Quarterly, 43,* 749–780

Chattopadhyay, P. (1999). Beyond direct and symmetrical effects: The influence of demographic dissimilarity on organizational citizenship behavior. *Academy of Management Journal, 42,* 273–287.

Chemers, M. M. (2001). Leadership effectiveness: An integrative review. In M. A. Hogg & R. S. Tindale (Eds.), *Blackwell handbook of social psychology: Group processes* (pp. 376–399). Oxford, UK: Blackwell.

Chemers, M. M., Oskamp, S., & Costanzo, M. A. (Eds.). (1995). *Diversity in organizations: New perspectives for a changing workplace.* London: Sage.

Cheney, G. (1983). On the various and changing meanings of organizational membership: A field study of organizational identification. *Communication Monographs, 50,* 342–362.

Cheney, G. (1991). *Rhetoric in an organizational society: Managing multiple identities.* Columbia, SC: Unversity of South Carolina Press.

Cole, R. E. (1979) *Work, mobility and participation: A comparative study of American and Japanese industry.* Los Angeles, CA: University of California Press.

Cole, R. E., Kalleberg, A. L., & Lincoln, J. R. (1993). Assessing commitment in the United States and Japan: A comment on Besser. *American Sociological Review, 59,* 882–885.

Coleman, J. (1990). *Foundations of social theory.* Cambridge, MA: Harvard University Press.

Collinson, D. L. (1992). *Managing the shopfloor: Subjectivity, masculinity and workplace culture.* Berlin: Walter de Gruyter.

Comer, D. R. (1991). Organizational newcomers' acquisition of information from peers. *Management Communication Quarterly, 5,* 64–89.

Conger, J. A., & Kanungo, R. N. (1987). Towards a behavioral theory of charismatic leadership in organizational settings. *Academy of Management Review, 12,* 637–647.

Conger, J. A., & Kanungo, R. N. (1988). Behavioral dimensions of charismatic leadership. In J. A. Conger, & R. N. Kanungo (Eds.), *Charismatic leadership: The elusive factor on organizational effectiveness* (pp. 78–97). San Francisco, CA: Jossey-Bass.

Cook, S. W. (1962). The systematic analysis of socially significant events. *Journal of Social Issues, 18,* 66–84.

Cook, S. W. (1984). Cooperative interaction in multiethnic contexts. In N. Miller & M. B. Brewer (Eds.), *Groups in contact: The psychology of desegregation* (pp.155–185). Orlando, FL: Academic Press.

Cooley, C. H. (1902). *Human nature and the social order.* New York: Scribner's.

Cota, A. A., & Dion, K. L. (1986). Salience of gender and sex composition of ad hoc groups: An experimental test of distinctiveness theory. *Journal of Personality and Social Psychology, 50,* 770–776.

Cousin, S. D. (1989). Culture and self-perception in Japan and in the United States. *Journal of Personality and Social Psychology, 56,* 124–131.

Covin, T. J, Sightler, K. W., Kolenko, T. A., & Tudor, K. R. (1996). An investigation of postacquisition satisfaction with the merger. *Journal of Applied Behavioral Science, 32,* 125–142.

Cox, T., & Blake, S. (1991). Managing cultural diversity: Implications for organizational competitiveness. *Academy of Management Executive, 5,* 45–56.

Cox, T. H., & Finley, J. A. (1995). An analysis of work specialization and organization level as dimensions of workforce diversity. In M. Chemers, S. Oskamp, & M. A. Costanzo (Eds.), *Diversity in organizations: New perspectives for a changing workplace* (pp. 62–90). Thousand Oaks, CA: Sage.

Creed, W. D., & Miles, R. E. (1996). Trust in organizations: A conceptual framework linking organizational forms, managerial philosophies, and the opportunity costs of controls. In R. M. Kramer & T. R. Tyler (Eds.), *Trust in organizations* (pp. 16–38). Thousand Oaks, CA: Sage.

Creed, W. E. D., & Scully, M. S. (2000). Songs of ourselves: Employees' deployment of social identity in workplace encounters. *Journal of Management Inquiry, 9,* 391–412.

Crisp, R. J. & Hewstone, M. (1999). Crossed categorization and intergroup bias: Context, process and social consequences. *Group Processes and Intergroup Relations, 2,* 307–333.

Crisp, R. J., & Hewstone, M. (2000a). Crossed categorization and intergroup bias: The moderating roles of intergroup and affective context. *Journal of Experimental Social Psychology, 36,* 357–383.

Crisp, R. J., & Hewstone, M. (2000b). Multiple categorization and social identity. In D. Capozza & R. Brown (Eds.). *Social identity theory: Trends in theory and research* (pp. 149–166). London, UK & Thousand Oaks, CA: Sage.

Crisp, R. J., Hewstone, M., & Rubin, M. (2001). Does multiple categorization reduce intergroup bias? *Personality and Social Psychology Bulletin, 27,* 76–89.

Crocker, J., & Major, B. (1989). Social stigma and self-esteem: The self-protective properties of stigma. *Psychological Review, 96,* 608–630.

Crosbie-Burnett, M. (1984). The centrality of the step relationship: A challenge to family theory and practice. *Family Relations, 33,* 459–463.

Crosby, F. J., Ferdman, B. M., & Wingate, B. R. (2001). Addressing and redressing discrimination: Affirmative action in social psychological perspective. In R. Brown & S. Gaertner (Eds.), *Blackwell handbook of social psychology: Intergroup processes* (pp. 495–513). Oxford, UK & Cambridge, MA: Blackwell.

Crosby, F. J., & VanDeVeer, C. (Eds.) (2000). *Sex, race, and merit: Debating affirmative action in education and employment.* Ann Arbor, MI: University of Michigan Press.

Csikszentmihalyi, M., & Sawyer, K. (1995). Creative insight: The social dimension of a solitary moment. In R. J. Sternberg & J. E. Davidson (Eds.), *The nature of insight* (pp. 329–363). Cambridge, MA: MIT Press.

Czarniawska, B. (1997). *Narrating the organization: Dramas of institutional identity.* Chicago: University of Chicago Press.

Dachler, H. P., & Hosking, D. (1995). The primacy of relations in socially constructing organizational realities. In D. Hosking, H. P. Dachler, & K. J. Gergen (Eds.), *Management and organizations: Relationship alternatives to individualism* (pp. 1–28). Aldershot, UK: Avebury.

Dalessio, A., & Imada, A. S. (1984). Relationships between interview selection decisions and perceptions of applicant similarity to an ideal employee and self: A field study. *Human Relations, 37,* 67–80.

Dansky, K. H. (1996). The effect of group mentoring on career outcomes. *Group and Organization Management, 21,* 5–21.

Darrah, C. (1994). Skill requirements at work: Rhetoric versus reality. *Work and Occupations, 21,* 64–84.

David, B., & Turner, J. C. (1996). Studies in self-categorization and minority conversion: Is being a member of the outgroup an advantage? *British Journal of Social Psychology, 35,* 179–199.

David, B., & Turner, J. C. (1999). Studies in self-categorization and minority conversion: The ingroup minority in intragroup and intergroup contexts. *British Journal of Social Psychology, 38,* 115–134.

Dawes, R. M., van de Kragt, A. J. C., & Orbell, J. M. (1988). Not me or thee but we: The importance of group identity in eliciting cooperation in dilemma situations: Experimental manipulations. *Acta Psychologica, 68,* 83–97.

Dawes, R. M., van de Kragt, A. J. C., & Orbell, J. M. (1990). Cooperation for the benefit of us—not me, or my conscience. In J. Mansbridge (Ed.), *Beyond self-interest* (pp. 97–110). Chicago: University of Chicago Press.

Day, D. V., Cross, W. E., Jr., Ringseis, E. L., & Williams, T. L. (1999). Self-categorization and identity construction associated with managing diversity. *Journal of Vocational Behavior, 54,* 188–195.

De Cremer, D., & van Vugt, M. (in press). Why do people cooperate with leaders in managing social dilemmas? Instrumental and relational aspects of structural cooperation. *Journal of Experimental Social Psychology.*

De Vries, N. K., & De Dreu, C. K. W. (in press). *Group consensus and innovation.* Oxford: Blackwell.

De Vries, N. K., De Dreu, C. K. W., Gordijn, E., & Schuurman, M. (1996). Majority and minority influence: A dual interpretation. In W. Stroebe & M. Hewstone (Eds.), *European review of social psychology* (Vol. 7, pp. 145–172). Chichester, UK: John Wiley.

Deaux, K. (1996). Social identification. In E. Tory Higgins and A. W. Kruglanski (Eds.), *Social Psychology* (pp. 777–798). New York, NY: Guilford.

Deaux, K., Reid, A., Mizrahi, K., & Cotting, D. (1999). Connecting the person to the social: The functions of social identification. In T. Tyler, R. M. Kramer, & O. P. John (Eds.), *The psychology of the social self* (pp. 91–113). Mahwah, NJ: Lawrence Erlbaum Associates.

DeDreu, C. K. W., & De Vries, N. K. (1997). Minority dissent in organizations. In C. K. W. De Dreu & E. Van De Vliert (Eds.). *Using conflict in organizations* (pp. 72–86). London: Sage.

DeSanctis, G., & Poole, M. S. (1997). Transitions in teamwork in new organizational forms. In B. Markovsky, M. J. Lovaglia, & E. J. Lawler (Eds.), *Advances in Group Processes* (Vol. 14. pp. 157–176). London: JAI Press.

Deschamps, J.-C., & Devos, T. (1998). Regarding the relationship between social identity and personal identity. In S. Worchel, J. F. Morales, D. Páez, & J.-C. Deschamps (Eds.), *Social identity: International perspectives* (pp. 1–12). London: Sage.

Deutsch, M. (1986). The malignant (spiral) process of hostile interaction. In R. K. White (Ed.), *Psychology and the prevention of nuclear war* (pp. 131–154). New York: New York University Press.

Devine, P. G., Hamilton, D. L., & Ostrom, T. M. (Eds.). (1994). *Social cognition: Impact on social psychology.* San Diego, CA: Academic Press.

Devos, T., Comby, L., & Deschamps, J.-C. (1996). Asymmetries in judgements of ingroup and out-group variability. In W. Stroebe & M. Hewstone (Eds.), *European Review of Social Psychology* (Vol. 7, pp. 95–144). Chichester, UK: J. Wiley.

Diehl, M. (1990). The minimal group paradigm: Theoretical explanations and empirical findings. In W. Stroebe & M. Hewstone (Eds.), *European review of social psychology* (Vol. 1, pp. 263–292). Chichester, UK: Wiley.

Diekmann, K. A., Samuels, S. M., Ross, L., & Bazerman, M. H. (1997). Self-interest and fairness in problems of resource allocation: Allocators versus recipients. *Journal of Personality and Social Psychology, 72,* 1061–1074.

Dietz, B. E., & Ritchey, P. N. (1996). The relative influence of individual identities, identity accumulation, and identity combinations on facets of psychological well-being. *Sociological Spectrum, 16,* 1–25.

Dirsmith, A. J., & Covaleski, M. A. (1985). Informal communications, nonformal communications, and mentoring in public accounting firms. *Accounting, Organizations, and Society, 10,* 149–169.

Doise, W. (1978). *Groups and individuals: Explanations in social psychology.* Cambridge, UK: Cambridge University Press.

Doise, W., & Sinclair, A. (1973). The categorization process in intergroup relations. *European Journal of Social Psychology, 9,* 281–289.

Doosje, B., & Ellemers, N. (1997). Stereotyping under threat: The role of group identification. In R. Spears, P. J. Oakes, N. Ellemers, & S. A. Haslam (Eds.), *The social psychology of stereotyping and group life* (pp. 257–272). Oxford, UK: Blackwell.

Drucker, P. F. (1986). *The frontiers of management: Where tomorrow decisions are being shaped today.* New York: J. P. Dutton.

Dovidio, J. F., Gaertner, S. L., Validzic, A., Matoka, K., Johnson, B., & Frazier, S. (1997). Extending the benefits of re-categorization: Evaluations, self-disclosure and helping. *Journal of Experimental Social Psychology, 33,* 401–420.

Dovidio, J. F., Gaertner, S. L., & Validzic, A. (1998). Intergroup bias: Status, differentiation, and a common ingroup identity. *Journal of Personality and Social Psychology, 75,* 109–120.

Dubrovsky, V. J., Kiesler, S., & Sethna, B. N. (1991). The equalization phenomenon: Status effects in computer-mediated and face-to-face decision making groups. *Human-Computer Interaction, 6,* 119–146.

Duck, J. M., & Fielding, K. S. (1999). Leaders and sub-groups: One of us or one of them? *Group Processes and Intergroup Relations, 2,* 203–230.

Dukerich, J. M., Golden, B. R., & Jacobson, C. K. (1996). Nested cultures and identities: A comparative study of nation and profession/occupation status effects on resource allocation decisions. *Research in the Sociology of Organizations, 14,* 35–89.

Dukerich, J., Kramer, R., & Parks, J. M. (1998). The dark side of organizational identification. In D. Whetten, and P. Godfrey (Eds.), *Identity in organizations: Developing theory through conversations* (pp. 245–256). Thousand Oaks, CA: Sage.

Dunbar, K. (1997). How scientists think: Online creativity and conceptual change in science. In T. B. Ward, S. M. Smith, & J. Vaid (Eds.), *Creative thought: An investigation of conceptual structures and processes* (pp. 461–493). Washington, DC: American Psychological Association.

Dunphy, D., & Stace, D. (1990). Transformation and coercive strategies for planned organizational change: Beyond the OD model. In F. Massarik (Ed.), *Advances in organization development* (Vol. 1, pp. 85–104). Norwood, NJ: Ablex Publishing Corp.

Dutton, J. E., & Dukerich, J. M. (1991). Keeping an eye on the mirror: Image and identity in organizational adaptation. *Academy of Management Journal, 34,* 517–554.

Dutton, J. E., Dukerich, J. M., & Harquail, C. V. (1994). Organizational images and member identification. *Administrative Science Quarterly, 39,* 239–263.

Eagly, A.H. (1987). *Sex differences in social behavior. A social-role interpretation.* Hillsdale, NJ: Erlbaum.

Eagly, A. H., Karau, S. J., & Makhijani, M. G. (1995). Gender and the effectiveness of leaders: A meta-analysis. *Psychological Bulletin, 117,* 125–145.

Eagly, A. H., Makhijani, M. G., & Klonsky, B. G. (1992). Gender and the evaluation of leaders: A meta-analysis. *Psychological Bulletin, 111,* 3–22.

Eagly, A. H., & Mladinic, A. (1994). Are people prejudiced against women? Some answers from research on attitudes, gender stereotypes, and judgements of competence. In W. Stroebe & M. Hewstone (Eds.), *European Review of Social Psychology* (Vol. 5, pp. 1–36). Chichester, UK: Wiley.

Earley, P. C. (1989). Social loafing and collectivism: A comparison of the United States and the People's Republic of China. *Administrative Science Quarterly, 34,* 565–581.

Eby, L. T., Freeman, D. M., Rush, M. C., & Lance, C. E. (1999). Motivational bases of affective organizational commitment: A partial test of an integrative theoretical model. *Journal of Occupational and Organizational Psychology, 72,* 463–483.

Edmondson, A. (1998). Psychological safety and learning behavior in work teams. *Administrative Science Quarterly, 44,* 350–383.

Eisenberger, R., Huntington, R., Hutchinson, S., & Sowa, D. (1986). Perceived organizational support. *Journal of Applied Psychology, 71,* 500–507.

Ellemers, N. (1993). The influence of socio-structural variables on identity management strategies. In W. Stroebe & M. Hewstone (Eds.), *European Review of Social Psychology* (Vol. 4, pp. 27–58). New York: Wiley.

Ellemers, N., Barreto, M., & Spears, R. (1999). Commitment and strategic responses to social context. In N. Ellemers, R. Spears, & B. Doosje, (Eds.), *Social identity: Context, commitment, content* (pp. 127–146). Oxford, UK: Blackwell.

Ellemers, N., De Gilder, D., & Van den Heuvel, H. (1998). Career-oriented versus team-oriented commitment and behavior at work. *Journal of Applied Psychology, 83,* 683–692.

Ellemers, N., Doosje, B. J., van Knippenberg, A., & Wilke, H. (1992). Status protection in high status minority groups. *European Journal of Social Psychology, 22,* 123–140.

Ellemers, N., Kortekaas, P., & Ouwerkerk, J. W. (1999). Self-categorization, commitment to the group, and group self-esteem as related but distinct aspects of social identity. *European Journal of Social Psychology, 29,* 371–389.

Ellemers, N., Spears, R., & Doosje, B. J. (Eds). (1999). *Social identity: Context, commitment, content.* Oxford, UK: Blackwell.

Ellemers, N., van Knippenberg, A., de Vries, N., & Wilke, H. (1988). Social identification and permeability of group boundaries. *European Journal of Social Psychology, 18,* 497–513.

Ellemers, N., van Knippenberg, A., & Wilke, H. (1990). The influence of permeability of group boundaries and stability of group status on strategies of individual mobility and social change. *British Journal of Social Psychology, 29,* 233–246.

Ellemers, N., & van Rijswijk, W. (1997). Identity needs versus social opportunities: The use of group-level and individual-level management strategies. *Social Psychology Quarterly, 60,* 52–65.

Ellemers, N., Van Rijswijk, W., Bruins, J., & De Gilder, D. (1998). Group commitment as a moderator of attributional and behavioural responses to power use. *European Journal of Social Psychology, 28,* 555–573.

Ellemers, N., Van Rijswijk, W., Roefs. M., & Simons, C. (1997). Bias in intergroup perceptions: Balancing ingroup identity with social reality. *Personality and Social Psychology Bulletin., 23,* 186–198.

Ellemers, N., Wilke, H., & van Knippenberg, A. (1993). Effects of the legitimacy of low group or individual status on individual and collective status-enhancement strategies. *Journal of Personality and Social Psychology, 64,* 766–778.

Ellis, D. J., & Pekar, P. P. (1978). Acquisitions: Is 50/50 good enough? *Planning Review, 6,* 15–19.

Elsbach, K. (1999). An expanded model of organizational identification. In R. Sutton & B. Staw (Eds), *Research in Organizational Behavior* (Vol. 21, pp. 163–199). Stanford, CA: JAI Press.

Elsbach, K. D. (2000). Coping with hybrid organizational identities: Evidence from California Legislative Staff. In J. Wagner (Ed.), *Advances in Qualitative Organizational Research, Vol. 3.* Forthcoming.

Elsbach, K. D., & Bhattacharya, C. B. (2000). *Organizational disidentification: A study of social identity and the national rifle association.* Unpublished manuscript, Emory University.

Elsbach, K. D., & Glynn, M. A. (1996). Believing your own "PR": Embedding identification in strategic reputation. *Advances in Strategic Management, 13,* 65–90.

Elsbach, K.D., & Kramer, R. (1996). Members' responses to organizational identity threats: Encountering and countering the Business Week ratings. *Administrative Science Quarterly, 41,* 442–476.

Erber, R., & Fiske, S. T. (1984). Outcome dependency and attention to inconsistent information. *Journal of Personality and Social Psychology, 47,* 709–726.

Fairhurst, G. T., & Snavely, B. K. (1983a). Majority and token minority group relationships: Power acquisition and communication. *Academy of Management Review, 8,* 292–300.

Fairhurst, G. T., & Snavely, B. K. (1983b). A test of the social isolation of male tokens. *Academy of Management Review, 26,* 353–361.

Farh, J.-L., Dobbins, G. H., & Cheng, B.-S. (1991). Cultural relativity in action: A comparison of self-ratings made by Chinese and U.S. workers. *Personnel Psychology, 44,* 129–147.

Farh, J.-L., Tsui, A. S., Xin, K., & Cheng, B.-S. (1998). The influence of relational demography and Guanxi: The Chinese case. *Organization Science, 9*(4), 471–488.

Farley, J. (1982). *Majority-minority relations.* Englewood, NJ: Prentice-Hall.

Farrell, D., & Rusbult, C.E. (1981). Exchange variables as predictors of job satisfaction, job commitment, and turnover: The impact of rewards, costs, alternatives and investments. *Organizational Behavior and Human Decision Processes, 28,* 78–95.

Feldman, D. C. (1981). The multiple socialization of organization members. *Academy of Management Review, 6,* 309–318.

Feldman, D. C. (1989). Careers in organizations: Recent trends and future directions. *Journal of Management, 15,* 135–156.

Feldman, M. S. (1991). The meanings of ambiguity: Learning from stories and metaphors. In P. J. Frost, L. F. Moore, M. R. Louis, C. C. Lundberg and J. Martin (Eds.), *Reframing Organizational Culture* (pp. 145–156). Newbury Park: Sage Publications.

Feldman, S. D. (1979). Nested identities. *Studies in Symbolic Interaction, 2,* 399–418.

Fenigstein, A. (1984). Self-consciousness and self as target. *Journal of Personality and Social Psychology, 47,* 860–870.

Fenigstein, A., & Vanable, P. A. (1992). Paranoia and self-consciousness. *Journal of Personality and Social Psychology, 62,* 129–138.

Festinger, L. (1954). A theory of social comparison processes. *Human Relations, 7,* 117–140.

Fiedler, F. E. (1965). A contingency model of leadership effectiveness. In L. Berkowitz (Ed.), *Advances in experimental social psychology* (Vol. 1, pp. 149–190). New York: Academic Press.

Fiedler, F. E. (1971). *Leadership.* Morristown, NJ: General Learning Press.

Fiedler, F. E. (1978). The contingency model and the dynamics of the leadership process. In L. Berkowitz (Ed.), *Advances in experimental social psychology* (Vol. 11, pp. 60-112). New York: Academic Press.

Fielding, K. S., & Hogg, M. A. (1997). Social identity, self-categorization, and leadership: A field study of small interactive groups.

*Group Dynamics: Theory, Research, and Practice, 1,* 39–51.

Fielding, K. S., & Hogg, M. A. (2000). Working hard to achieve self-defining group goals: A social identity analysis. *Zeitschrift für Sozialpsychologie, 31,* 191–203.

Fine, G., & Holyfield, L. (1996). Secrecy, trust, and dangerous leisure: Generating group cohesion in voluntary organizations. *Social Psychology Quarterly, 59,* 22–38.

Fine, M. A., McKenry, P. C., Donnelly, B. W., & Voydanoff, P. (1992). Perceived adjustment of parents and children: Variations by family structure, race, and gender. *Journal of Marriage and the Family, 54,* 118–127.

Fishbein, M., & Ajzen, I. (1975). *Belief, attitude, intention and behavior: An introduction to theory and research.* Reading, MA: Addison-Wesley

Fishbein, M., & Stasson, M. (1990). The role of desires, self-predictions, and perceived control in the prediction of training session attendance. *Journal of Applied Social Psychology, 20,* 173–198.

Fisher, C. D. (1986). Organizational socialization: An integrative review. In G. R. Ferris & K. M. Rowland (Eds.), *Research in personnel and human resources management* (Vol. 4, pp. 101–145). Greenwich, CT: JAI Press.

Fisher, R.J., Maltz, E., & Jaworski, B.J. (1997). Enhancing communication between marketing and engineering: The moderating role of relative functional identification. *Journal of Marketing, 61*(3), 54–70.

Fiske, S. T. (1993). Controlling other people: The impact of power on stereotyping. *American Psychologist, 48,* 621–628.

Fiske, S. T. (1998). Stereotyping, prejudice, and discrimination. In D.T. Gilbert, S.T. Fiske, & G. Lindzey (Eds.), *Handbook of social psychology* (4th ed., pp. 357–411). Boston, MA: McGraw-Hill.

Fiske, S. T., & Dépret, E. (1996). Control, interdependence and power: Understanding social cognition in its social context. *European Review of Social Psychology, 7,* 31–61.

Fiske, S. T., & Neuberg, S. L. (1990). A continuum of impression formation, from category-based to individuating processes: Influences of information and motivation on attention and interpretation. In M. Zanna (Ed.), *Advances in experimental social psychology* (Vol. 23, pp. 1–74). Orlando, FL: Academic Press.

Fiske, S. T., & Ruscher, J.B. (1993). Negative interdependence and prejudice: Whence the affect? In D. Mackie & D. Hamilton (Eds.), *Affect, cognition and stereotyping* (pp. 239–268). San Diego: Academic Press.

Fiske, S. T., & Taylor, S.E. (1991). *Social cognition* (2nd ed.). New York: McGraw-Hill.

Fleishman, E. A., & Peters, D. A. (1962). Interpersonal values, leadership attitudes, and managerial success. *Personnel Psychology, 15,* 43–56.

Floge, L., & Merrill, D. (1986). Tokenism reconsidered: Male nurses and female physicians in a hospital setting. *Social Forces, 64,* 925–947.

Foddy, M., & Hogg M. A. (1999). Impact of leaders on resource consumption in social dilemmas: The intergroup context. In M. Foddy, M. Smithson, S. Schneider, & M. A. Hogg (Eds.), *Resolving social dilemmas: Dynamic, structural, and intergroup aspects* (pp. 309–330). Philadelphia: Psychology Press.

Foddy, M., Smithson, M., Schneider, S., & Hogg, M. (1999). *Resolving social dilemmas: Dynamic, structural, and intergroup aspects.* Philadelphia: Psychology Press.

Folger, R., & Kanovsky, M.A. (1989). Effects of procedural and distributive justice on reactions to pay raise decisions. *Academy of Management Journal, 32,* 115–130.

Foster, M .D., & Matheson, K. (1998). Perceiving and feeling discrimination: Motivation or inhibition for collective action. *Group Processes and Intergroup Relations, 1,* 165–174.

Fox, A. (1974). *Beyond contract: Power and trust relations.* London: Faber & Faber.

Frable, D. E. S. (1993). Dimensions of marginality: Distinctions among those who are different. *Personality and Social Psychology Bulletin, 19,* 370–380.

Frable, D. E. S., Blackstone, T., & Scherbaum, C. (1990). Marginal and mindful: Deviants in social interactions. *Journal of Personality and Social Psychology, 59,* 140–149.

Frank, R. (1985). *Choosing the right pond: The quest for status.* New York: Oxford University Press.

Fukuyama, F. (1995). *Trust: The social virtues and the creation of prosperity.* New York: Free Press.

Fulk, J. (1993). Social construction of communication technology. *Academy of Management Journal, 36,* 921–950.

Furstenberg, F. F., Jr. (1987). The new extended family: The experience of parents and children after remarriage. In K. Pasley & M. Ihinger-Tallman (Eds.), *Remarriage and stepparenting: Current research and theory* (pp. 42–61). New York: Guilford.

Furstenberg, F. F., Jr., & Spanier, G. (1984). The risk of dissolution in remarriage: An examination of Cherlin's Hypothesis of Incomplete Institutionalization. *Family Relations, 33*, 433–441.

Gaertner, S. L., & Dovidio, J. F. (2000). *Reducing intergroup bias: The Common Ingroup Identity Model.* Philadelphia: Psychology Press.

Gaertner, S. L., Dovidio, J. F., Anastasio, P. A., Bachman, B. A., & Rust, M. C. (1993). The common ingroup identity model: Recategorization and the reduction of intergroup bias. In: W. Stroebe & M. Hewstone (Eds.), *The European review of Ssocial psychology* (Vol. 4, pp. 1–126). London: Wiley.

Gaertner, S. L., Dovidio, J. F., & Bachman, B. A. (1996). Revisiting the contact hypothesis: The induction of a common ingroup identity. *Journal of Intercultural Relationships, 20*, 271–290.

Gaertner, S. L., Dovidio, J. F., Nier, J. A., Banker, B. S., Ward, C. M., Houlette, M., & Loux, S. (2000). The common ingroup identity model for reducing intergroup bias: Progress and challenges. In D. Capozza & R. Brown (Eds.), *Social identity processes* (pp 133–148). London, UK & Thousand Oaks, CA: Sage.

Gaertner, S. L., Dovidio, J. F., Rust, M. C., Nier, J. A., Banker, B. S., Ward, C. M., Mottola, G. R., & Houlette, M. (1999). Reducing intergroup bias: Elements of intergroup cooperation. *Journal of Personality and Social Psychology, 76*, 388–402.

Gaertner, S. L., Mann, J. A., Dovidio, J. F., Murrell, A. J., & Pomare, M. (1990). How does cooperation reduce intergroup bias? *Journal of Personality and Social Psychology, 59*, 692–704.

Gaertner, S. L., Mann, J., Murrell, A., & Dovidio, J. F. (1989). Reducing intergroup bias: The benefits of recategorization. *Journal of Personality and Social Psychology, 57*, 239–249.

Gaertner, S. L., Rust, M. C., Dovidio, J. F., Bachman, B. A., & Anastasio, P.A. (1994). The contact hypothesis: The role of a common ingroup identity on reducing intergroup bias. *Small Group Research, 25*, 224–249.

Gaertner, S. L., Rust, M. C., Dovidio, J. F., Bachman, B. A., & Anastasio, P. A. (1996). The Contact Hypothesis: The role of a common ingroup identity on reducing intergroup bias among majority and minority group members. In J. L. Nye & A. M. Brower (Eds.), *What's social about social cognition?* (pp. 230–360). Newbury Park, CA: Sage.

Geis, F. L. (1993). Self-fulfilling prophecies: A social-psychological view of gender. In A. E. Beall & R. J. Sternberg (Eds.), *The psychology of gender* (pp. 9–54). New York: Guilford Press.

George, J. M. (1990). Personality, affect, and behavior in groups. *Journal of Applied Psychology, 75*, 107–116.

George, J. M., & Bettenhausen, K. (1990). Understanding prosocial behavior, sales performance, and turnover: A group-level analysis in a service context. *Journal of Applied Psychology, 75*, 698–709.

Gergen, K. J. (1991). *The saturated self: Dilemmas of identity in contemporary life.* New York: Basic Books.

Gergen, K. (1994). *Reality and relationships.* Cambridge: Harvard University Press.

Gergen, K. J., & Gergen, M. M. (1988). Narrative and the self as relationship. In L. Berkowitz (Ed.), *Advances in experimental social psychology* (Vol. 21, pp.17–56). New York: Academic Press.

Gilbert, D. T., Fiske, S. T., & Lindzey, G. (Eds.). (1998). *The handbook of social psychology* (4th ed.). New York: McGraw-Hill.

Gilbert, D. T., & Jones, E. E. (1986). Perceiver-induced constraint: Interpretations of self-generated reality. *Journal of Personality and Social Psychology, 50*, 269–280.

Gilbert, D. T., & Malone, P. S. (1995). The correspondence bias. *Psychological Bulletin, 117*, 21–38.

Glick, P. (1991). Trait-based and sex-based discrimination in occupational prestige, occupational salary, and hiring. *Sex Roles, 25*, 351–378.

Glick, P., & Fiske, S. T. (1996). The ambivalent sexism inventory: Differentiating hostile and benevolent sexism. *Journal of Personality and Social Psychology, 70*, 491–512.

Glick, P., & Fiske, S. T. (2001). Ambivalent stereotypes as legitimizing ideologies: Differentiating paternalistic and envious prejudice. In J. T. Jost & B. Major (Eds.), *The psychology of legitimacy: Emerging perspectives on ideology, justice, and intergroup relations.* Cambridge, UK: Cambridge University Press.

Goffman, E. (1959). *The presentation of self in everyday life.* New York: Doubleday.

Goffman, E. (1963). *Stigma: Notes on the management of a spoiled identity.* Englewood Cliffs, NJ: Prentice-Hall.

Golden-Biddle, K., & Rao, H. (1997). Breaches in the boardroom: Organizational identity and conflict of commitment in a non-profit organization. *Organization Science, 8,* 593–611.

Goldstein, I. L, & Gilliam, P. (1990). Training system issues in the year 2000. *American Psychologist, 45,* 134–145.

Gordon, M. E., & Ladd, R. T. (1990). Dual allegiance: Renewal, reconsideration, and recantation. *Personnel Psychology, 43,* 37–69.

Gouldner, A. W. (1957). Cosmopolitans and locals: Toward an analysis of latent social roles— I. *Administrative Science Quarterly, 2,* 281–306.

Granovetter, M. (1985). Economic action and social structure: The problem of embeddedness. *American Journal of Sociology, 91,* 481–510

Grant, P. R., & Brown, R. (1995). From ethnocentrism to collective protest. *Social Psychology Quarterly, 58,* 195–211.

Graves, D. (1981). Individual reactions to a merger of two small firms of brokers in the re-insurance industry: A total population survey. *Journal of Management Studies, 18,* 89–113.

Greene, C. N. (1978). Identification modes of professionals: Relationship with formalization, role strain, and alienation. *Academy of Management Journal, 21,* 486–492.

Greenwald, A. G. (1980). The totalitarian ego: Fabrication and revision of personal history. *American Psychologist, 35,* 603–618.

Gregersen, H. B. (1993). Multiple commitments at work and extra-role behavior during three stages of organizational tenure. *Journal of Business Research, 26,* 31–47.

Gregory, K. L. (1983). Native-view paradigms: Multiple cultures and culture conflicts in organizations. *Administrative Science Quarterly, 28,* 359–376.

Griffeth, R. W., Hom, P. W., Fink, L. S., & Cohen, D. J. (1997). Comparative tests of multivariate models of recruiting sources effects. *Journal of Management, 23,* 19–36.

Gruenfeld, D. H., Martorana, P. V., & Fan, E. T. (2000). What do groups learn from their worldliest members? Direct and indirect influence in dynamic teams. *Organizational Behavior and Human Decision Processes, 82,* 45–49.

Guetzkow, H. (1955). *Multiple loyalties.* Princeton, NJ: Princeton University Press.

Guild, W. (1999). *Order, authority & identity: A comparative study of ski patrollers and lift operators at a California Ski Resort.* Unpublished dissertation, Massachusetts Institute of Technology, Cambridge.

Gutek, B. A. (1993). Asymmetric changes in men's and women's roles. In B. C. Long & S. E. Kahn (Eds.), *Women, work, and coping* (pp. 11–31). Montreal: McGill-Queen's University Press.

Hackett, R. D., Bycio, P., & Hausdorf, P. A. (1994). Further assessments of Meyer and Allen's (1991) three-component model of organizational commitment. *Journal of Applied Psychology, 79,* 15–23,

Hains, S. C., Hogg, M. A., & Duck, J. M. (1997). Self-categorization and leadership: Effects of group prototypicality and leader stereotypicality. *Personality and Social Psychology Bulletin, 23,* 1087–1099.

Hall, D. T., Schneider, B., & Nygren, H. T. (1970). Personal factors in organizational identification. *Administrative Science Quarterly, 15,* 176–190.

Hall, R. J., & Lord, R. G. (1995). Multi-level information processing explanations of followers' leadership perceptions. *Leadership Quarterly, 6,* 265–287.

Hallier, J., & James, P. (1999). Group rites and trainer wrongs in employee experiences of job change. *Journal of Management Studies, 36,* 45–67.

Hambrick, D. C., & Cannella, A. A. (1993). Relative standing: A framework for understanding departures of acquired executives. *Academy of Management Journal, 36,* 733–762.

Hamburger, Y. (1994). The contact hypothesis reconsidered: Effects of the atypical outgroup member on the outgroup stereotype. *Basic and Applied Social Psychology, 15,* 339–358.

Hamilton, D. L., & Sherman, S. J. (1996). Perceiving persons and groups. *Psychological Review, 103,* 336–355.

Hardin R. (1992). The street-level epistemology of trust. *Analyse & Kritik, 14,* 152–176.

Harquail, C.V. (1998). Organizational identification and the « whole person » : Integrating affect, behavior, and cognition. In D. Whetten & P. Godfrey (Eds.), *Identity in organizations: Developing theory through conversations* (pp. 223–231). Thousand Oaks, CA: Sage.

Haslam, S. A. (2000). Going the extra mile: Social identity and the link between leadership and followership. *Keeping Managers Up-to-date.* Australian Graduate School of Management: January–March, 2–4.

Haslam, S. A. (2001). *Psychology in organizations: The social identity approach.* London: Sage.

Haslam, S. A., McGarty, C., Brown, P. M., Eggins, R. A, Morrison, B. E., & Reynolds, K. J. (1998). Inspecting the emperor's clothes: Evidence that randomly-selected leaders can enhance group performance. *Group Dynamics: Theory, Research and Practice, 2,* 168–184.

Haslam, S. A., Oakes, P. J., McGarty, C., Turner, J. C., & Onorato, S. (1995). Contextual changes in the prototypicality of extreme and moderate outgroup members. *European Journal of Social Psychology, 25,* 509–530.

Haslam, S. A. & Platow, M. J. (in press). Social identity and the link between leadership and followership: How affirming a social identity translates personal vision into group action. *Personality and Social Psychology Bulletin.*

Haslam, S. A., Platow, M. J., Turner, J. C., Reynolds, K. J., McGarty, C., Oakes, P. J., Johnson, S., Ryan, M. K., & Veenstra, K. (in press). Social identity and the romance of leadership: The importance of being seen to be 'doing it for us.' *Group Processes and Intergroup Relations.*

Haslam, S. A., Powell, C., & Turner, J. C. (2000). Social identity, self-categorization and work motivation: Rethinking the contribution of the group to positive and sustainable organizational outcomes. *Applied Psychology: An International Review, 49,* 319–339.

Haslam, S. A., Turner, J. C., & Oakes, P. J. (1999). *Contextual variation in leader prototypes.* Manuscript undergoing revision.

Haunschild, P. R., Moreland, R. L., & Murrell, A. J. (1994). Sources of resistance to mergers between groups. *Journal of Applied Social Psychology, 24,* 1150–1178.

Heikes, E. J. (1991). When men are the minority: The case of men in nursing. *The Sociological Quarterly, 32,* 389–401.

Heilman, M. E. (1980). The impact of situational factors on personnel decisions concerning women: Varying the sex composition of the applicant pool. *Organizational Behavior and Human Performance, 26,* 386–395.

Henderson, G. (1994). *Cultural diversity in the workplace: Issues and strategies.* Westport, CT: Praeger.

Henson, K. D. (1996). *Just a temp.* Philadelphia: Temple University Press.

Herek, G. M., & Capitanio, J. P. (1996). "Some of my best friends": Intergroup contact, concealable stigma, and heterosexuals' attitudes toward gay men and lesbians. *Personality and Social Psychology Bulletin, 22,* 412–424.

Hewstone, M. (1992). The 'ultimate attribution error'? A review of the literature on intergroup causal attribution. *European Journal of Social Psychology, 20,* 311–335.

Hewstone, M. (1996). Contact and categorization: Social psychological interventions to change intergroup relations. In C. N. Macrae, C. Stagnor, & M. Hewstone (Eds.), *Foundations of stereotypes and stereotyping* (pp. 323–368). New York: Guilford.

Hewstone, M., & Brown, R. (1986). Contact is not enough: An intergroup perspective on the "contact hypothesis." In M. Hewstone & R. Brown (Eds.), *Contact and conflict in intergroup encounters* (pp. 1–44). Oxford, UK: Basil Blackwell.

Hewstone, M., & Crisp, R. J. (2000). *Perceptions of gender group variability in majority and minority contexts: Two field studies with nurses and police officers.* Manuscript submitted for publication.

Hewstone, M., Crisp, R., Contarello, A., Conway, L., Voci, A., Marletta, G., & Willis, H. (2000). *Perceptual processes and interaction dynamics in settings with 'skewed', 'tilted' and 'balanced' sex ratios: Two field studies of women and men in academia.* Manuscript submitted for publication.

Hewstone, M., Crisp, R. J., Richards, Z., Voci, A., & Rubin, M. (2000). *Gender, group size and perceived group variability.* Manuscript submitted for publication.

Hewstone, M., & Hamberger, J. (2000). Perceived variability and stereotype change. *Journal of Experimental Social Psychology, 36,* 103–124.

Hewstone, M., Islam, M. R., & Judd, C. M. (1993). Models of crossed categorization and intergroup relations. *Journal of Personality and Social Psychology, 64,* 779–793.

Hewstone, M., & Jaspars, J. (1984). Social dimensions of attribution. In H. Tajfel (Ed.), *The social dimension: European developments in social psychology* (Vol. 2, pp. 379–404). Cambridge, UK: Cambridge University Press.

Hewstone, M., & Ward, C. (1985). Ethnocentrism and causal attribution in southeast Asia. *Journal of Personality and Social Psychology, 48,* 614–623.

Higgins, E. T. (1996). Knowledge activation: Accessibility, applicability, and salience. In E. T. Higgins & A. W. Kruglanski (Eds.), *Social psychology: Handbook of basic principles* (pp. 133–168). New York: Guilford.

Higgins, E. T., & King, G. (1981). Accessibility of social constructs: Information-processing consequences of individual and contextual variability. In N. Cantor & J. F. Kihlstrom (Eds.), *Personality, cognition, and social interaction* (pp. 69–121). Hillsdale, NJ: Erlbaum.

Hinkle, S., & Brown, R. J. (1990). Intergroup comparisons and social identity: Some links and lacunae. In D. Abrams & M. A. Hogg (Eds.), *Social identity theory: Constructive and critical advances* (pp. 48–70). New York: Harvester Wheatsheaf.

Hinkle, S., Fox-Cardamone, L., Haseleu, J. A., Brown, R., & Irwin, L. M. (1996). Grassroots political action as an intergroup phenomenon. *Journal of Social Issues, 52,* 39–52.

Hinkle, S., & Schopler, J. (1986). Bias in the evaluation of in-group and out-group performance. In S. Worchel & W. G. Austin (Eds.), *Psychology of intergroup relations* (pp. 196–212). Chicago: Nelson-Hall.

Hinkle, S., Taylor, L. A., Fox-Cardamone, D. L., & Crook, K. F. (1989). Intragroup identification and intergroup differentiation: A multi-component approach. *British Journal of Social Psychology, 28,* 305–317.

Hinz, V.B., & Nelson, L.C. (1990). Testing models of turnover intentions with university faculty. *Journal of Applied Social Psychology, 20,* 68-84.

Hofstede, G. (1980) *Culture's consequences.* Beverly Hills: Sage

Hofstede, G. (1991). *Cultures and organizations: Software of the mind.* New York: McGraw-Hill.

Hogan, E. A., & Overmyer-Day, L. (1994). The psychology of mergers and acquisitions. In C. L. Cooper & L. T. Robertson (Eds), *International review of industrial and organizational psychology* (Vol. 9, pp. 247–281). Chichester, UK: Wiley.

Hogg, M. A. (1992). *The social psychology of group cohesiveness: From attraction to social identity.* Hemel Hempstead, UK: Harvester Wheatsheaf, and New York: New York University Press.

Hogg, M. A. (1993). Group cohesiveness: A critical review and some new directions. *European Review of Social Psychology, 4,* 85–111.

Hogg, M. A. (1996a). Intragroup processes, group structure and social identity. In W. P. Robinson (Ed.), *Social groups and identities: The developing legacy of Henri Tajfel* (pp. 65–93). Oxford, UK: Butterworth-Heineman.

Hogg, M. (1996b). Social identity, self-categorization, and the small group. In J. Davis and E. Witte (Eds.), *Understanding Group Behavior: Vol. 2. Small group processes and interpersonal relations* (pp. 227–254). Hillsdale, NJ: Earlbaum.

Hogg, M. A. (2000a, July). *It's a long way to the top: Social identity and the "glass ceiling".* Invited paper presented at the European Association of Experimental Social Psychology small group meeting on Social Identity Processes in Organizations. Amsterdam, The Netherlands.

Hogg, M. A. (2000b). Self-categorization and subjective uncertainty resolutions: Cognitive and motivational facets of social identity and group membership. In J. P. Forgas, K. D. Williams, & L. Wheeler (Eds.), *The social mind: Cognitive and motivational aspects of interpersonal behavior* (pp. 323–349). New York: Cambridge University Press.

Hogg, M. A. (2000c). Social identity and social comparison. In J. Suls & L. Wheeler (Eds.), *Handbook of social comparison: Theory and research* (pp. 401–421). New York: Kluwer/Plenum.

Hogg, M. A. (2000d). Subjective uncertainty reduction through self-categorization: A motivational theory of social identity processes. *European Review of Social Psychology, 11,* 223–255.

Hogg, M. A. (2001). Social categorization, depersonalization, and group behavior. In M. A. Hogg & R. S. Tindale, (Eds.), *Blackwell handbook of social psychology: Group processes* (pp. 56–85). Oxford, UK: Blackwell.

Hogg, M. A. (2001). From prototypicality to power: A social identity analysis of leadership. In S. R. Thye, E. Lawler, M. Macy, & H. Walker (Eds.), *Advances in group processes* (Vol. 18, pp. 1–30). Oxford, UK: Elsevier.

Hogg, M. A. (in press c). Social identity and the sovereignty of the group: A psychology of belonging. In C. Sedikides & M. B. Brewer (Eds.), *Individual self, relational self, and collective self* (pp. 123–143). Philadelphia, PA: Psychology Press.

Hogg, M. A. (in press c). A social identity theory of leadership. *Personality and Social Psychology Review.*

Hogg, M. A. & Abrams, D. (1988) *Social identifications: A social psychology of intergroup relations and group processes.* London & New York: Routledge.

Hogg, M. A., & Abrams, D. (1993). Towards a single-process uncertainty-reduction model of social motivation in groups. In M. A. Hogg & D. Abrams (Eds.), *Group motivation: Social psychological perspectives* (pp. 173–190). London: Harvester-Wheatsheaf, & New York: Prentice-Hall.

Hogg, M. A., & Abrams, D. (1999). Social identity and social cognition: Historical background and current trends. In D. Abrams & M. A. Hogg (Eds.), *Social identity and social cognition* (pp. 1–25). Oxford, UK: Blackwell.

Hogg, M. A., Cooper-Shaw, L., & Holtzworth, D. W. (1993). Group prototypicality and depersonalized attraction in small interactive groups. *Personality and Social Psychology Bulletin, 19,* 452–465.

Hogg, M. A., & Hains, S. C. (1996). Intergroup relations and group solidarity: Effects of group identification and social beliefs on depersonalized attraction. *Journal of Personality and Social Psychology, 70,* 295–309.

Hogg, M. A., & Hains, S. C. (1998). Friendship and group identification: A new look at the role of cohesiveness in groupthink. *European Journal of Social Psychology, 28,* 323–341.

Hogg, M. A., Hains, S. C., & Mason, I. (1998). Identification and leadership in small groups: Salience, frame of reference, and leader stereotypicality effects on leader evaluations. *Journal of Personality and Social Psychology, 75,* 1248–1263.

Hogg, M. A., & Hardie, E. A. (1991). Social attraction, personal attraction, and self-categorization: A field study. *Personality and Social Psychology Bulletin, 17,* 175–180.

Hogg, M. A., & Hardie, E. A. (1992). Prototypicality, conformity, and depersonalized attraction: A self-categorization analysis of group cohesiveness. *British Journal of Social Psychology, 31,* 41–56.

Hogg, M. A., Hardie, E. A., & Reynolds, K. J. (1995). Prototypical similarity, self-categorization, and depersonalized attraction: A perspective on group cohesiveness. *European Journal of Social Psychology, 25,* 159–177.

Hogg, M. A., & Mullin, B. A. (1999). Joining groups to reduce uncertainty: Subjective uncertainty reduction and group identification. In D. Abrams & M. A. Hogg, (Eds.), *Social identity and social cognition* (pp. 249–279). Malden, MA: Blackwell.

Hogg, M. A., & Reid, S. (in press). Social identity, leadership, and power. In J. Bargh & A. Lee-Chai (Eds.), *The use and abuse of power: Multiple perspectives on the causes of corruption.* Philadelphia: Psychology Press.

Hogg, M., & Terry, D. (2000). Social identity and self-categorization processes in organizational contexts. *Academy of Management Review, 25,* 121–140.

Hogg, M. A., Terry, D. J., & White, K. M. (1995). A tale of two theories: a critical comparison of identity theory with social identity theory. *Social Psychology Quarterly, 58,* 255–269.

Hogg, M., & Turner, J. (1987). Intergroup behavior, self-stereotyping, and the salience of social categories. *British Journal of Social Psychology, 26,* 325–340.

Hogg, M. A., & Williams, K. D. (2000). From I to we: Social identity and the collective self. *Group Dynamics: Theory, Research, and Practice, 4,* 81–97.

Hollander, E. P. (1958). Conformity, status, and idiosyncracy credit. *Psychological Review, 65,* 117–127.

Hollander, E. P. (1985). Leadership and power. In G. Lindzey & E. Aronson (Eds.), *The handbook of social psychology* (3rd ed., Vol. 2, pp. 485–537). New York: Random House.

Hollander, E. P. (1995). Organizational leadership and followership. In P. Collett & A. Furnham (Eds.), *Social psychology at work: Essays in honour of Michael Argyle* (pp. 69-87). London: Routledge.

Hollander, E. P., & Julian, J. W. (1969). Contemporary trends in the analysis of leadership processes. *Psychological Bulletin, 71,* 387–391.

Hollander, E. P., & Julian, J. W. (1970). Studies in leader legitimacy, influence, and innovation. In L. Berkowitz (Ed.), *Advances in experimental social psychology* (Vol. 5, pp. 34–69). New York: Academic Press.

Holson, L. M. (1999, January 4). After 2.5 trillion in combinations in 1998, the sky's the limit in 1999. *New York Times.*

Hom, P. W., Katerberg, R., & Hullin, C. L. (1979). Comparative examination of three approaches to the prediction of turnover. *Journal of Applied Psychology, 64,* 280–290.

Hornsey, M. J., & Hogg, M. A. (2000a). Assimilation and diversity: An integrative model of subgroup relations. *Personality and Social Psychology Review, 4,* 143–156.

Hornsey, M. J., & Hogg, M. A. (2000b). Subgroup relations: A comparison of mutual intergroup differentiation and common ingroup identity models of prejudice reduction. *Personality and Social Psychology Bulletin, 26,* 242–256.

House, R. J., Spangler, W. D., & Woycke, J. (1991). Personality and charisma in the U.S. presidency: A psychological theory of leader effectiveness. *Administrative Science Quarterly, 36,* 364–396.

Howell, D.C. (1987). *Statistical methods for Psychology* (2nd ed.). Boston: Duxbury Press.

Hrebiniak, L. G., & Alutto, J. A. (1972). Personal and role-related factors in the development of organizational commitment. *Administrative Science Quarterly, 17,* 555–573.

Hughes, E. (1951). Work and self. In J. Rohrer, & M. Sherif (Eds.), *Social psychology at the cross-roads* (pp. 313–323). New York: Harper & Brothers.

Hunt, S. A., & Benford, R. D. (1994). Identity talk in the peace and justice movement. *Journal of Contemporary Ethnography, 22,* 488–517.

Hunt, S. D., & Morgan, R. M. (1994). Organizational commitment: One of many commitments or key mediating construct? *Academy of Management Journal, 37,* 1568–1587.

Huo, Y. J., Smith, H. J., Tyler, T. R., & Lind, E. A. (1996). Superordinate identification, subgroup identification, and justice concerns: Is separatism the problem; is assimilation the answer? *Psychological Science, 7,* 40–45.

Ibarra, H. (1999). Provisional selves: Experimenting with image and identity in professional adaptation. *Administrative Science Quarterly, 44,* 764–791.

Insko, C. A., & Schopler, J. (1998). Differential distrust of groups and individuals. In C. Sedikides, J. Schopler, & C. Insko (Eds.), *Intergroup cognition and intergroup behavior* (pp. 75–107). Hillsdale, NJ: Erlbaum.

Insko, C. A., Schopler, J., Hoyle, R., Dardis, G., & Graetz, K. (1990). Individual-group discontinuity as a function of fear and greed. *Journal of Personality and Social Psychology, 58,* 68–79.

Islam, M. R., & Hewstone, M. (1993). Dimensions of contact as predictors of intergroup anxiety, perceived outgroup variability and outgroup attitude: An integrative model. *Personality and Social Psychology Bulletin, 19,* 700–710.

Jackson, S. E., Brett, J. F., Sessa, V. I., Cooper, D. M., Julin, J. A., & Peyronnin, K. (1991). Some differences make a difference: Individual dissimilarity and group heterogeneity as correlates of recruitment, promotion, and turnover. *Journal of Applied Psychology, 76,* 675–689.

Jacobs, J. A., & Powell, B. (1985). Occupational prestige: A sex-neutral concept? *Sex Roles, 12,* 1061–1071.

James, K., Lavato, C., & Khoo, G. (1994). Social identity correlates of minority workers' health. *Academy of Management Journal, 37*(2), 383–396.

James, S. D., & Johnson, D. W. (1987). Social interdependence, psychological adjustment, and marital satisfaction in second marriages. *Journal of Social Psychology, 128,* 287–303.

Janis, I. L. (1972). *Victims of groupthink: A psychological study of foreign policy decisions and fiascoes.* Boston, MA: Houghton-Mifflin.

Janoff-Bulman, R. (1992). *Shattered assumptions: Towards a new psychology of trauma.* New York: Free Press.

Jehn, K. A., Northcraft, G. B., & Neale, M. A. (1999). Why differences make a difference: A field study of diversity, conflict, and performance in workgroups. *Administrative Science Quarterly, 44(4),* 741–763.

Jensen, M. C., & Meckling, W. H. (1976). Theory of the firm: Managerial behavior, agency costs, and ownership structure. *Journal of Financial Economics, 3,* 305–360.

Jetten, J., Spears, R., & Manstead, A. S. R. (1996). Intergroup norms and intergroup discrimination: Distinctive self-categorization and social identity effects. *Journal of Personality and Social Psychology, 71,* 1222–1233.

Jetten, J., Spears, R., & Manstead, A. S. R. (1998). Intergroup similarity and group variability: The effects of group distinctiveness on the expression of ingroup bias. *Journal of Personality and Social Psychology, 74,* 1481–1492.

Jinnett, K., & Alexander, J.A. (1999). The influence of organizational context on quitting intention: An examination of treatment staff in long-term mental health care settings. *Research on Aging, 21,* 176–204.

Johns, G., & Nicholson, N. (1982). The meaning of absence: New strategies for theory and research. In B. M. Staw & L. L. Cummings (Eds.), *Research in organizational behavior* (Vol. 4, pp. 127–172). Greenwich, CT: JAI Press.

Johnson, D. W., Johnson, R., & Maruyama, G. (1984). Goal interdependence and interpersonal attraction in heterogeneous classrooms: A meta-analysis. In N. Miller & M. B. Brewer (Eds.), *Groups in contact: The psychology of desegregation* (pp. 187–212). Orlando, FL: Academic Press.

Johnson, S. A. (2001). *Employment externalization in a service environment: The impact of identification with multiple targets.* Unpublished doctoral dissertation, Arizona State University.

Jones, E. E., Wood, G. C., & Quattrone, G. A. (1981). Perceived variability of personal characteristics in in-groups and out-groups: The role of knowledge and evaluation. *Personality and Social Psychology Bulletin, 7,* 523–528.

Jost, J. T. (1997). An experimental replication of the depressed entitlement effect among women. *Psychology of Women Quarterly, 21,* 387–393.

Jost, J. T. (in press). Outgroup favoritism and the theory of system justification: An experimental paradigm for investigating the effects of socio-economic success on stereotype content. In G. Moskowitz (Ed.), *Cognitive social psychology: On the tenure and future of social cognition.* Hillsdale, NJ: Erlbaum.

Jost, J. T., & Banaji, M. R. (1994). The role of stereotyping in system-justification and the production of false consciousness. *British Journal of Social Psychology, 33,* 1–27.

Jost, J. T., & Burgess, D. (2000). Attitudinal ambivalence and the conflict between group and system justification motives in low status groups. *Personality and Social Psychology Bulletin, 26,* 293–305.

Jost, J. T., Pelham, B. W., & Carvallo, M. (2000). *Non-conscious forms of system justification: Cognitive, affective, and behavioral preferences for higher status groups.* Unpublished manuscript, Stanford University.

Jost, J. T., & Ross, L. (1999). Fairness norms and the potential for mutual agreements involving majority and minority groups. In E. Mannix, M. Neale, & R. Wageman (Eds.), *Research on managing groups and teams: Vol. 2. Context* (pp. 93-114). Greenwich, CT: JAI Press.

Jost, J. T., & Thompson, E. P. (2000). Group-based dominance and opposition to equality as independent predictors of self-esteem, ethnocentrism, and social policy attitudes among African Americans and European Americans. *Journal of Experimental Social Psychology, 36,* 209–232.

Joyce, W. F., & Slocum, J. W. (1984). Collective climate: Agreement as a basis for defining aggregate climates in organizations. *Academy of Management Journal, 27,* 721–742

Kanter, R.M. (1977a). Some effects of proportions on group life: Skewed sex ratios and responses to token women. *American Journal of Sociology, 82,* 965–990.

Kanter, R. M. (1977b). *Men and women of the corporation.* New York: Basic Books.

Katz, R. (1985). Organizational stress and early socialization experiences. In T. Beehr & R. Bhagat (Eds.), *Human stress and cognition in organizations: An integrative perspective* (pp. 117–139). New York: Wiley.

Kawakami, K., & Dion K. (1995). Social identity and affect as determinants of collective action. *Theory and Psychology, 5(4),* 551–577.

Keizai Koho Center. (1987). *Japan 1987: An*

*international Comparison.* Tokyo: Japan Institute for Social and Economic Affairs

Kelley, H. H. (1973). Causal schemata and the attribution process. *American Psychologist, 28,* 107–123.

Kelly, C., & Kelly, J. (1994). Who gets involved in collective action? *Human Relations, 47,* 63–88.

Kelman, H. C. (1961). Processes of opinion change. *Public Opinion Quarterly, 25,* 57–78.

Kelman, H. C., & Hamilton, V. L. (1989). *Crimes of obedience.* New Haven, CT: Yale University Press.

Kiesler, S., & Sproull, L. (1992). Group decision making and communication technology. *Organizational Behavior and Human Decision Processes, 52*(1), 96–123.

Kihlstrom, J. F., Cantor, N., Albright, J. S., Chew, B. R., Klein, S. B., & Niedenthal, P. M. (1988). Information processing and the study of the self. In L. Berkowitz (Ed.), *Advances in experimental social psychology* (Vol. 21, pp. 145–180). New York: Academic Press.

King, N., & Anderson, N. (1995). *Innovation and change in organizations.* London: Routledge.

Kitching, J. (1967). Why do mergers miscarry? *Harvard Business Review, 45,* 84–100.

Knez, M., & Camerer, C. F. (1994). Creating "expectational assets" in the laboratory: 'Weakest link' coordination games. *Strategic Management Journal, 15,* 101–120.

Koch, J. T., & Steers, R. M. (1978) Job attachment, satisfaction, and turnover among public sector employees. *Journal of Vocational Behavior, 12,* 119–128.

Kohn, A. (1993). Why incentive plans cannot work. *Harvard Business Review, Sept–Oct,* 54–63.

Korn, P. (1996). *Lovejoy: A year in the life of an abortion clinic.* New York: Atlantic Monthly Press.

Kram, K. E. (1988). *Mentoring at work: Developmental relationships in organizational life.* Lanham, MD: University Press of America.

Kram, K. E., & Isabella, L. A. (1985). Mentoring alternatives: The role of peer relationships in career development. *Academy of Management Journal, 28,* 110–132.

Kramer, M. W. (1993a). Communication after job transfers: Social exchange processes in learning new roles. *Human Communication Research, 20,* 147–174.

Kramer, M. W. (1993b). Communication and uncertainty reduction during job transfers: Learning and joining processes. *Communication Monographs, 60,* 178–198.

Kramer, R. M. (1989). Windows of vulnerability or cognitive illusions? Cognitive processes and the nuclear arms race. *Journal of Experimental Social Psychology, 25,* 79–100.

Kramer, R. M. (1991). Intergroup relations and organizational dilemmas: The role of categorization processes. In L. L. Cummings & B. M. Staw (Eds.), *Research in organizational behavior* (Vol. 13, pp. 191–228). Greenwich, CT: JAI Press.

Kramer, R. M. (1993). Cooperation and organizational identification. In J. K. Murnighan (Ed.), *Social psychology in organizations: Advances in theory and research* (pp. 244–268). Englewood Cliffs, NJ: Prentice-Hall.

Kramer, R. M. (1994). The sinister attribution error: Origins and consequences of collective paranoia. *Motivation and Emotion, 18,* 199–231.

Kramer, R. M. (1995). Distrust and suspicion within groups: A social categorization perspective. In B. Markovsky, M. Lovaglia, R. Simon (Eds.), *Advances in group process* (Vol. 13, pp. 1–32). Greenwich, CT: JAI Press.

Kramer, R. M. (1996a). Divergent realities and convergent disappointments in the hierarchic relation: The intuitive auditor at work. In R. M. Kramer & T. R. Tyler (Eds.), *Trust in organizations: Frontiers of Theory and Research.* Thousand Oaks, CA: Sage.

Kramer, R. M. (1996b). Paranoia, distrust and suspicion within social groups: A social categorization perspective. *Advances in group process, 13,* 1–32.

Kramer, R. M. (1998). Paranoid cognition in social systems: Thinking and acting in the shadow of doubt. *Personality and Social Psychology Review, 2,* 251–275.

Kramer, R. M. (1999). Trust and distrust in organizations: Emerging perspectives, enduring questions. *Annual Review of Psychology, 50,* 569–598.

Kramer, R. M., & Brewer, M. B. (1984). Effects of group identity on resource use in a simulated commons dilemma. *Journal of Personality and Social Psychology, 46,* 1044–1057.

Kramer, R. M., & Brewer, M. B. (1986). Social group identity and the emergence of cooperation in resource conservation dilemmas. In H. Wilke, C. Rutte, & D. Messick (Eds.), *Experimental studies of social dilemmas.* Frankfurt, Germany: Peter Lang Publishing Company.

Kramer, R. M., Brewer, M. B., & Hanna, B. (1996). Collective trust and collective action in organizations: The decision to trust as a social decision. In R. M. Kramer and T. R. Tyler (Eds.), *Trust in organizations: Frontiers of Theory and Research* (pp. 357–389). Thousand Oaks, CA: Sage.

Kramer, R. M., & Goldman, L. (1995). Helping the group or helping yourself? Determinants of cooperation in resource conservation dilemmas. In D. A. Schroeder (Ed.), *Social dilemmas.* New York: Praeger.

Kramer, R. M., & Messick, D. M. (1998). Getting by with a little help from our enemies: Collective paranoia and its role in intergroup relations. In C. Sedikides, J. Schopler, and C. Insko (Eds.), *Intergroup cognition and intergroup behavior* (pp. 233–255). Hillsdale, NJ: Erlbaum.

Kramer, R. M., Pommerenke, P., & Newton, E. (1993). The social context of negotiation: Effects of social identity and accountability on negotiator judgment and decision making. *Journal of Conflict Resolution, 37,* 633–654.

Kramer, R. M., Pradhan-Shah, P., & Woerner, S. (1995). Why ultimatums fail: Social identity and moralistic aggression in coercive bargaining. In R. M. Kramer & D. M. Messick (Eds.), *Negotiation as a social process* (pp. 285–308). Thousand Oaks, CA: Sage.

Kramer, R. M., & Tyler, T. R. (1996). *Trust in organizations: Frontiers of theory and research.* Thousand Oaks, CA: Sage.

Kramer, R. M.& Wei, J. (1999). Social uncertainty and the problem of trust in social groups: The social self in doubt. In T. Tyler, R. M. Kramer, & O. P. John (Eds.), *The psychology of the social self* (pp. 145–168). Mahwah, NJ: Erlbaum.

Krueger, J., & Rothbart, M. (1988). Use of categorical and individuating information in making inferences about personality. *Journal of Personality and Social Psychology, 55,* 187–195.

Kunda, G. (1992). *Engineering culture: Control and commitment in a high-tech corporation.* Philadelphia: Temple University Press,

Kunda, G., Barley, S. R., & Evans, J. (1999). *Why do contractors contract? The theory and reality of high-end contingent labor.* Unpublished manuscript, Stanford University.

Lalonde, R. N. (1992). The dynamics of group differentiation in the face of defeat. *Personality and Social Psychology Bulletin, 18,* 336–342.

LaLonde, R. N., & Silverman, R. A. (1994). Behavioral preferences in response to social injustice. *Journal of Personality and Social Psychology, 66,* 78–85.

Lane, C., & Bachmann, R. (1998). *Trust within and between organizations: Conceptual issues and empirical applications.* New York: Oxford University Press.

Lane, I. M., Mathews, R. C., & Presholdt, P.H. (1988). Determinants of nurses' intentions to leave their profession. *Journal of Organizational Behavior, 9,* 367–372.

Lant, T. K., Hewlin, P. F., & Rindova, V. U. (2000). *Identity at the interfaces: The dynamic construction of identity in organizational fields.* Symposium presented at the annual meeting of the Academy of Management, Toronto, Canada, August.

Lanzetta, J. T., & Englis, B. G. (1989). Expectations of cooperation and competition and their effects on observers' vicarious emotion responses. *Journal of Personality and Social Psychology, 56,* 543–554.

La Piere, R. T. (1934). Attitudes vs. actions. *Social Forces, 13,* 230–237.

Lau, D. C., & Murnighan, J. K. (1998). Demographic diversity and faultlines: The compositional dynamics of organizational groups. *Academy of Management Review, 23,* 325–340.

Lautsch, B. (2000). *Boundary labor markets: Toward a theory explaining variance in the features and outcomes of contingent work.* Unpublished manuscript, paper, Simon Fraser University,

Lawler, E. J. (1992). Affective attachments to nested groups: A choice process theory. *American Sociological Review, 57,* 327–339.

Laws, J. L. (1975). The psychology of tokenism: An analysis. *Sex Roles, 1,* 51–67.

Lea, M., & Spears, R. (1992). Paralanguage and social perception in computer-mediated communication. *Journal of Organizational Computing, 2,* 321–324.

Leary, M. R. (1990). Responses to social exclusion: Social anxiety, jealousy, loneliness, depression, and low self-esteem. *Journal of Social and Clinical Psychology, 9,* 221–229.

LeBon, G. (1895 trans. 1947). *The crowd: A study of the popular mind.* London: Ernsest Benn.

Lebra, T.S. (1976). *Japanese patterns of behavior.* Honolulu: University of Hawaii Press.

Lee, Y.-T., & Duenas, G. (1997). Stereotype accuracy in multicultural business. In Y.-T. Lee, L. J. Jussim, & C. R. McCauley (Eds.), *Stereotype accuracy: Toward appreciating group differences* (pp. 157–186). Washington, DC: American Psychological Association.

Lemaine, G. (1974). Social differentiation and social originality. *European Journal of Social Psychology, 4,* 17–52.

Lemyre, L., & Smith, P. M. (1985). Intergroup discrimination and self-esteem in the minimal group paradigm. *Journal of Personality and Social Psychology, 49,* 660–670.

Lerner, M. J. (1980). *The belief in a just world: A fundamental delusion.* New York: Plenum Press.

Levine, J. M., & Moreland, R. L. (1990). Progress in small group research. *Annual Review of Psychology, 41,* 585–634.

Levine, J. M., & Moreland, R. L. (1991). Culture and socialization in work groups. In L. B. Resnick, J. M. Levine, & S. D. Teasley (Eds.), *Perspectives on socially shared cognition* (pp. 257–279). Washington, DC: APA Press.

Levine, J. M., & Moreland, R. L. (1994). Group socialization: Theory and research. In W. Stroebe & M. Hewstone (Eds.), *European review of social psychology* (Vol. 5, pp. 305–336). Chichester, UK: Wiley.

Levine, J. M., & Moreland, R. L. (1995). Group processes. In A. Tesser (Ed.), *Advanced social psychology* (pp. 419–465). New York: McGraw-Hill.

Levine, J. M., & Moreland, R. L. (1999). Knowledge transmission in work groups: Helping newcomers to succeed. In L. Thompson, J. Levine, & D. Messick (Eds.), *Shared cognition in organizations: The management of knowledge* (pp. 267–296). Mahwah, NJ: Erlbaum.

Levine, J. M., Moreland, R. L., & Choi, H.-S.

(2001). Group socialization and newcomer innovation. In M. Hogg & S. Tindale (Eds.), *Blackwell handbook in social psychology: Vol. 3: Group processes* (pp. 86–106). Oxford, UK: Blackwell.

Levine, J.M., Resnick, L. D., & Higgins, E. T. (1993). Social foundations of cognition. *Annual Review of Psychology, 44,* 585–612.

LeVine, R. A., & Campbell, D. T. (1972). *Ethnocentrism: Theories of conflict, ethnic attitude and group behavior.* New York: Wiley.

Lewicki, R., & Bunker, B. (1995). Trust in relationships: A model of trust development and decline. In B. B. Bunker & J. Z. Rubin (Eds.), *Conflict, cooperation, and justice* (pp. 131–145). San Francisco: Jossey-Bass.

Lewin, K. (1943). Defining the "field at a given time." *Psychological Review, 50,* 292–310.

Lewin, K. (1997). *Field theory in social sciences.* Washington, DC: American Psychological Association.

Lincoln, J. R., & Kalleberg, A. L. (1985). Work organization and workforce commitment: A study of plants and employees in the U.S. and Japan. *American Sociological Review, 50,* 738–760.

Lincoln, J. R., & Kalleberg, A. L. (1990). *Culture, control, and commitment: A study of work organization and work attitudes in the United States and Japan.* New York: Cambridge University Press.

Lind, E. A., & Tyler, T. R. (1988). *The social psychology of procedural justice.* New York: Plenum.

Lindskold, S. (1978). Trust development, the GRIT proposal, and the effects of conciliatory acts on trust and cooperation. *Psychological Bulletin, 85,* 772–793.

Linville, P.W. (1998). The heterogeneity of homogeneity. In J. Cooper & J. Darley (Eds.), *Attribution processes and social interaction: The legacy of Edward E. Jones* (pp. 423–487). Washington, DC: American Psychological Association.

Lipnack, J., & Stamps, J. (1997). *Virtual teams: Reaching across space, time, and organizations with technology.* New York: Wiley.

Lippitt, R., & White, R. (1943). The 'social climate' of children's groups. In R. G. Barker, J. Kounin, & H. Wright (Eds.), *Child behavior and development* (pp. 485–508). New York: McGraw-Hill.

Long, K., & Spears, R. (1997). The self-esteem hypothesis revisited: Differentiation and the disaffected. In R. Spears, P. J. Oakes, N. Ellemers, & S. A. Haslam (Eds.), *The social psychology of stereotyping and group life* (pp. 296–317). Oxford, UK: Blackwell.

Lord, C. G., & Saenz, D. S. (1985). Memory deficits and memory surfeits: Differential cognitive consequences of tokenism for tokens and observers. *Journal of Personality and Social Psychology, 49,* 918–926.

Lord, R. G., Brown, D. J., & Harvey, J. L. (2001). System constraints on leadership perceptions, behavior and influence: An example of connectionist level processes. In M. A. Hogg & R. S. Tindale (Eds.), *Blackwell handbook of social psychology: Group processes* (pp. 283–310). Oxford, UK: Blackwell.

Lord, R. G., Foti, R., & De Vader, C. L. (1984). A test of leadership categorization theory: Internal structure, information processing and leadership perceptions. *Organizational Behaviour and Human Performance, 34,* 343–378.

Lord, R. G., & Maher, K. J. (1991). *Leadership and information processing: Linking perceptions and performance.* Winchester, MA: Unwin Hyman.

Lorenzi-Cioldi, F., Eagly, A. H., & Stewart, T. L. (1995). Homogeneity of gender groups in memory. *Journal of Experimental Social Psychology, 31,* 193–217.

Losocco, K. A., & Kalleberg, A. L. (1988). Age and the meaning of work in the United States and Japan. *Social Forces, 67,* 337–356.

Louis, M. R. (1980). Surprise and sense-making: What newcomers experience in entering unfamiliar organizational settings. *Administrative Science Quarterly, 25,* 226–251.

Louis, M. R. (1983). Organizations as culture-bearing milieux. In L. R. Pondy, P. J. Frost, G. Morgan, & T. C. Dandridge (Eds.), *Organizational symbolism* (pp. 39–54). Greenwich, CT: JAI Press.

Louis, M. R. (1990). Acculturation in the workplace: Newcomers as lay ethnographers. In B. Schneider (Ed.), *Organizational climate and culture* (pp. 85–129). San Francisco: Jossey-Bass.

Louis, M. R., Posner, B. Z., & Powell, G. N. (1983). The availability and helpfulness of socialization practices. *Personnel Psychology, 36,* 857–866.

Lusch, R. F., Boyt, T., & Schuler, D. (1996). Employees as customers: The role of social controls and employee socialization in de-veloping patronage. *Journal of Business Research, 35,* 179–187.

Luthans, F., McCaul, H. S., & Dodd, N. G. (1985). Organizational commitment: A comparison of American, Japanese and Korean employees. *Academy of Management Journal, 28,* 213–219.

Lyon, E. (1974). Work and play: Resource constraints in a small theater. *Urban Life and Culture, 3,* 71–97.

MacKenzie, S. B., Podsakoff, P. M., & Fetter, R. (1991). Organizational citizenship behavior and objective productivity as determinants of managerial evaluations of salespersons' performance. *Organizational Behavior and Human Decision Processes, 50,* 123–150.

Mael, F. (1988). *Organizational identification: Construct redefinition and a field application with organizational alumni.* Unpublished doctoral Dissertation, Wayne State University, Detroit, MI.

Mael, F. A. (1991). A conceptual rationale for the domain and attributes of biodata items. *Personnel Psychology, 44,* 763–792.

Mael, F., & Ashforth, B. E. (1992). Alumni and their alma mater: A partial test of the reformulated model of organizational identification. *Journal of Organizational Behavior, 13,* 103–123.

Mael, F., & Ashforth, B. E. (1995). Loyal from day one: Biodata, organizational identification, and turnover among newcomers. *Personnel Psychology, 48,* 309–333.

Mael, F. A., & Tetrick. L. E. (1992) Identifying organizational identification. *Educational and Psychological Measurement, 52,* 813–824.

Major, B. (1994). From social inequality to personal entitlement: The role of social comparisons, legitimacy appraisals, and group memberships. *Advances in Experimental Social Psychology, 26,* 293–355.

Major, B., & Crocker, J. (1993). Social stigma: The consequences of attributional ambiguity. In D. M. Mackie & D. L. Hamilton (Eds.), *Affect, cognition, and stereotyping: Interactive processes in group perception* (pp. 345–370). New York: Academic Press.

Major, B., & Schmader, T. (2001). Legitimacy and the construal of social disadvantage. In J. T. Jost & B. Major (Eds.), *The psychology of legitimacy: Emerging perspectives on ideology, justice, and intergroup relations.*

Cambridge, UK: Cambridge University Press.

Major, D. A., Kozlowski, S. W., Chao, G. T., & Gardner, P. D. (1995). A longitudinal investigation of newcomer expectations, early socialization outcomes, and the moderating effects of role development factors. *Journal of Applied Psychology, 80,* 418–431.

Manning, F. J., & Ingraham, L. H. (1987). An investigation into the value of unit cohesion in peacetime. In G. Belenky (Ed.), *Contemporary studies in combat psychiatry: Contributions in military studies, No. 62* (pp. 47–67). Westport, CT: Greenwood Press.

March, J. G. (1994). *A primer on decision making.* New York: Free Press.

March, J. G., & Simon, H. A. (1958). *Organizations.* New York: Wiley.

Marcus-Newhall, A., Miller, N., Holtz, R., & Brewer, M. B. (1993). Cross-cutting category membership with role assignment: A means of reducing intergroup bias. *British Journal of Social Psychology, 32,* 125–146.

Markham, S. E., & McKee, G. H. (1995). Group absence behavior and standards: A multilevel analysis. *Academy of Management Journal, 38,* 1174–1190

Marks, M. L. (1988, January/February). The merger syndrome: The human side of corporate combinations. *Journal of Buyouts and Acquisitions,* 18–23.

Marks, S. R., & MacDermid, S. M. (1996). Multiple roles and the self: A theory of role balance. *Journal of Marriage and the Family, 58,* 417–432.

Markus, H. R., & Kitayama, S. (1991). Culture and the self: Implications for cognition, emotion, and motivation. *Psychological Review, 98,* 224–253.

Markus, H. R., & Kitayama, S. (1994). A collective fear of the collective: implications for selves and theories of selves. *Personality and Social Psychology Bulletin, 20,* 568–579.

Marques, J. M., Abrams, D., Paez, D., & Martinez-Taboada, C. (1998). The role of categorization and in-group norms in judgments of groups and their members. *Journal of Personality and Social Psychology, 75,* 976–988.

Marques, J. M., & Paez, D. (1994). The 'black sheep effect': Social categorization, rejection of ingroup deviates and perception of group variability. *European Review of Social Psychology, 5,* 37–68.

Martin, J. (1986). The tolerance of injustice. In J. Olson, C. P. Herman, & M. P. Zanna (Eds.), *Relative deprivation and social comparison: The Ontario symposium: Volume IV* (pp. 217–242). Hillsdale, NJ: Erlbaum.

Martin, P. Y. (1985). Group sex composition in work organizations: A structural-normative model. *Research in the Sociology of Organizations, 4,* 311–349.

Martin, R. (1996). Minority influence and argument generation. *British Journal of Social Psychology, 35,* 91–103.

Martin, R., & Hewstone, M. (1999). Minority influence and optimal problem-solving. *European Journal of Social Psychology, 29,* 825–832.

Martin, R., & Hewstone, M. (2001). Conformity and independence in groups: Majorities and minorities. In M. A. Hogg & R. S. Tindale (Eds.), *Blackwell handbook of social psychology: Group processes* (pp. 209–234). Oxford, UK: Blackwell.

Martin, R., & Hewstone, M. (in press). Determinants and consequences of cognitive processes in majority and minority influence. In J. P. Forgas & K. Williams (Eds.), *Social influence: Direct and indirect processes.* Philadelphia: Psychology Press.

Martocchio, J. J. (1994). The effects of absence culture on individual absence. *Human Relations, 47,* 243–262.

Maslyn, J. M., & Fedor, D. B. (1998). Perceptions of politics: Does measuring different foci matter? *Journal of Applied Psychology, 84,* 645–653.

Mathieu, J. E. (1991). A cross-level nonrecursive model of the antecedents of organizational commitment and satisfaction. *Journal of Applied Psychology, 76,* 607–618.

Mathieu, J. E., & Kohler, S. S. (1990). A cross-level examination of group absence influences on individual absence. *Journal of Applied Psychology, 75,* 217–220.

Mathieu, J. E., & Zajac, D. (1990). A review and meta-analysis of the antecedents, correlates, and consequences of organizational commitment. *Psychological Bulletin, 108,* 171–194.

McGrath, J.E. (1997). Small group research, that once and future field: An interpretation of the past with an eye to the future. *Group Dynamics: Theory, Research, and Practice, 1,* 7–27.

McGregor, D. (1960). *The human side of en-*

*terprise.* New York: McGraw-Hill.

McKinlay, A., Potter, J., & Wetherell, M. (1993). Discourse analysis and social representation. In G. M. Breakwell (Ed.), *Empirical approaches to social representations* (pp. 134–156). Oxford, England: Clarendon Press/Oxford University Press.

Mead, G. H. (1934). *Mind, self, and society.* Chicago: University of Chicago Press.

Mehra, A., Kilduff, M., & Brass, D. J. (1998). At the margins: A distinctiveness approach to the social identity and social networks of underrepresented groups. *Academy of Management Journal, 41,* 441–452.

Meindl, J. R., Ehrlich, S. B., & Dukerich, J. M. (1985). The romance of leadership. *Administrative Science Quarterly, 30,* 78–102.

Mellor, S. (1996). Gender composition and gender representation in local unions: Relationships between women's participation in local office and women's participation in local activities. *Journal of Applied Psychology, 80,* 706–720.

Messick, D. M., Wilke, H., Brewer, M. B., Kramer, R. M., Zemke, P. E., & Lui, L. (1983). Individual adaptations and structural change as solutions to social dilemmas. *Journal of Personality and Social Psychhlology, 44,* 294–309.

Meyer, J. P., & Allen, N. J. (1984). Testing the "side-bet theory" of organizational commitment: Some methodological considerations. *Journal of Applied Psychology, 69,* 372–378.

Meyer, J. P., & Allen, N. J. (1988). Links between work experiences and organizational commitment during the first year of employment: A longitudinal analysis. *Journal of Occupational Psychology, 61,* 195–209.

Meyer, J. P., & Allen, N. J. (1991). A three-component conceptualization of organizational commitment. *Human Resource Management Review, 1,* 61–89.

Meyer, J. P., & Allen, N. J. (1997). *Commitment in the workplace: Theory, research and application.* Thousand Oaks, CA: Sage.

Meyer, J. P., Allen, N. J., & Smith, C. A. (1993). Commitment to organizations and occupations: Extension and test of a three-component conceptualization. *Journal of Applied Psychology, 78,* 538–551.

Meyer, J. P., Paunonen, S. V., Gellatly, I. H., Goffin, R. D., & Jackson, D. N. (1989). Organizational commitment and job performance: It's the nature of the commitment that counts. *Journal of Applied Psychology, 74,* 152–156.

Meyerson, D. E. (1991). Normal ambiguity? A glimpse of an occupational structure. In P. J. Frost, L. F. Moore, M. R. Louis, C. C. Lundberg, & J. Martin (Eds.), *Reframing Organizational Culture* (pp. 131–144). Newbury Park, CA: Sage.

Meyerson, D. E., & Fletcher, J. K. (2000, January/February). A modest manifesto for shattering the glass ceiling. *Harvard Business Review,* 127–136.

Micklethwait, J., & Wooldridge, A. (1997). *The witch doctors: What the management gurus are saying, why it matters and how to make sense of it.* London: Random House.

Migdal, M., Hewstone, M., & Mullen, B. (1998). The effects of crossed categorization on intergroup evaluations: A meta-analysis. *British Journal of Social Psychology, 69,* 1203–1215.

Miller, G. J. (1992). *Managerial dilemmas: The political economy of hierarchies.* New York: Cambridge University Press

Miller, N., & Brewer, M. B. (1986). Categorization effects on ingroup and outgroup perception. In J. F. Dovidio & S. L. Gaertner (Eds.), *Prejudice, discrimination, and racism* (pp. 209–230). Orlando, FL: Academic Press.

Miller, N., Brewer, M. B., & Edwards, K. (1985). Cooperative interaction in desegregated settings: A laboratory analogue. *Journal of Social Issues, 41,* 63–79.

Miller, N., & Davidson-Podgorny, G. (1987). Theoretical models of intergroup relations and the use of cooperative teams as an intervention for desegregated settings. In C. Hendrick (Ed.), *Group processes and intergroup relations: Review of personality and social psychology* (Vol. 9, pp. 41–67). Beverly Hills, CA: Sage.

Miller, N., & Harrington, H. J. (1992). Social categorization and intergroup acceptance: Principles for the design and development of cooperative learning teams. In R. Hertz-Lazarowitz & N. Miller (Eds.), *Interaction in cooperative groups—the theoretical anatomy of group learning* (pp. 203–227). New York: Cambridge University Press.

Miller, N., Urban, L. M., & Vanman, E. J. (1998). A theoretical analysis of crossed social categorization effects. In C. Sedikides, J. Schopler, & C. A. Insko (Eds.), *Intergroup cognition and intergroup behavior* (pp. 393–420). Mahwah, NJ: Erlbaum.

Milliken, F. J., & Martins, L. L. (1996). Searching for common threads: Understanding the multiple effects of diversity in organizational groups. *Academy of Management Review, 21*, 402–433.

Mirvis, P. H., & Marks, M. L. (1986). The human side of merger planning: Assessing and analyzing "fit." *Human Resource Planning, 15*, 69–92.

Mobley, W. H, Griffeth, R. W., Hand, H. H., & Meglino, B. M. (1979). Review and conceptual analysis of the employee turnover process. *Psychological Bulletin, 86*, 493–522.

Moghaddam, F. M., & Perreault, S. (1991). Individual and collective mobility strategies among minority group members. *Journal of Social Psychology, 132*(3), 343–357.

Moore, D., Kurtzberg, T., Thompson, L., & Morris, M. (1999). Long and short routes to success in electronically mediated negations: Group affiliations and good vibrations. *Organizational Behavior and Human Decision Processes, 77*, 22–43.

Moorman, R.H., & Blakely, G.L. (1995). Individualism/collectivism as an individual difference predictor of organizational citizenship behavior. *Journal of Organizational Behavior, 16*, 127–142.

Moreland, R. L., Argote, L., & Krishnan, R. (1998). Training people to work in groups. In R. S. Tindale, L. Heath, J. Edwards, E. J. Posavac, F. B. Bryant, Y. Suarez-Balcazar, E. Henderson-King, & J. Myers (Eds.), *Theory and research on small groups* (pp. 37–60). New York: Plenum Press.

Moreland, R. L., & Beach, S. R. (1992). Exposure effects in the classroom: The development of affinity among students. *Journal of Experimental Social Psychology, 28*, 255–276.

Moreland, R. L., Hogg, M. A., & Hains, S. C. (1994). Back to the future: Social psychological research on groups. *Journal of Experimental Social Psychology, 30*, 527–555.

Moreland, R. L., & Levine, J. M. (1982). Group socialization: Temporal changes in individual-group relations. In L. Berkowitz (Ed.), *Advances in experimental social psychology* (Vol. 15, pp. 137–192). New York: Academic Press.

Moreland, R. L., & Levine, J. M. (1992). The composition of small groups. In E. Lawler,

B. Markovsky, C. Ridgeway, & H. Walker (Eds.), *Advances in group processes* (Vol. 9, pp. 237–280). Greenwich, CT: JAI Press.

Moreland, R. L., & Levine, J.M. (2000). Socialization in organizations and work groups. In M. Turner (Ed.), *Groups at work: Advances in theory and research* (pp. 69–112). Mahwah, NJ: Erlbaum.

Moreland, R. L., & Levine, J. M. (1989). Newcomers and oldtimers in small groups. In P. Paulus (Ed.), *Psychology of group influence* (2nd ed., pp. 143–186). Hillsdale, NJ: Erlbaum.

Moreland, R. L., Levine, J. M., & Wingert, M. L. (1996). Creating the ideal group: Composition effects at work. In E. H. Witte & J. H. Davis (Eds.), *Understanding group behavior: Vol. 2. Small group processes and interpersonal relations* (pp. 11–35). Mahwah, NJ: Erlbaum.

Morris, L., Hulbert, L. G., & Abrams, D. (2000). An experimental investigation of group members' perceived influence over leader decisions. *Group Dynamics: Theory, Research, and Practice, 4*, 157–167.

Morrison, E. W. (1993). Newcomer information seeking: Exploring types, modes, sources, and outcomes. *Academy of Management Journal, 36*, 557–589.

Moscovici, S. (1976). *Social influence and social change.* London: Academic Press.

Moscovici, S. (1980). Toward a theory of conversion behavior. In L. Berkowitz (Ed.), *Advances in experimental social psychology* (Vol. 13, pp. 209–239). New York: Academic Press.

Moscovici, S. (1985). Social influence and conformity. In G. Lindsey & E. Aronson (Eds.), *The handbook of social psychology* (3rd ed., Vol. 2, pp. 347–412). New York: Random House.

Moss, M. K., & Frieze, I. H. (1993). Job preferences in the anticipatory socialization phase: A comparison of two matching models. *Journal of Vocational Behavior, 42*, 282–297.

Mottola, G. R., Bachman, B. A., Gaertner, S. L., & Dovidio, J. F. (1997). How groups merge: The effects of merger integration patterns on anticipated commitment to the merged organization. *Journal of Applied Social Psychology, 27*, 1335–1358.

Mowday, R. T., Steers, R. M., & Porter, L. W. (1979). The measurement of organizational commitment. *Journal of Vocational Behavior, 14,* 224–247.

Mowday, R. T., & Sutton, R. I. (1993). Organizational behavior: Linking individuals and groups to organizational contexts. *Annual Review of Psychology, 44,* 195–229.

Mudrack, P. E. (1989). Group cohesiveness and productivity: A closer look. *Human Relations, 42,* 771–785.

Mueller, C. W., & Lawler, E. J. (1999). Commitment to nested organizational units: Some basic principles and preliminary findings. *Social Psychological Quarterly, 62,* 325–346.

Mugny, G. (1982). *The power of minorities.* London: Academic Press.

Mugny, G., & Pérez, J. (1991). *The social psychology of minority influence.* Cambridge: Cambridge University Press.

Mullen, B., Brown, R. J., & Smith, C. (1992). Ingroup bias as a function of salience, relevance, and status: An integration. *European Journal of Social Psychology, 22,* 103–122.

Mullen, B., & Copper, C. (1994). The relation between group cohesiveness and performance: An integration. *Psychological Bulletin, 115,* 210–227.

Mullen, B., Johnson, C., & Salas, E. (1991). Productivity loss in brainstorming groups: A meta-analytic integration. *Basic and Applied Social Psychology, 12,* 3–23.

Mummendey, A., & Schreiber, H. J. (1983). Better or just different? Positive social identity by discrimination against or differentiation from outgroups. *European Journal of Social Psychology, 13,* 389–397.

Murray, A.I. (1989). Top management group heterogeneity and firm performance. *Strategic Management Journal, 10,* 125–141.

Mussen, P., & Eisenberg-Berg, N. (1977). *Roots of caring, sharing, and helping: The development of prosocial behavior in children.* San Francisco: Freeman.

Nadler, D. A., & Tushman, M. L. (1990). Beyond the charismatic leader: Leadership and organizational change. *California Management Review, 32,* 77–97.

Nahavandi, A., & Malekzadeh, A. R. (1988). Acculturation in mergers and acquisitions. *Academy of Management Review, 13,* 79–90.

Near, J. P. (1989). Organizational commitment among Japanese and U.S. workers. *Organizational studies, 10,* 281–300.

Nelson, D. L. (1987). Organizational socialization: A stress perspective. *Journal of Organizational Behavior, 8,* 311–324.

Nelson, D. L., & Quick, J. C. (1991). Social support and newcomer adjustment in organizations: Attachment theory at work? *Journal of Organizational Behavior, 12,* 543–554.

Nelson, D. L., Quick, J. C., & Eakin, M. E. (1988). A longitudinal study of newcomer role adjustment in U.S. organizations. *Work & Stress, 2,* 239–253.

Nelson, D. L., Quick, J. C., & Joplin, J. R. (1991). Psychological contracting and newcomer socialization: An attachment theory foundation. *Journal of Social Behavior and Personality, 6,* 55–72.

Nemeth, C. (1986). Differential contributions of majority and minority influence. *Psychological Review, 93,* 23–32.

Nemeth, C. (1995). Dissent as driving cognition, attitudes and judgements. *Social Cognition, 13,* 273–291.

Nemeth, C. J., & Kwan, J. (1985). Originality of word associations as a function of majority and minority influence. *Social Psychology Quarterly, 48,* 277–282.

Nemeth, C. J., & Kwan, J. (1987). Minority influence, divergent thinking and detection of correct solutions. *Journal of Applied Social Psychology, 17,* 788–799.

Nemeth, C., Mosier, K., & Chiles, C. (1992). When convergent thought improves performance: Majority vs. minority influence. *Personality and Social Psychology Bulletin, 18,* 139–144.

Nemeth, C., & Owens, P. (1996). Making work groups more effective: The value of minority dissent. In M. A. West (Ed.), *Handbook of work group psychology* (pp. 125–142). Chichester, UK: John Wiley.

Nemeth, C. J., & Staw, B. M. (1989). The tradeoffs of social control and innovation in groups and organizations. In L. Berkowitz (Ed.), *Advances in experimental social psychology* (Vol. 22, pp. 175–209). New York: Academic Press.

Nemeth, C. J., & Wachtler, J. (1983). Creative problem solving as a result of majority versus minority influence. *European Journal of Social Psychology, 13,* 45–55.

Newman, P.R., & Newman, B. M. (1976). Early adolescence and its conflict: Group identity versus alienation. *Adolescence, 11,* 261–274.

Niedenthal, P. M., Cantor, N., & Kihlstrom, J.

F. (1985). Prototype matching: A strategy for social decision making. *Journal of Personality and Social Psychology, 48,* 575–584.

Niemann, Y. F., & Dovidio, J. F. (1998). Relationship of solo status, academic rank, and perceived distinctiveness to job satisfaction of racial/ethnic minorities. *Journal of Applied Psychology, 83,* 55–71.

Nieva, V. F., & Gutek, B. A. (1981). *Women and work: A psychological perspective.* New York: Praeger.

Nippert-Eng, C. E. (1996). *Home and work: Negotiating boundaries through everyday life.* Chicago: University of Chicago Press.

Nkomo, S. M., & Cox, T., Jr. (1996). Diverse identities in organizations. In S. R. Clegg, C. Hardy, & W. R. Nord, (Eds.), *Handbook of Organizational Studies* (pp. 338–356). London, UK & Thousand Oaks, CA: Sage.

Noon, M., & Blyton, P. (1997). *The realities of work.* Basingstoke, UK: Macmillan Business Press.

Noon, M., & Delbridge, R. (1993). News from behind my hand: Gossip in organizations. *Organization Studies, 14,* 23-36.

Norton, A. J., & Miller, L. F. (1992). *Marriage, divorce and remarriage in the 1990s* (U.S. Bureau of the Census, Current Population Reports. Series P-23, No. 180). Washington, DC: U.S. Government Printing Office.

Nulty, P. (1995, November 13). Incentive pay can be crippling. *Fortune,* p. 235.

Nye, J.L., & Forsyth, D.R. (1991). The effects of prototype-based biases on leadership appraisals: A test of leadership categorization theory. *Small Group Research, 22,* 360-379.

Nye, J. L., & Simonetta, L. G. (1996). Followers' perceptions of group leaders: The impact of recognition-based and inference-based processes. In J. L. Nye, & A. M. Bower, (Eds.), *What's social about social cognition: Research on socially shared cognition in small groups* (pp. 124–153). Thousand Oaks, CA: Sage.

Oaker, G., & Brown, R. (1986). Intergroup relations in a hospital setting: A further test of social identity theory. *Human Relations, 39,* 767–778.

Oakes, P. J. (1987). The salience of social categories. In J. C. Turner, M. A. Hogg, P. J. Oakes, S. D. Reicher, & M. S. Wetherell, *Rediscovering the social group: A self-categorization theory* (pp. 117–141). Oxford, UK: Blackwell.

Oakes, P. J., Haslam, S. A., & Turner, J. C. (1994). *Stereotyping and social reality.* Oxford, UK: Blackwell.

Oakes, P., Haslam, S. A., & Turner, J. C. (1998). The role of prototypicality in group influence and cohesion: Contextual variation in the graded structure of social categories. In S. Worchel, J. F. Morales, D. Paez, & J. C. Deschamps (Eds.), *Social identity: International perspectives* (pp. 75–92). London: Sage.

Oakes, P., & Turner, J. C. (1980). Social categorization and intergroup behaviour: Does minimal intergroup discrimination make social identity more positive? *European Journal of Social Psychology, 10,* 295–302.

Oakes, P. J., & Turner, J. C. (1990). Is limited information processing the cause of social stereotyping. *European Review of Social Psychology, 1,* 111–135.

Organ, D. W. (1988). *Organizational citizenship behavior: The good soldier syndrome.* Lexington, MA: Lexington.

Organ, D. W., & Ryan, K. (1995). A meta-analytic review of attitudinal and dispositional predictors of organizational citizenship behavior. *Personnel Psychology, 48,* 775–802.

Ostroff, C., & Kozlowski, S. W. J. (1993). The role of mentoring in the information-gathering processes of newcomers during early organizational socialization. *Journal of Vocational Behavior, 42,* 170–183.

Ostrom, T. M., & Sedikides, C. (1992). Outgroup homogeneity effects in natural and minimal groups. *Psychological Bulletin, 112,* 536–552.

Ott, E. M. (1989). Effects of the male-female ratio at work: Policewomen and male nurses. *Psychology of Women Quarterly, 13,* 41–58.

Ouchi, W. G. (1980). Markets, bureaucracies, and clans. *Administrative Science Quarterly, 25,* 129–141.

Ouwerkerk, J. W., Ellemers, N., & De Gilder, D. (1999). Group commitment and individual effort in experimental and organisational contexts. In N. Ellemers, R. Spears, & B. Doosje (Eds.), *Social identity: Context, commitment, content* (pp. 184–204). Oxford, UK: Blackwell.

Palich, L. E., & Hom, P. W. (1992). The impact of leader power and behavior on leadership perceptions: A lisrel test of an expanded categorization theory of leadership model. *Group and Organization Management, 17,* 279–296.

Park, B., & Judd, C. M. (1990). Measures and models of perceived group variability. *Journal of Personality and Social Psychology, 59,* 173–191.

Paulus, P. B. (2000). Groups, teams and creativity: The creative potential of idea generating groups. *Applied Psychology: An International Review, 49,* 237–262.

Paulus, P. B., Leggett Dugosh, K., Dzindolet, M. T., Putman, V. L., & Coskun, H. (in press). Social and cognitive influences in group brainstorming: Predicting production gains and losses. In W. Stroebe & M. Hewstone (Eds.), *European Review of Social Psychology* (Vol. 12). Chichester, UK: Wiley.

Pawar, B. S., & Eastman, K. (1997). The nature and implications of contextual influences on transformational leadership. *Academy of Management Review, 22,* 80–109.

Pelled, L. H. (1996). Demographic diversity, conflict, and work group outcomes: An intervening process theory. *Organizational Science, 7,* 615–631.

Pemberton, M. J., Insko, C. A., & Schopler, J. (1996). Experience of and memory for differential distrust of individuals and groups. *Journal of Personality and Social Psychology, 71,* 953–966.

Pepels., J. (1999). *The myth of the positive crossed categorization effect.* ERCOMER Monograph. Amsterdam: Netherlands School for Social and Economic Policy Research.

Pérez, J. A., & Mugny, G. (1998). Categorization and social influence. In S. Worchel & J. M. Francisco (Eds.), *Social identity: International perspectives* (pp. 142–153). London: Sage.

Perry, E. (1984). A prototype-matching approach to understanding the role of applicant gender and age in the evaluation of job applicants. *Journal of Applied Social Psychology, 24,* 1433–1473.

Peterson, R., & Nemeth, C. J. (1996). Focus versus flexibility: Majority and minority influence can both improve performance. *Personality and Social Psychology Bulletin, 22,* 14–23.

Pettigrew, T. F. (1979). The ultimate attribution error: Extending Gordan Allport's cognitive analysis of prejudice. *Personality and Social Psychology Bulletin, 5,* 461–477.

Pettigrew, T. F. (1997). Generalized intergroup contact effects on prejudice. *Personality and Social Psychology Bulletin. 23,* 173–185.

Pettigrew, T. F. (1998). Intergroup contact theory. *Annual Review of Psychology, 49,* 65–85.

Pettigrew, T. F., & Martin, J. (1987). Shaping the organizational context for black American inclusion. *Journal of Social Issues, 43,* 41–78.

Pettigrew, T. F., & Tropp, L. R. (2000). Does intergroup contact reduce prejudice? Recent meta-analytic findings. In S. Oskamp (Ed.), *Reducing prejudice and discrimination* (pp. 93–114). Mahwah, NJ: Erlbaum

Pfeffer, J. (1981). Management as symbolic action: The creation and maintenance of organizational paradigms. *Research in Organizational Behavior, 3,* 1–52.

Pfeffer, J. (1982). *Organizations and organization theory.* Boston, MA: Pitman.

Pfeffer, J. (1997). *New directions for organizational theory: Problems and prospects.* New York: Oxford University Press.

Pfeffer, J., & Davis-Blake, A. (1987). The effect of the proportion of women on salaries: The case of college administrators. *Administrative Science Quarterly, 32,* 1–24.

Pfeffer, J., & Sutton, R. I. (2000). *The knowing-doing gap.* Boston: MA: Harvard University Press.

Philips, K. (2000). *Disentangling the complex effects of diversity: The interplay of expectations, process, and performance in groups.* Working paper. Northwestern University, Evanston, IL.

Platow, M. J., Hoar, S., Reid, S., Harley, K., & Morrison, D. (1997). Endorsement of distributively fair or unfair leaders in interpersonal and intergroup situations. *European Journal of Social Psychology, 27,* 465–494.

Platow, M. J., Mills, D., & Morrison, D. (2000). The effects of social context, source fairness, and perceived self-source similarity on social influence: A self-categorisation analysis. *European Journal of Social Psychology, 30,* 69–81.

Platow, M., Reid, S., & Andrew, S. (1998). Leadership endorsement: The role of distributive and procedural behavior in interpersonal and intergroup contexts. *Group Processes and Intergroup Relations, 1,* 35–47.

Platow, M. J., & van Knippenberg, D. (1999, July). *The impact of a leader's in-group prototypicality and normative fairness on leadership endorsements in an intergroup context.* Paper presented at the 12th General meeting of the European Association of Experimental Social Psychology, Oxford, UK.

Podsakoff, P. M., Ahearne, M., & MacKenzie, S. B. (1997). Organizational citizenship behavior and the quantity and quality of work group performance. *Journal of Applied Psychology, 82,* 262–270.

Polzer, J.T ., Stewart, K. J., & Simmons, J. L. (1999). A social categorization explanation for framing effects in nested social dilemmas. *Organizational Behavior and Human Decision Processes, 79,* 154–178.

Porter, L. W., Crampon, W. F., & Smith, F. J. (1976). Organizational commitment and managerial turnover: A longitudinal study. *Organizational Behavior and Human Performance, 15,* 87–98.

Porter, L. W., & Steers, R. M. (1973). Organizational, work, and personal factors in employee turnover and absenteeism. *Psychological Bulletin, 80,* 151–176.

Porter, L. W., Steers, R. M., Mowday, R. T., & Boulian, P. V. (1974). Organizational commitment, job satisfaction, and turnover among psychiatric technicians. *Journal of Applied Psychology, 59,* 603–609.

Porter, M. (1987). From competitive advantage to corporate strategy. *Harvard Business Review, 67,* 43–49.

Postmes, T., Spears, R., & Lea, M. (1998). Breaching or building social boundaries?: SIDE-effects of computer mediated communication. *Communication Research, 25,* 689–715.

Potter, J., & Wetherell, M. (1998). Social representations, discourse analysis, and racism. In U. Flick (Ed.), *The psychology of the social* (pp. 138–155). New York: Cambridge University Press.

Pratt, M. G. (1998). To be or not to be? Central questions in organizational identification. In D. A. Whetten & P. C. Godfrey (Eds.), *Identity in Organizations: Building theory through conversations* (pp. 171–207). Thousand Oaks, CA: Sage.

Pratt, M. G. (2000). Building an ideological fortress: The role of spirituality, encapsulation, and sensemaking. *Studies in Cultures, Organizations, and Societies, 6,* 35–69.

Pratt, M. G. (100a). The good, the bad, and the ambivalent: Managing identification among Amway distributors. *Administrative Science Quarterly, 45,* 456–493.

Pratt, M. G., & Doucet, L. (2000). Ambiva-lent feelings in organizational relationships. In S. Fineman (Ed.), *Emotions in Organizations, Vol. II* (pp. 204–226). London: Sage.

Pratt, M.G., & Foreman, P. O. (2000). Classifying Managerial Responses to Multiple Organizational Identities. *Academy Management Review, 25,* 18–42.

Pratt, M. G., Fuller, M., & Northcraft, G.B. (2000). Media selection and identification in distributed groups: The potential cost of "rich" media. In T. Griffith, E. Mannix, & M. Neale (Eds.), *Research on Managing Groups and Teams: Vol. III* (pp. 231–254). Stamford, CT: JAI Press.

Pratt, M. G., & Rafaeli, A. (1997). Organizational dress as a symbol of multilayered social identities. *Academy of Management Journal, 40,* 862–898.

Pratt, M. G. & Rafaeli, A. (2000). *Symbols and relating work in organizations.* Unpublished manuscript, University of Illinois, Urbana-Champaign.

Presholdt, P. H., Lane, I. M., & Mathews, R. C. (1987). Nurse turnover as reasoned action: Development of a process model. *Journal of Applied Psychology, 72,* 221–227.

Pruitt, D. G. (1987). Conspiracy theory in conflict escalation. In C. F. Graumann & S. Moscovici (Eds.), *Changing conceptions of conspiracy* (pp. 191–202). New York: Springer-Verlag.

Prus, R. (1996). *Symbolic interaction and ethnographic research.* Albany, NY: State University of New York Press.

Putnam, R. D. (1993). *Making democracy work: Civic traditions in modern Italy.* Princeton, NJ: Princeton University Press.

Pyszczynski, T., & Greenberg, J. (1987). Toward an integration of cognitive and motivational perspectives on social inference: A biased hypothesis-testing model. In L. Berkowitz (Ed.), *Advances in experimental social psychology* (Vol. 20, pp. 297–340). San Diego, CA: Academic Press.

Quick, D. S., McKenry, P. C., & Newman, B. M. (1994). Stepmothers and their adolescent children: Adjustment to new family roles. In K. Pasley & M. Ihinger-Tallman (Eds.), *Stepfamilies: Issues in theory, research and practice* (pp. 105–126). Westport, CT: Greenwood.

Quinn, R. P., & Shepard, L. J. (1974). *The 1972–73 quality of employment survey: Descriptive statistics with comparison data from the 1969–70 survey of working conditions.* Ann Arbor, MI: University of Michigan, Institute of Social Research.

Rabbie, J. M., & Bekkers, F. (1978). Threatened leadership and intergroup competition. *European Journal of Social Psychology, 8,* 9–20.

Rafaeli, A. (1997). What is an organization? Who are the members? In C. L. Cooper and S. E. Jackson (Eds.), *Creating tomorrow's organizations* (pp. 121–138). Chichester, UK: Wiley.

Rafaeli, A., Dutton, J. E., Harquail, C. V., & Mackie-Lewis, S. (1997). Navigating by attire: The use of dress by female administrative employees. *Academy of Management Journal, 40,* 9–46.

Rafaeli, A., & Pratt, M. G. (1993). Tailored meanings: On the meaning and impact of organizational dress. *Academy of Management Journal, 18,* 32–55.

Randall, D. M., & Cote, J. (1991). Interrelationships of work commitment constructs. *Work & Occupations, 18,* 194–211.

Raven, B.H. (1965). Social influence and power. In I.D. Steiner & M. Fishbein (Eds.), *Current studies in social psychology* (pp. 371–382). New York: Holt, Rinehart & Winston.

Reicher, S. (1995). Three dimensions of the social self. In A. Oosterwegel (Ed.), *The self in European and North American culture: Development and processes* (pp. 277–290). Dordrecht, the Netherlands: Kluwer.

Reicher, S. D. (2001). The psychology of crowd dynamics. In M. A. Hogg & R. S. Tindale (Eds.), *Blackwell handbook of social psychology: Group processes* (pp. 182–208). Oxford, UK: Blackwell.

Reicher, S. D., Drury, J., Hopkins, N. & Stott, C. (in press). A model of crowd prototypes and crowd leadership. In C. Barker (Ed.), *Leadership and social movements.* Manchester, UK: Manchester University Press.

Reicher, S. D., & Hopkins, N. (1996a). Seeking influence through characterising self-categories: An analysis of anti-abortionist rhetoric. *British Journal of Social Psychology, 35,* 297–311.

Reicher, S. D., & Hopkins, N. (1996b). Self-category constructions in political rhetoric: An analysis of Thatcher's and Kinnock's speeches concerning the British Miners' Strike (1984–5). *European Journal of Social Psychology, 26,* 353–372.

Reicher, S., & Levine R. (1994). Deindividuation, power relations between groups and the expression of social identity: The effects of visibility to the out-group. *British Journal of Social Psychology, 33,* 145–163.

Reicher, S., Levine R., & Gordijn, E. (1998). More on deindividuation, power relations between groups and the expression of social identity: Three studies on the effects of visibility to the in-group. *British Journal of Social Psychology, 37,* 15–40.

Reicher, S., Spears, R., & Postmes, T. (1995). A social identity model of deindividuation phenomena . *European Review of Social Psychology, 6,* 161–198.

Reichers, A. E. (1985). A review and reconceptualization of organizational commitment. *Academy of Management Review, 10,* 465–476.

Reichers, A. E. (1986). Conflict and organizational commitments. *Journal of Applied Psycohlogy, 71,* 508–514.

Reichl, A. J. (1997). Ingroup favouritism and outgroup favouritism in low status minimal groups: Differential responses to status-related and status-unrelated measures. *European Journal of Social Psychology, 27,* 617–633.

Rentsch, J. R. (1990). Climate and culture: Interaction and qualitative differences in organizational meanings. *Journal of Applied Psychology, 75,* 668-681.

Rentsch, J. R., & Schneider, B. (1991). Expectations for postcombination organizational life: A study of responses to merger and acquisition scenarios. *Journal of Applied Social Psychology, 21,* 233–252.

Reskin, B. F., & Roos, P. A. (1990). *Job cues, gender cues: Explaining women's inroads into male occupations.* Philadelphia: Temple University Press.

Richards, Z., & Hewstone, M. (in press). Subtyping and subgrouping: Processes for the prevention and promotion of stereotype change. *Personality and Social Psychology Review.*

Ridgeway, C. (1991). The social construction of status value: Gender and other nominal characteristics. *Social Forces, 70,* 367–386.

Ridgeway, C.L., & Diekema, D. (1992). Are gender differences status differences? In C.L. Ridgeway (Ed.), *Gender, interaction, and inequality* (pp. 157–180). New York: Springer-Verlag.

Riordan, C. M., & Shore, L. M. (1997). Demographic diversity and employee attitudes: An empirical examination of relational demography within work units. *Journal of Applied Psychology, 82,* 342–358.

Ritchie, R. J., & Moses, J. L. (1983). Assessment center correlates of women's advancement into middle-management. *Journal of Applied Psychology, 68,* 227–231.

Rizzo, J., House, R. J., & Lirtzman, S. I. (1970). Role conflict and ambiguity in complex organizations. *Administrative Science Quarterly, 15,* 150–163.

Robinson, S. L. (1996). Trust and breach of the psychological contract. *Administrative Science Quarterly, 41,* 574–99.

Robinson, S. L., & Rousseau, D. M. (1994). Violating the psychological contract: Not the exception but the norm. *Journal of Organizational Behavior, 15,* 245–259.

Robinson, W. P. (Ed.) (1996). *Social groups and identities: Developing the legacy of Henri Tajfel.* Oxford, UK: Butterworth-Heinemann.

Rohlen, T. P. (1974). *For harmony and strength: Japanese white-collar organization in anthropological perspective.* Berkeley, CA: University of California Press.

Rosenthal, R., & Jacobson, L. (1968). *Pygmalion in the classroom: Teacher expectations and pupils' intellectual development.* New York: Rinehart and Winston.

Ross, L. (1977). The intuitive psychologist and his shortcomings. In L. Berkowitz (Ed.), *Advances in experimental social psychology* (Vol. 10, pp. 174–220). New York: Academic Press.

Rosse, J. G., & Hulin, C. L. (1985). Adaptation to work: An analysis of employee health, withdrawal and change. *Organizational Behavior and Human Decision Processes, 36,* 324–347.

Rothbart, M., & Hallmark, W. (1988). Ingroup-outgroup differences in the perceived efficacy of coercion and conciliation in resolving social conflict. *Journal of Personality and Social Psychology, 55,* 248–257.

Rothbart, M., & John, O. P. (1985). Social categorization and behavioral episodes: A cognitive analysis of the effects of intergroup contact. *Journal of Social Issues, 41,* 81–104.

Rotondi, T., Jr. (1975). Organizational identification: Issues and implications. *Organizational Behavior and Human Performance, 13,* 95–109.

Rotter, J. B. (1980). Interpersonal trust, trust-worthiness, and gullibility. *American Psychologist, 35,* 1–7.

Rousseau, D. M. (1998).Why workers still identify with organizations. *Journal of Organizational Behavior, 19,* 217–233.

Rousseau, D. M., Sitkin, S. B., Burt, R. S., & Camerer, C. (1998). Not so different after all: A cross-discipline view of trust. *Academy of Management Review, 23,* 393–404.

Rousseau, D. M., & Wade-Benzoni, K. A. (1995). Changing individual-organization attachments: A two-way street. In A. Howard (Ed.), *The changing nature of work* (pp. 290–322). San Francisco: Jossey-Bass.

Rowe, P. M. (1984). Decision processes in personnel selection. *Canadian Journal of Behavioral Science, 16,* 326–337.

Rubin, M., & Hewstone, M. (1998). Social identity theory's self-esteem hypothesis: A review and some suggestions for clarification. *Personality and Social Psychology Review, 2,* 40–62.

Rusbult, C. E., Farrell, D., Rogers, G., & Mainous, A.G. (1988). Impact of exchange variables on exit, voice, loyalty and neglect: An integrative model of responses to declining job satisfaction. *Academy of Management Journal, 31,* 599–627.

Rusbult, C., & Van Lange, P. (1996). Interdependence processes. In E. T. Higgins & A. W. Kruglanski (Eds.), *Social psychology* (pp. 564–596). New York: Guilford.

Rush, M. C., & Russell, J. E. A. (1988). Leader prototypes and prototype-contingent consensus in leader behavior descriptions. *Journal of Experimental Social Psychology, 24,* 88–104.

Russo, T. C. (1998). Organizational and professional identification: A case of newspaper journalists. *Management Communication Quarterly, 12,* 72–111.

Rustad, M. (1982). *Women in khaki: The American enlisted woman.* New York: Praeger.

Ryan, C. S., Judd, C. M., & Park, B. (1996). Effects of racial stereotypes on judgments of individuals: The moderating role of perceived group variability. *Journal of Experimental Social Psychology, 32,* 71–103.

Sachdev, I., & Bourhis, R. Y. (1984). Minimal majorities and minorities. *European Journal of Social Psychology, 14,* 35–52.

Sachdev, I., & Bourhis, R. Y. (1987). Status differentials and intergroup behavior. *Euro-*

pean *Journal of Social Psychology, 17,* 277–293.

Sachdev, I., & Bourhis, R. Y. (1991). Power and status differentials in minority and majority group relations. *European Journal of Social Psychology, 21,* 1–24.

Sackett, P. R., DuBois, C. L. Z., & Noe, A. W. (1991). Tokenism in performance evaluation: The effects of work group representation on male-female and white-black differences in performance ratings. *Journal of Applied Psychology, 76,* 263–267.

Sackman, S. A. (1992). Culture and subcultures: An analysis of organizational knowledge. *Administrative Science Quarterly, 37,* 140–161.

Saks, A. M., & Ashforth, B. E. (1997). Organizational socialization: Making sense of the past and present as a prologue for the future. *Journal of Vocational Behavior, 51,* 234–279.

Sales, A. L., & Mirvis, P. H. (1984). Acquisition and the collision of cultures. In R. Quinn & J. Kimberly (Eds.), *Managing organizational transitions* (pp. 107–133). New York: Dow-Jones.

Sampson, E. (1993). *Celebrating the other: A dialogical account of human nature.* Boulder, CO: Westview Press.

Sanna, L. J., & Parks, C. D. (1997). Group research trends in social and organizational psychology: Whatever happened to intragroup research? *Psychological Science, 8,* 261-267.

Sarros, J. C., & Butchatsky, O. (1996). *Leadership: Australia's top CEOs—Finding out what makes them the best.* Sydney, Australia: HarperCollins.

Sauer, L. E., & Fine, M. A. (1988). Parent-child relationships in stepparent families. *Journal of Family Psychology, 1,* 434–451.

Scarberry, N. C., Ratcliff, C. D., Lord, C. G., Lanicek, D. L., & Desforges, D. M. (1997). Effects of individuating information on the generalization part of Allport's contact hypothesis. *Personality and Social Psychology Bulletin, 23,* 1291–1299.

Schaubroeck, J., & Ganster, D. C. (1991). Beyond the call of duty: A field study of extra-role behavior in voluntary organizations. *Human Relations, 44,* 569–582.

Schaubroek, J., May, D. R., & Brown, F. W. (1994). Procedural justice explanations and employee reactions to economic hardship: A field experiment. *Journal of Applied Psychology, 79,* 455–460.

Schlenker, B. R. (1985). Identity and self-identification. In B. R. Schlenker (Ed.), *The self in social life* (pp. 65–99). New York: McGraw-Hill.

Schmitt, N. (1976). Social and situational determinants of interview decisions: Implications for the employment interview. *Personnel Psychology, 29,* 79–101.

Schmitz, J., & Fulk, J. (1991). Organizational colleagues, media richness, and electronic mail: A test of the social influence model of technology use. *Communication Research, 18,* 487–523.

Schneider, B., Goldstein, H. W., & Smith, D. B. (1995). The ASA framework: An update. *Personnel Psychology, 48,* 747–773.

Schneider, S. K., & Northcraft, G. B. (1999). Three social dilemmas of workforce diversity in organizations: A social identity perspective. *Human Relations, 52,* 1445–1467.

Schopler, J., & Insko, C. A. (1992). The discontinuity effect in interpersonal and intergroup relations: Generality and mediation. In W. Stroebe & M. Hewstone (Eds.), *European review of social psychology* (Vol. 3, pp. 121–151). Chichester, UK: Wiley.

Schweiger, D. L., & Ivancevich, J. M. (1985). Human resources: The forgotten factor in mergers and acquisitions. *Personnel Administrator, 30,* 47–61.

Schweiger, D. M., & Walsh, J. P. (1990). Mergers and acquisitions: An interdisciplinary view. *Research in Personnel and Human Resources Management, 8,* 41–107.

Schweiger, D. M., & Weber, Y. (1989). Strategies for managing human resources during mergers and acquisitions: An empirical investigation. *Human Resource Planning, 12,* 69–86.

Scott, C. R. (1997). Identification with multiple targets in a geographically dispersed organization. *Management Communication Quarterly, 10,* 491–522.

Scott, C. R. (1999). The impact of physical and discursive anonymity on group members' multiple identifications during computer-supported decision making. *Western Journal of Communication, 63,* 456–487.

Scott, C. R., Corman, S. R., & Cheney, G. (1998). Development of a structurational model of identification in the organization. *Communication Theory, 8,* 298–336.

Sengoku, T. (1985). *Willing workers: The work ethics in Japan, England, and the United States.* Westport, CT: Quorum Books.

Settles, B. H. (1993). The illusion of stability in family life: The reality of change and mobility. *Marriage and Family Review, 19,* 5–29.

Shaffer, D.R., Gresham, A., Clary, E. G., & Theilman, T. J. (1986). Sex ratios as a basis for occupational evaluations: A contemporary view. *Social Behavior and Personality, 14,* 77–83.

Shaw, M. E. (1981). *Group dynamics: The psychology of small group behavior* (2nd ed.). New York: McGraw-Hill.

Sherif, M. (1962). *Intergroup relations and leadership: Approaches and research in industrial, ethnic, and political areas.* New York: Wiley.

Sherif, M. (1966). *In common predicament: Social psychology of intergroup conflict and cooperation.* Boston, MA: Houghton-Mifflin.

Sherif, M., & Sherif, C. W. (1969). *Social psychology.* New York: Harper & Row.

Sherif, M., Harvey, L. J., White, B. J., Hood, W. R., & Sherif, C. W. (1961). *Intergroup cooperation and competition: The Robber's Cave experiment.* Norman, OK: University Book Exchange.

Sherman, S. J., Hamilton, D. L., & Lewis, A. C. (1999). Perceived entitativity and the social identity value of group memberships. In D. Abrams & M. A. Hogg (Eds.), *Social identity and social cognition* (pp. 80–110). Oxford, UK: Blackwell.

Shook, R. L. (1988) *Honda: An American Success Story.* New York: Prentice Hall.

Shrivastava, P. (1986). Postmerger integration. *Journal of Business Strategy, 7,* 65–76.

Sidanius, J., & Pratto, F. (1999). *Social dominance.* New York: Cambridge University Press.

Simon, B. (1992). The perception of in-group and out-group homogeneity: Reintroducing the intergroup context. In W. Stroebe & M. Hewstone (Eds.), *European Review Of Social Psychology* (Vol. 3, pp. 1–30). Chichester, UK: J. Wiley.

Simon, B., Aufderheide, B., & Kampmeier, C. (2001). The social psychology of minority-majority relations. In R. Brown & S.L. Gaertner (Eds.), *Blackwell handbook of social psychology: Intergroup processes* (pp. 303–323). Oxford, UK & Cambridge, MA: Blackwell.

Simon, B., & Brown, R. (1987). Perceived intragroup homogeneity in minority-majority contexts. *Journal of Personality and Social Psychology, 53,* 703–711.

Simon, B., Loewy, M., Sturmer, S., Wever, U., Freytey, P., Habig, C., Kempmeier, C., and Spahlinger, P. (1998). Collective identification and social movement participation. *Journal of Personality and Social Psychology, 74,* 646–658.

Simon, H. A. (1991). Organizations and markets. *Journal of Economic Perspectives, 5,* 34–38.

Simonton, D.K. (1999). *The origins of genius: Darwinian perspectives on creativity.* New York, NY: Oxford University Press.

Skevington, S. (1981). Intergroup relations and nursing. *European Journal of Social Psychology, 11,* 43–59.

Slovic, P. (1993). Perceived risk, trust, and democracy. *Risk Analysis, 13,* 675–682.

Slugoski, B. R., Marcia, J. E., & Koopman, R. F. (1984). Cognitive and social interactional characteristics of ego identity statuses in college males. *Journal of Personality and Social Psychology, 47,* 646–661.

Smith, H. J., & Tyler, T. R. (1996). Justice and power: When will justice concerns encourage the advantaged to support policies which redistribute economic resources and the disadvantaged to willingly obey the law. *European Journal of Social Psychology, 26,* 171–200.

Smith, H. J., & Tyler, T. R. (1997). Choosing the right pond: The impact of group membership on self-esteem and group-oriented behavior. *Journal of Experimental Social Psychology, 33,* 146–170.

Smith, H. J., Tyler, T. R., Huo, Y. J., Ortiz, D. J., & Lind, E. A. (1998). The self-relevant implications of the group-value model: Group membership, self-worth, and treatment quality. *Journal of Experimental Social Psychology, 34,* 470–493.

Smith, V. (1997). New forms of work organization. *Annual Review of Sociology, 23,* 315–339.

Snow, D. A., & Anderson, L. (1987). Identity work among the homeless: The verbal construction and avowal of personal identities. *American Journal of Sociology, 92,* 1336–1371.

Sobel, M. E. (1982). Asympotic confidence intervals for indirect effects in structural equation models. In S. Leinhardt (Ed.), *Sociological methodology 1982* (pp. 290–312). Washington, DC: American Sociological Association.

Somers, M. R. (1994). The narrative construction of identity: A relational and network approach. *Theory and Society, 23,* 605–649.

South, S. J., Bonjean, C. M., Markham, W. T., & Corder, J. (1982). Social structure and intergroup interaction: Men and women of the federal bureaucracy. *American Sociological Review, 47,* 587–599.

Spears, R., & Lea, M. (1994). Panacea or panopticon? The hidden power in computer-mediated communication. *Communication Research, 21,* 427–459.

Spears, R., & Manstead, A. S. R. (1989). The social context of stereotyping and differentiation. *European Journal of Social Psychology, 19,* 101–121.

Spears, R., Oakes, P. J., Ellemers, N., & Haslam, S. A. (Eds.). (1997). *The social psychology of stereotyping and group life.* Oxford, UK: Blackwell.

Spencer, D. G., & Steers, R. M. (1981). Performance as a moderator of the job satisfaction-turnover relationship. *Journal of Applied Psychology, 66,* 511–514.

Staw, B., McKechnie, P. I., & Puffer, S. M. (1983). The justification of organizational performance. *Administrative Science Quarterly, 28,* 582–600.

Steel, R. P., & Ovalle, N. K. (1984). A review and meta-analysis of research on the relationship between behavioral intentions and employee turnover. *Journal of Applied Psychology, 69,* 673–686.

Steele, C. M. (1997). A threat in the air: How stereotypes shape intellectual identity and performance. *American Psychologist, 52,* 613–629.

Steele, C. M., & Aronson, J. (1995). Stereotype threat and the intellectual test performance of African Americans. *Journal of Personality and Social Psychology, 69,* 797–811.

Steiner, I. D. (1974). Whatever happened to the group in social psychology? *Journal of Experimental Social Psychology, 10,* 94–108.

Steiner, I. D. (1986). Paradigms and groups. *Advances in Experimental Social Psychology, 19,* 251–289.

Stephan, W. G., & Stephan, C. W. (1984). The role of ignorance in intergroup relations. In N. Miller & M. B. Brewer (Eds.), *Groups in contact: The psychology of desegregation* (pp. 229–257). Orlando, FL: Academic Press.

Stephan, W. G., & Stephan, C. W. (1985). Intergroup anxiety. *Journal of Social Issues, 41,* 157–175.

Stern, S. (1988). Symbolic representation of organizational identity: The role of emblem at the Garrett Corporation. In M. O. Jones, M. D. Moore, & R. C. Snyder (Eds.), *Inside organizations: Understanding the human dimension* (pp. 281–295). Newbury Park, CA: Sage.

Stevens, L. E., & Fiske, S. T. (1995). Motivation and cognition in social life: A social survival perspective. *Social Cognition, 13,* 189–214.

Stogdill, R. M. (1948). Personal factors associated with leadership: A survey of the literature. *Journal of Psychology, 25,* 35–71.

Stogdill, R. (1974). *Handbook of leadership.* New York: Free Press.

Stroebe, W., & Diehl, M. (1994). Why groups are less effective than their members: On productivity losses in idea-generating groups. In W. Stroebe & M. Hewstone (Eds.), *European review of social psychology* (Vol. 5, pp. 271–303). Chichester, UK: Wiley.

Stroh, L. K., Brett, J. M., & Reilly, A. H. (1994). A decade of change: Managers' attachment to their organizations and their jobs. *Human Resource Management, 33,* 531–548.

Stryker, S. (1980). *Symbolic interactionism: A social structural version.* Menlo Park, CA: Benjamin/Cummings.

Stryker, S., & Serpe, R. (1982). Commitment, identity salience, and role behavior: Theory and research example. In W. Ickers & E. Knowles (Eds.), *Personality, roles and social behavior* (pp. 199–219). New York: Springer-Verlag.

Sullivan, S. E. (1999). The changing nature of careers: A review and research agenda. *Journal of Management, 25,* 457–484.

Surrey, J. L. (1991). The self-in-relation: A theory of women's development. In J. V. Jordan, A. G. Kaplan, J. B. Miller, I. P. Stiver & J. L. Surrey (Eds.), *Women's growth in connection: Writings from the Stone Center.* New York: Guilford Press.

Sutton, R. I., & Callaghan (1987). The stigma

of bankruptcy: Spoiled organizational image and its management. *Academy of Management Journal, 30,* 405–436.

Sutton, R. I., & Galunic, D. C. (1996). Consequences of public scrutiny for leaders and their organizations. In B. M. Staw & L. L. Cummings (Eds.), *Research in organizational behavior* (Vol. 18, pp. 201–250). Greenwich, CT: JAI Press.

Sutton, R. I., & Hargadon, A. (1996). Brainstorming groups in context. *Administrative Science Quarterly, 41,* 685–718.

Swan, S., & Wyer, R. S. (1997). Gender stereotypes and social identity: How being in the minority affects judgments of self and others. *Personality and Social Psychology Bulletin, 23,* 1265–1277.

Swann, W. B. (1987). Identity negotiation: Where two roads meet. *Journal of Personality and Social Psychology, 53,* 1038–1051.

Swann, W. B., Jr. (1990). To be adored or to be known? The interplay of self-enhancement and self-verification. In E.T. Higgins & R.M. Sorrentino (Eds.), *Handbook of motivation and cognition: Vol. 2* (pp. 408–448). New York: Guilford Press.

Swann, W. B., Jr. (1996). *Self-traps: The elusive quest for higher self-esteem.* New York: Freeman.

Swann, W. B., Jr., Griffin, J. J., Jr., Predmore, S. C., & Gaines, B. (1987). The cognitive-affective crossfire: When self-consistency confronts self-enhancement. *Journal of Personality and Social Psychology, 52,* 881–889.

Tabachnick, B. G., & Fidell, L. S. (1989). *Using multivariate statistics* (2nd ed.). New York: Harper and Row.

Tajfel, H. (1959). Quantitative judgment in social perception. *British Journal of Psychology, 50,* 16–29.

Tajfel, H. (1969). Cognitive aspects of prejudice. *Journal of Social Issues, 25,* 79–97.

Tajfel, H. (1970). Experiments in intergroup discrimination. *Scientific American, 223,* 96–102.

Tajfel, H. (1972). Social categorization. English manuscript of 'La catégorisation sociale.' In S. Moscovici (Ed.) *Introduction à la Psychologie Sociale* (Vol. 1, pp. 272–302). Paris: Larousse.

Tajfel, H. (1974a). *Intergroup behaviour, social comparison and social change.* Unpublished Katz-Newcomb Lectures, University of Michigan, Ann Arbor.

Tajfel, H. (1974b). Social identity and intergroup behaviour. *Social Science Information, 13,* 65–93.

Tajfel, H. (1975). The exit of social mobility and the voice of social change. *Social Science Information, 14,* 101–118.

Tajfel, H. (1978a). *Differentiation between social groups: Studies in the social psychology of intergroup relations.* London: Academic Press.

Tajfel, H. (1978b). Interindividual behaviour and intergroup behaviour. In H. Tajfel (Ed.), *Differentiation between social groups: Studies in the social psychology of intergroup relations* (pp. 27–60). London: Academic Press.

Tajfel, H. (1978c). Social categorization, social identity and social comparison. In H. Tajfel (Ed.), *Differentiation between social groups: Studies in the social psychology of intergroup relations* (pp. 61–76). London: Academic Press.

Tajfel, H. (1981). Social stereotypes and social groups. In J. C. Turner and H. Giles (Eds.), *Intergroup behavior* (pp. 144–167). Oxford, UK: Blackwell.

Tajfel, H. (1982). Social psychology of intergroup relations. *Annual Review of Psychology, 33,* 1–39.

Tajfel, H., & Turner, J. C. (1979). An integrative theory of intergroup conflict. In W. G. Austin & S. Worchel (Eds.), *The social psychology of intergroup relations* (pp. 33–47). Monterey, CA: Brooks-Cole.

Tajfel, H., & Turner, J. C. (1986). The social identity theory of intergroup behaviour. In S. Worchel & W. G. Austin (Eds.), *Psychology of intergroup relations* (pp. 7–24). Chicago: Nelson-Hall

Tajfel, H., & Wilkes, A. L. (1963). Classification and quantitative judgment. *British Journal of Psychology, 54,* 101–114.

Takezawa, S., & Whitehill, A. M. (1981). *Work ways: Japan and America.* Tokyo: The Japan Institute of Labor.

Taylor, D. M., & Brown, R.J. (1979). Towards a more social social psychology? *British Journal of Social and Clinical Psychology, 18,* 173–179.

Taylor, D. M., & McKirnan, D.J. (1984). A five-stage model of intergroup relations. *British Journal of Social Psychology, 23,* 291–300.

Taylor, D. M., Moghaddam, F. M., Gamble, I., & Zellerer, E. (1987). Disadvantaged group responses to perceived inequality: From passive acceptance to collective action. *Journal of Social Psychology, 127,* 259–272.

Taylor, S. E. (1981). A categorization approach to stereotyping. In D. L. Hamilton (Ed.), *Cognitive processes in stereotyping and intergroup behavior* (pp. 83–114). Hillsdale, NJ: Erlbaum.

Taylor, S. E., & Fiske, S. T. (1975). Point-of-view and perceptions of causality. *Journal of Personality and Social Psychology, 32,* 439–445.

Taylor, S. E., & Fiske, S. T. (1978). Salience, attention, and attribution: Top of the head phenomena. In L. Berkowitz (Ed.), *Advances in experimental social psychology* (Vol. 11, pp. 249–288). New York: Academic Press.

Taylor, S. E., Fiske, S. T., Etcoff, N. L., & Ruderman, A. J. (1978). Categorical bases of person memory and stereotyping. *Journal of Personality and Social Psychology, 36,* 778–793.

Terry, D. J., & Callan, V. J. (1998). In-group bias in response to an organizational merger. *Group Dynamics: Theory, Research, and Practice, 2,* 67–81.

Terry, D. J., Callan, V. J., & Sartori, G. (1996). A test of a stress-coping model of adjustment to large-scale organizational change. *Stress Medicine, 12,* 105–122.

Terry, D. J., Carey, C. J., & Callan, V. J. (in press). Employee adjustment to an organizational merger: An intergroup perspective. *Personality and Social Psychology Bulletin.*

Terry, D. J., & Hogg, M. A. (1996). Group norms and the attitude-behavior relationship: A role for group identification. *Personality and Social Psychology Bulletin, 22,* 776–793.

Terry, D. J., & Hogg, M. A. (Eds.) (1999). *Attitudes, behavior, and social context: The role of norms and group membership.* Mahwah, NJ: Erlbaum.

Terry, D. J., & O'Brien, A. T. (2000). *Status, legitimacy, and ingroup bias in the context of an organizational merger.* Manuscript submitted for publication.

Thibaut, J., & Kelley, H.H. (1959). *The social psychology of groups.* New York: Wiley.

Thoits, P. A., & Virshup, L. K. (1997). Me's and we's: Forms and functions of social identities. In R. D. Ashmore & L. Jussim (Eds.), *Self and identity: Fundamental issues* (pp.

106–133). New York: Oxford University Press.

Thomas, R. R., Jr. (1990). From affirmative action to affirming diversity. *Harvard Business Review, March-April,* 107–117.

Thompson, L., Valley, K. L., & Kramer, R. M. (1995). The bittersweet feeling of success: An examination of social perception in negotiation. *Journal of Experimental Social Psychology, 31,* 467–492.

Thompson, P., & Warhurst, C. (Eds.) (1998). *Workplaces of the future.* Houndmills, UK: Macmillan.

Tindale, R. S., & Anderson, E. M. (1998). Small group research and applied social psychology: An introduction. In R. S. Tindale, L. Heath, J. Edwards, E. J. Posavac, F. B. Bryant, Y. Suarez-Balcazar, E. Henderson-King, & J. Myer (Eds.), *Social psychological applications to social issues: Theory and research on small groups* (Vol. 4, pp. 1–8). New York: Plenum Press.

Toren, N. (1990). Would more women make a difference? Academic women in Israel. In S. S. Lie & V. E. O'Leary (Eds.), *Storming the tower: Women in the academic world* (pp. 74–85). New York: Nichols G/P Publishing.

Triandis, H. C. (1995). *Individualism and collectivism.* Boulder, CO: Westview Press.

Triandis, H. C., Bontempo, R., Villareal, M. J., Asai, M., & Lucca, N. (1988). Individualism and collectivism: Cross-cultural perspectives on self-ingroup relationships. *Journal of Personality and Social Psychology, 54,* 323–338.

Trice, H. M., & Beyer, J. M. (1984). Studying organizational cultures through rites and ceremonials. *Academy of Management Review, 9,* 653–669.

Trope, Y., & Liberman, A. (1993). The use of trait conceptions to identify other people's behavior and to draw inferences about their personalities. *Personality and Social Psychology Bulletin, 19,* 553–562.

Tsui, A. S., Egan, T. D., & O'Reilly, C. (1992). Being different: Relational demography and organizational attachment. *Administrative Science Quarterly, 37,* 549–579.

Tsui, A. S., & O'Reilly, C. A. (1989). Beyond simple demographic effects: The importance of relational demography in superior-subordinate dyads. *Academy of Management Journal, 32,* 402–423.

Tsui, A. S., Pearce, J. L., Porter, L. W., & Hite, J. (1995). Choice of employee-organization relationship: Influence of external and internal organizational factors. In G. R. Ferris (Ed.), *Research in personnel and human resources management* (Vol. 13, pp. 117–151). Greenwich, CT: JAI Press.

Turner, J. C. (1975). Social comparison and social identity: Some prospects for intergroup behavior. *European Journal of Social Psychology, 5,* 5–24.

Turner, J. C. (1982). Toward a cognitive redefinition of the social group. In H. Tajfel (Ed.), *Social identity and intergroup relations* (pp. 15–40). Cambridge, UK: Cambridge University Press.

Turner, J. C. (1984). Social identification and psychological group formation. In H. Tajfel (Ed.), *The social dimension: European developments in social psychology: Vol. 2* (pp. 518–538). Cambridge, UK: Cambridge University Press.

Turner, J. C. (1985). Social categorization and the self-concept: A social-cognitive theory of group behavior. In E. J. Lawler (Ed.), *Advances in group processes: Theory and research* (Vol. 2, pp. 77–122). Greenwich, CT: JAI Press.

Turner, J. C. (1987a). A self-categorization theory. In J. C. Turner, M. A. Hogg, P. J. Oakes, S. Reicher & M. S. Wetherell. *Rediscovering the social group: A self-categorization theory.* (pp. 42–67). Oxford, UK: Blackwell.

Turner, J. C. (1987b). The analysis of social influence. In J. C. Turner, M. A. Hogg, P. J. Oakes, S. D. Reicher, & M. S. Wetherell, *Rediscovering the social group: A self-categorization theory* (pp. 68–88). Oxford, UK: Blackwell.

Turner, J. C. (1991). *Social influence.* Buckingham, UK: Open University Press.

Turner, J. C. (1999). Some current issues in research on social identity and self-categorization theories. In N. Ellemers, R. Spears, & B. Doosje (Eds.), *Social identity* (pp. 6–34). Oxford, UK: Blackwell.

Turner, J. C., & Brown, R. (1978). Social status, cognitive alternatives, and intergroup relations. In H. Tajfel (Ed.), *Differentiation between social groups* (pp. 201–234). London: Academic Press.

Turner, J. C., & Haslam, S. A. (2001). Social identity, organizations and leadership. In M.

E. Turner (Ed.) *Groups at work: Advances in theory and research* (pp. 25–65). Hillsdale, NJ: Erlbaum.

Turner, J. C., Hogg, M. A., Oakes, P. J., Reicher, S. D., & Wetherell, M. (1987). *Rediscovering the social group: A self-categorization theory.* Oxford, UK: Blackwell.

Turner, J. C., & Oakes, P. (1989). Self-categorization theory and social influence. In P. Paulus (Ed.), *Psychology of group influence* (2nd ed., pp. 233–275). Hillsdale, NJ: Erlbaum.

Turner, J. C., Oakes, P. J., Haslam, S. A., & McGarty, C. A. (1994). Self and collective: Cognition and social context. *Personality and Social Psychology Bulletin, 20,* 454–463.

Turner, M.E., Pratkanis, A.R., Probasco, P., & Leve, C. (1992). Threat, cohesion, and group effectiveness: Testing a social identity maintenance perspective on groupthink. *Journal of Personality and Social Psychology, 63,* 781–796.

Tyler, T. R. (1993). The social psychology of authority. In J. K. Murnighan (Ed.), *Social psychology in organizations: Advances in theory and practice* (pp. 141–160). Englewood Cliffs, NJ: Prentice-Hall.

Tyler, T. R. (1994). Psychological models of the justice motive: Antecedents of distributive and procedural justice. *Journal of Personality and Social Psychology, 67,* 850–863.

Tyler, T.R. (1997). The psychology of legitimacy: A relational perspective on voluntary deference to authorities. *Personality and Social Psychology Review, 1,* 323–345.

Tyler, T. R. (1999). Why people co-operate with organizations: An identity-based perspective. In R. I. Sutton & B. M. Staw (Eds.), *Research in organizational behavior* (Vol. 21, pp. 201–246). Greenwich, CT: JAI Press.

Tyler, T. R. (in press b). Social justice. In R. Brown and S. Gaertner (Eds.), *Blackwell Handbook of Social Psychology: Vol. 4. Intergroup processes* (pp. 344–366).

Tyler, T. R., & Blader, S. (2000). *Cooperation in groups.* Philadelphia: Psychology Press.

Tyler, T. R., & Degoey, P. (1995). Collective restraint in social dilemmas: Procedural justice and social identification effects on support for authorities. *Journal of Personality and Social Psychology, 69,* 482–497.

Tyler, T. R., Degoey, P., & Smith, H. (1996). Understanding why the justice of group procedures matters. *Journal of Personality and Social Psychology, 70,* 913–930.

Tyler, T. R., & Lind, E. A. (1992). A relational model of authority in groups. In M. Zanna (Ed.), *Advances in experimental social psychology* (Vol. 25, pp. 115–192). New York: Academic Press.

Tyler, T. R., & Smith, H. J. (1999). Justice, social identity, and group processes. In T. R. Tyler, R. Kramer, & O. P. John (Eds.), *The psychology of the social self* (pp. 223–264). Mahwah, NJ: Erlbaum.

Urban, L. M., & Miller, N. M. (1998). A meta-analysis of crossed categorization effects. *Journal of Personality and Social Psychology, 74,* 894–908.

Uzzi, B. (1997). Social structure and competition in interfirm networks: The paradox of embeddedness. *Administrative Science Quarterly, 42,* 35–67.

van Knippenberg, A. F. M. (1978). Intergroup differences in group perceptions. In H. Tajfel (Ed.), *The social dimension: European developments in social psychology,* (pp. 560–578). Cambridge, UK: Cambridge University Press.

van Knippenberg, A., & Ellemers, N. (1993). Strategies in intergroup relations. In M. A. Hogg & D. Abrams (Eds.), *Group motivation: Social psychological perspectives* (pp. 17–23). London: Harvester Wheatsheaf, and New York: Prentice-Hall.

van Knippenberg, A., van Knippenberg, B., van Knippenberg, C., & van Knippenberg, D. (2000). *Identificatie met de organisatie: Een meetinstrument.* Gedrag & organisatie. Manuscript submitted for publication.

van Knippenberg, D. (2000). Work motivation and performance: A social identity perspective. *Applied Psychology: An International Review, 49,* 357–371.

van Knippenberg, D., & Groeneveld, M. (1999). *Work group identification after organizational merger: Sense of continuity and work group entitativity.* Unpublished manuscript, University of Amsterdam.

van Knippenberg, D., van Knippenberg, B., Monden, L., & de Lima, F. (in press). Organizational identification after a merger: A social identity perspective. *British Journal of Social Psychology.*

van Knippenberg, D., & van Schie, E. C. M. (2000). Foci and correlates of organizational identification. *Journal of Occupational and Organizational Psychology, 73,* 137–147.

van Leeuwen, E., & van Knippenberg, D. (1999). *Social value orientations and group performance: The role of expectations of other group members' effort.* Manuscript submitted for publication.

van Leeuwen, E., van Knippenberg, D., & Ellemers, N. (2000a). *Continuing and changing group identities: The effects of merging on post-merger identification and ingroup bias.* Unpublished manuscript, Leiden University.

van Leeuwen, E., van Knippenberg, D. & Ellemers, N. (2000). *Preserving identity in times of change: The dynamics of post-merger group identification.* Working paper. Leiden University.

Van Maanen, J. (1998). *Identity work: Notes on the personal identity of police officers.* Paper presented at the annual meeting of the Academy of Management, San Diego, CA, August.

Van Maanen, J., & Barley, S. R. (1985). Cultural organization: Fragments of a theory. In P. J. Frost, L. F. Moore, M. R. Louis, C. C. Lundberg, & J. Martin (Eds.), *Organizational culture* (pp. 31–53). Beverly Hills, CA: Sage.

Van Maanen, J., & Schein, E. H. (1979). Toward a theory of organizational socialization. In B. M. Staw (Ed.), *Research in Organizational Behavior* (Vol. 1, pp. 209–264). Greenwich, CT: JAI Press.

van Oudenhoven, J. P., & deBoer, T. (1995). Complementarity and similarity of partners in international mergers. *Basic and Applied Social Psychology, 17,* 343–356.

Van Oudenhoven, J.-P., Groenewoud, J. T., & Hewstone, M. (1996). Cooperation, ethnic salience and generalization of interethnic attitudes. *European Journal of Social Psychology, 26,* 649–661.

Van Vianen, A. E. M. (2000). Person-organization fit: The match between newcomers' and recruiters' preferences for organizational cultures. *Personnel Psychology, 53,* 113–149.

van Vugt, M., & de Cremer, D. (1999). Leadership in social dilemmas: The effects of group identification on collective actions to provide public goods. *Journal of Personality and Social Psychology, 76,* 587–599.

Vanbeselaere, N. (1991). The different effects of simple and crossed categorisations: A result of the category differentiation process or of differential category salience? In W.

Stroebe & M. Hewstone (Eds.), *European review of social psychology* (Vol. 2, pp. 247–278). Chichester, UK: Wiley.

Veenstra, K. & Haslam, S. A. (2000). Willingness to participate in industrial protest: Exploring social identification in context. *British Journal of Social Psychology, 39,* 153–172.

Vescio, T. K., Hewstone, M., Crisp, R. J., & Rubin, J. M. (1999). Perceiving and responding to multiply categorizable individuals: Cognitive processes and affective intergroup bias. In D. Abrams & M. A. Hogg (Eds.), *Social identity and social cognition* (pp. 111–140). Oxford, UK and Cambridge, MA: Blackwell.

Voci, A. (2000). Perceived group variability and the salience of personal and social identity. In W. Stroebe & M. Hewstone (Eds.), *European Review of Social Psychology* (Vol. 11, pp. 177–222). Chichester, UK: Wiley.

Wallace, J. E. (1993). Professional and organizational commitment: Compatible or incompatible? *Journal of Vocational Behavior, 42,* 333–349.

Walther, J., Anderson, J., & Park, D. (1994). Interpersonal effects in computer-mediated interaction: A meta-analysis of social and antisocial communication. *Communication Research, 21,* 460–487.

Wan-Huggins, V. N., Riordan, C. M., & Griffeth, R. W. (1998). The development and longitudinal test of a model of organizational identification. *Journal of Applied Social Psychology, 28,* 724–749.

Wanous, J. P., & Youtz, M. A. (1986). Solution diversity and the quality of group decisions. *Academy of Management Journal, 29,* 149–158.

Weber, R., & Crocker, J. (1983). Cognitive processes in the revision of stereotypic beliefs. *Journal of Personality and Social Psychology, 45,* 961–77.

Weber, Y., & Schweiger, D. (1989). *Implementing mergers and acquitions: the role of cultural differences and the level of integration.* Unpublished manuscript, University of South Carolina.

Wech, B. A., Mossholder, K. W., Steel, R. P., & Bennett, N. (1998). Does work group cohesiveness affect an individual's performance and organizational commitment: A cross-level examination. *Small Group Research, 29,* 472–494.

Weiner, B. (1985). "Spontaneous" causal thinking. *Psychological Bulletin, 97,* 74–84.

Werbel, J. D., & Landau, J. (1996). The effectiveness of different recruitment sources: A mediating variable analysis. *Journal of Applied Social Psychology, 23,* 19–36.

West, M. A. (in press). Creativity and innovation implementation in work groups. *Applied Psychology: An International Review.*

West, M. A., Borrill, C. S., & Unsworth, K. L. (1998). Team effectiveness in organizations. In C. L. Cooper & I. T. Robertson (Eds.), *International Review of Industrial Organizational Psychology* (Vol. 13, pp. 1–48). Chichester, UK: Wiley.

Wharton, A. S. (1992). The social construction of gender and race in organizations: A social identity and group mobilization perspective. *Research in the Sociology of Organizations, 10,* 55–84.

Wharton, A. S., & Baron, J. N. (1987). So happy together? The impact of gender segregation on men at work. *American Sociological Review, 52,* 574–587.

White, L. K., & Booth, A. (1985). The quality and stability of remarriages: The role of stepchildren. *American Sociological Review, 50,* 689–698.

White, M. M., Parks, J. D., Gallagher, D. G., Tetrault, L. A., & Wakabayashi, M. (1995). Validity evidence for the organizational commitment questionnaire in the Japanese corporate culture. *Educational and Psychological Measurement, 55*(2), 278–290.

Wiesenfeld, B., Raghuram, S., & Garud, R. (2000). Communication patterns as determinants of organizational identification. Forthcoming in *Organizational Science.*

Wilder, D. A. (1984). Intergroup contact: The typical member and the exception to the rule. *Journal of Experimental Social Psychology, 20,* 177–94.

Williams, K., & O'Reilly, C. (1998). The complexity of diversity: A review of forty years of research. In B. Staw & R. Sutton (Eds.), *Research in organizational behavior* (Vol. 21, pp. 77–140). Greenwich, CT: JAI Press.

Williams, K. D. (1997). Social ostracism. In R. M. Kowalski (Ed.), *Aversive interpersonal behaviors* (pp. 133–170). New York: Plenum Press.

Williams, K. D., & Sommer, K. L. (1997). Social ostracism by coworkers: Does rejection lead to loafing or compensation? *Personal-*

*ity and Social Psychology Bulletin, 23,* 693–706.

Williamson, O. (1993). Calculativeness, trust, and economic organization. *Journal of Law and Economics, 34,* 453–502.

Wood, W., Lundgren, S., Ouellette, J. A., Busceme, S., & Blackstone, T. (1994). Minority influence: A meta-analytic review of social influence processes. *Psychological Bulletin, 115,* 323–345.

Worchel, S., Morales, J. F., Páez, D., & Deschamps, J.-C. (Eds.) (1998). *Social identity: International perspectives.* London: Sage.

Wright, P. L. (1990). Teller job satisfaction and organization commitment as they relate to career orientations. *Human Relations, 43,* 369–381.

Wright, S., Aron, A., McLaughlin-Volpe, T., & Ropp, S. A. (1997). The extended contact effect: Knowledge of cross-group friendships and prejudice. *Journal of Personality and Social Psychology, 73,* 73–90.

Wright, S., Taylor, D. M., & Moghaddam, F. M. (1990). Responding to membership in a disadvantaged group: From acceptance to collective protest. *Journal of Personality and Social Psychology, 58,* 994–1003.

Yamagishi, T. (1986). The provision of a sanctioning system as a public good. *Journal of Personality and Social Psychology, 51,* 110–116.

Yamagishi, T., & Yamagishi, M. (1994). Trust and commitment in the United States and Japan. *Motivation and Emotion, 18,* 129–166.

Yan, A., & Louis, M. R. (1999). The migration of organizational functions to the work unit level: Buffering, spanning, and bringing up boundaries. *Human Relations, 52,* 25–47.

Yoder, J. D. (1991). Rethinking tokenism: Looking beyond numbers. *Gender & Society, 5,* 178–192.

Yoder, J. D. (1994). Looking beyond numbers: The effects of gender status, job prestige, and occupational gender-typing on tokenism processes. *Social Psychology Quarterly, 57,* 150–159.

Yoder, J. D., & Sinnett, L. (1985). Is it all in the numbers? A case study of tokenism. *Psychology of Women Quarterly, 9,* 412–418.

Yoder, J. D., Adams, J., & Prince, H. (1983). The price of a token. *Journal of Political and Military Sociology, 11,* 325–337.

Yoon, J. K., Baker, M. R., & Ko, J. (1994). Interpersonal attachment and organizational commitment: Subgroup hypothesis revisited. *Human Relations, 47,* 329–351.

Young, C. J., Mackenzie, D. I., & Sherif, C.W. (1980). In search of token women in academia. *Psychology of Women Quarterly, 4,* 508–525.

Yu, J., & Murphy, K. R. (1993). Modesty bias in self-ratings of performance: A test of the cultural relativity hypothesis. *Personnel Psychology, 46,* 257–363.

Yukl, G. (1998). *Leadership in organizations.* New York: Prentice Hall.

Yukl, G. A., & Falbe, C. M. (1991). Importance of different power sources in downward and lateral relations. *Journal of Applied Psychology, 76,* 416–423.

Yukl, G., & Van Fleet, D. D. (1992). Theory and research on leadership in organizations. In M. D. Dunnette & L. M. Hough (Eds.), *Handbook of organizational psychology* (2nd ed., Vol. 3, pp. 147–197). Palo Alto, CA: Consulting Psychologists Press.

Zaccaro, S. J., & Dobbins, G. H. (1989). Contrasting group and organizational commitment: Evidence for differences among multilevel attachments. *Journal of Organizational Behavior, 10,* 267–273.

Zenger, T. R. (1992). Why do employers only reward extreme performance? Examining the relationships among performance, pay, and turnover. *Administrative Science Quarterly, 37,* 198–219.

Zimbardo, P. (1969). The human choice: Individuation, reason and order versus deindividuation, impulse and chaos. In W .J. Arnold & D. Levine (Eds.), *Nebraska Symposium on Motivation* (Vol. 17, pp. 237–307). Lincoln, NB: Nebraska University Press.

Zimbardo, P. G., Andersen, S. M., & Kabat, L. G. (1981). Induced hearing deficit generates experimental paranoia. *Science, 212,* 1529–1531.

Zucker, L. G. (1986). Production of trust: Institutional sources of economic structure. In B. M. Staw & L. L. Cummings (Eds.), *Research in organizational behavior* (Vol. 8, pp. 53–111). Greenwich, CT: JAI Press.

Zuckerman, M. (1979). Attribution of success and failure revisited, or: The motivational bias is alive and well in attributional theory. *Journal of Personality, 47,* 245–287.

Zurcher, L. A. (1982). The staging of emotion: A dramaturgical analysis. *Symbolic Interaction, 5,* 1–22.

# Author Index

# Subject Index